Second European Glaucoma Symposium

Documenta Ophthalmologica
Proceedings Series volume 43

Editor H. E. Henkes

Second European Glaucoma Symposium Helsinki, May 1984

E.L. Greve, W. Leydhecker and C. Raitta (Editors)

1985 **DR W. JUNK PUBLISHERS**
a member of the KLUWER ACADEMIC PUBLISHERS GROUP
DORDRECHT / BOSTON / LANCASTER

Distributors

for the United States and Canada: Kluwer Academic Publishers, 190 Old Derby Street, Hingham, MA 02043, USA

for the UK and Ireland: Kluwer Academic Publishers, MTP Press Limited, Falcon House, Queen Square, Lancaster LA1 1RN, UK

for all other countries: Kluwer Academic Publishers Group, Distribution Center, P.O. Box 322, 3300 AH Dordrecht, The Netherlands

Library of Congress Cataloging in Publication Data

European Glaucoma Symposium (2nd : 1984 : Helsinki,
    Finland)
    Second European Glaucoma Symposium, Helsinki, May
1984.

    (Documenta ophthalmologica. Proceedings series ;
v. 43)
    Includes index.
    1. Glaucoma--Congresses. 2. Perimetry--Congresses.
I. Greve, Erik L. II. Leydhecker, W. (Wolfgang)
III. Raitta, C. IV. Title. V. Series. [DNLM:
1. Glaucoma--congresses. 2. Glaucoma--therapy--con-
gresses. W3 D0637 v.43 / WW 290 E887 1984s]

RE871.E97 1984   617.7'41   85-4287

ISBN-13: 978-94-010-8934-0   e-ISBN-13: 978-94-009-5516-5
DOI:10.1007/ 978-94-009-5516-5

CONTENTS

PART TWO: MEDICAL THERAPY

PART THREE: LASER TREATMENT

PART FOUR: SURGICAL TREATMENT

IX

OPENING ADDRESS

Dear Professor Leydhecker, Ladies and Gentlemen, my dear friends,

I would first of all like to thank Professor Leydhecker and his Committee for having asked me to be the honorary president of this Glaucoma Congress. I am very honored at this token of esteem and friendship.

Some years ago the European Glaucoma Society was founded in Ghent. Professor Leydhecker became the president and Dr Greve the general secretary. The first congress took place in 1980 at Brighton and was a great success.

I am sure that the present congress will be at least as successful as the previous one, when one considers the great number of participants and the quality of the speakers. Glaucoma still remains at the forefront of clinical ophthalmology and the cases of blindness resulting from glaucoma are very numerous.

Although we have at the present time very good medical treatment thanks to the cholinergic and anticholinesterasic drugs, epinephrine, betablockers and inhibitors of carbonanhydrase, and similarly very good surgical treatment, including trabeculectomy, much basic research is still needed before we have the ideal therapeutics. In the present state of our knowledge, there are still several problems which have to be solved:

1. The pathogenesis of glaucoma is still imperfectly known.

2. The efficacy of trabeculoplasty by laser photocoagulation is still being discussed.

3. Computer assisted perimetry and some other psychophysical tests have to be brought up to data and improved.

These problems are precisely the main topics of this congress, which once more will demonstrate that research in glaucoma is a lively science.

Ladies and Gentlemen, my dear friends, we should thank Professor Leydhecker, Dr. Greve and Dr. Raitta, and her staff, the local organizers, for giving us the opportunity to contribute to the advancement of glaucoma research. I wish you all a fruitful, instructive and agreeable meeting.

Prof. Jules François (†)

INTRODUCTION

The European Glaucoma Society was founded in the spring of 1978 at the initiative of Drs François, Leydhecker and Greve. Representatives of most European countries met in Ghent and agreed to create a society that would promote the contacts and exchange of knowledge between European glaucomatologists.

The European Glaucoma Society serves to stimulate glaucoma research and diffuse specific knowledge to general ophthalmologists. The European Glaucoma Society would like to cooperate closely with similar glaucoma organizations in other continents.

The first symposium of the EGS was held in April 1980 in Brighton, England. No proceedings were published. The second symposium took place in May 1984 in Hyvinkää, Finland. A great number of participants enjoyed a well organized scientific programme of attractive quality.

The local organization was in the able hands of Raitta and her colleagues, Raivio and Lehto. The scientific programme was coordinated in Amsterdam where a great amount of work was done by Stella Ompi, secretary to the general secretary.

The contents of the meeting have been summarized in this book. This second symposium of the EGS, which took place in an atmosphere of great enthusiasm and friendship, has shown great promise for the future of the European glaucoma.

The Editors

SUMMARY OF THE SCIENTIFIC PROGRAMME OF THE SECOND SYMPOSIUM OF THE EUROPEAN GLAUCOMA SOCIETY

ERIK L. GREVE

In the section on *Visual Function* Greve opened with an overview of the developments in computer assisted perimetry. Techniques for measurements in the assessment phase were discussed. Analysis of fluctuation is necessary especially in relative defects. The numerical expression of defect volume will be extremely important for the evaluation of progression. Visual fatigue is a phenomenon that may be helpful in detecting early glaucomatous damage and may be a problem insofar as it increases fluctuation. It was stressed that psychological factors are more important in computer assisted perimetry than previously believed and that *semi*-automated procedures may be necessary for at least some glaucoma patients.

Flammer presented evidence that the visual function in glaucomatous disease is affected in two ways: a general diffuse reduction of sensitivity caused by the direct mechanical effect of intraocular pressure (IOP) and local defects caused by circulatory insufficiency. The latter may be caused by vascular risk factors and/or raised IOP. Several papers dealt with the relation between the optic disc and the visual function. Marré found no correlation between optic disc densitometry and VECP. Dimitrakos et al. found no good correlation between change of field loss and change of surface of the rim over the years. Interestingly Krakau found that saucerization of the disc was associated with general reduction of sensitivity whereas local notching was associated with local defects.

A method to quantify the results of computer assisted perimetry was presented by Etienne, while Mertz demonstrated a method using image analysis to display fluctuation and changes in the visual field.

The Humphrey Field Analyzer was introduced by Heijl.

Manual and computer assisted perimetry was performed in congenital glaucoma by Rolando et al. They demonstrated general reduction of sensitivity as an early sign of damage.

Gandolfo et al. showed a rapid screening programme combining static and kinetic automatic techniques.

From the land of Bjerrum came a comparative study on the Bjerrum screen and the Octopus computer assisted perimetry (Thygesen et al.). As expected the tangent screen detected about half of the "absolute defects" detected by the Octopus.

XV

E.L. Greve, W. Leydhecker & C. Raitta (eds.), Second European Glaucoma Symposium, Helsinki 1984.
© *1985, Dr. W. Junk Publishers, Dordrecht. ISBN 978-94-010-8934-0*

The section on *Medical Treatment* opened with some basic research reports.

Petounis et al. suggested that osmotic agents reduce IOP by a direct dehydrating effect on the bulbus oculi and not by central neural mechanisms.

The effect of ocular pigmentation on pilocarpine availability was studied by Salminen and Urtti. The same authors measured concentration of epinephrine, pilocarpine and timolol in the different parts of the eye.

The location of β-adrenergic receptors in the cornea and ciliary body (non-pigmented epithelial cells) was studied by Lehto et al.

Palkama et al. described the mechanism of action of adrenergic agonists and $\beta_1-\beta_2$ antagonists in the rabbit.

The effect of ophthalmic rods containing pilocarpine is comparable to that of pilocarpine eye drops according to Krieglstein et al. Many studies were devoted to the dominating antiglaucomatous drug of the eighties: the β-blockers.

Robert and Hendrickson measured the pallor of the disc in healthy subjects with and without the effect of the β-blockers timolol and pindolol. They could not demonstrate any effect of the drugs on the vascular behavior of the disc.

Propanolol does not seem to have an adrenergic neuronal blocking action according to Fleig and Krieglstein. The long duration of action of β-blockers might be explained by high-affinity binding to pigment cells.

Merté and Stryz compared propanol, timolol, metipropanolol, L-befunolol, befunolol and pindolol. The direct effects on IOP are highest for timolol, metipranolol, L-befunolol and befunolol. The authors concluded that in the long run the effects of these drugs are comparable. Hoskins et al. showed how the use of timolol is beneficial in the treatment of childhood glaucomas.

Pindolol was compared to timolol in a long-term study by Goethals et al. The authors conclude that although the direct effect of timolol is more pronounced than that of pinolol, the long-term effect of both drugs is comparable.

The effect of the addition of timolol to maximal medical therapy was once again shown by Sefić et al.

Krieglstein and Scoville used an eye-irritation score to evaluate carteolol and timolol. Three and ten minutes after application the irritation caused by carteolol and timolol was similar, while immediately after application timolol is somewhat more irritating.

In two studies of Long et al. and Berson et al. the effects of levobunolol were compared to timolol. No significant differences were found.

The section on *Laser and Glaucoma* was opened with a review by Pohjanpelto. The mean success rate of Laser trabeculoplasty (LTP) is 82%. LTP works well in capsular glaucoma, less well in post traumatic glaucoma, and glaucoma secondary to uveitis.

The complications of LTP were discussed. Pohjanpelto reported a success rate of 72% in primary open angle glaucoma at the end of six months and at the end of a longer follow-up period. The long-term results of pseudoexfoliation glaucoma seem to be somewhat less good than the immediate results (76% and 95% respectively).

Cases with a recurring high IOP appeared at a steady rate during the first three years of follow-up.

Deterioration of the visual field was reported to occur in 33% of cases with primary open angle glaucoma and 45% of cases with pseudoexfoliation. There was no evidence of a relation between immediate post-laser IOP rise and visual field deterioration. These high percentages of deterioration require further confirmation.

Holmin and Bauer measured the visual field in 48 eyes before and one month after LTP. These authors found no significant differences before and after LTP.

Traverso et al. described their LTP results: these were better in pseudo-exfoliation and pigment dyspersion glaucoma. Out of 113 cases with accept-able automated perimetry, 32 got worse, 19 got better and 62 remained unchanged (according to the criteria of these authors).

Kitazawa et al. varied several LTP parameters. These authors concluded that treatment of the posterior meshwork over 180° is preferable. Teräsvirta et al. made comparable variations of LTP parameters (180° and 360°; anterior and posterior trabecular meshwork) both in primary open angle suspects and pseudoexfoliation glaucoma. These authors stressed the reduc-tion of diurnal variation caused by LTP. They concluded that all four treat-ment modes used were equally acceptable.

Béchetoille and Jallet described the results of laser burns to the ciliary band, as compared to the trabecular meshwork (180°).

Laser coagulation of the ciliary band seemed to be at least as effective as LTP directed towards the trabecular meshwork. Similar good results of laser coagulation of the ciliary band were reported by Krasnov. It is my personal experience since 1981 that laser treatment of the ciliary band can be as effective as treatment of the meshwork. My colleagues Dake and Bos have demonstrated that coagulations directed to the scleral spur likewise have a good effect.

Ljubojević and Kuljača confirmed earlier findings of LTP: 74.6% of eyes controlled over almost two years.

Honrubia et al. described the beneficial effect of panretinal photo-coagulation in central retinal vein occlusion in preventing neovascular glaucoma.

The same group of authors treated 13 eyes of patients after failure of trabeculectomy and obtained a 25% reduction of IOP.

Schrems et al. found a significant dysfunction of the blood-aqueous barrier after neodynium-YAG laser iridotomy which could be prevented by topical indomethacin.

Long-lasting iridotomies were obtained by Brihaye et al. using a neodynium-YAG laser for perforation after precoagulation with an Argon laser.

Schrems et al. recorded IOP levels after neodynium-YAG laser iridotomies and found considerable IOP peaks.

In the section on *Surgical Treatment* Leydhecker presented his views on the indications, techniques and documentation of surgery of glaucoma. He stressed the importance of IOP in the pathogenesis of glaucomatous damage.

The requirements for correct evaluation of the effect of medical treatment were discussed. Patient compliance and the role of adequate information are considered.

Apart from a few cases where surgical treatment is the first choice, surgery is reserved for failures of medical (and laser) treatment. Both a high IOP or a visual field deterioration can be indications for surgery. A field defect close to fixation is no contraindication. As far as the surgical technique is concerned all modifications of trabeculectomy or goniotrephining work as external filtering operations. The author furthermore discusses peripheral iridenclysis, iridectomy, goniotomy, cyclodialysis, cryosurgery and laser treatment. Finally the importance of accurate documentation on preprinted computer sheets is stressed.

Roszíval and Řehák described the scanning electron microscopic effects of Scheie's diathermy and incision in rabbits.

Lambrou and Christakis evaluated those patients that could be followed for at least 10 years after goniotrephination (108 out of 493 operations; 69 patients). The mean IOP rose 2 mm during the follow-up period. At the end of 10 years 13 out of 108 eyes received extra medical treatment. Only three cases showed visual field deterioration, while only seven cases showed a reduction of visual acuity.

Greve et al. reported on a 10-year prospective study of a covered filtering operation. After 10 years almost half of the patients had died (20 out of 47; mean age at the beginning: 66). If an IOP of 21 mm or less and a stable visual field were taken as criteria then 45% of cases were controlled. If additional medical treatment and reoperations were included 93% were controlled. Thirteen out of 29 eyes showed an increase of cataract but only four had to be operated.

Vossen and Neubauer studied 29 eyes with defects close to fixation. They found no deterioration of visual acuity after filtering operations in the majority of cases. In some cases, the "residual visual field slowly melted away".

Modifications of filtering techniques were shown by Nesterov et al. Good results were reported for valve-trabeculotomy in open angle glaucoma and for filtering irido-cycloretraction in angle closure glaucoma. A goniotomy approach to cyclodialysis was reported by Draeger and Wirt, the advantage being the continuous visual control in addition to the use of hyaluronic acid. A similar approach to trabeculotomy also using healon was described by Quintana.

The effects of direct cyclodiathermy both in rabbits and in glaucoma patients were studied by Kontić et al. This method deserves further attention. Another operation for late stage glaucoma was demonstrated by Takáts: a modification of Cohan's filtering corneal trephination. Twelve out of 16 cases were reported successful (75%).

Bordeianu performed trabeculectomy using a corneal approach and showed that in this case the operation does not function, implying that permanent dehiscense of the scleral wound is necessary. He furthermore described the inclusion of a corneal strip under a scleral flat as part of a filtering procedure.

The fifth and last section contains *Miscellaneous* subjects. Clark and Mapstone measured anterior chamber volume after a pilocarpine phenylephrine provocation test in eyes with and without a peripheral iridectomy (p.i.). The anterior chamber volume decreased in the presence of a p.i. The thickness of the lens is the major difference in eyes with unilateral acute angle closure glaucoma as shown by Strasser and Hauff.

The value of limbal anterior chamber depth estimation with the slitlamp for the detection of angle closure glaucoma was illustrated by Alsbirk. Nasotemporal differences in limbal anterior chamber depth may not reflect gonioscopic differences.

Tarkkanen et al. discussed the use of ultrasonographic biometry in congenital glaucoma. Such measurements proved to be of great help in diagnosis and follow-up of this disease and made the indication for surgical intervention easier.

Prevention of amblyopia due to astigmatism in congenital glaucoma is important according to Tsamparlakis et al.

Valle and Kivelä presented a Finnish family with hereditary juvenile glaucoma being autosomally dominent with complex penetrance. The long-term prognosis of patients with pseudoexfoliation glaucoma is not different from those with primary open angle glaucoma as studied by Demailly and Gruber.

Patients with low-tension glaucoma, especially those classified as focal ischemic glaucoma, may have a significantly higher blood viscosity than matched cataract patients. Klaver et al. suggested that increased blood viscosity may be regarded as a risk factor in glaucoma.

Baring of the circumlinear vessels, as a sign of early glaucomatous damage was considered by Rolando et al. They found this sign in 10% of normals, 40% of ocular hypertensives and 88% of glaucomas. The difficulty of evaluating glaucomatous damage in myopic discs was pointed out by Miglior et al.

The aqueous dynamics in spontaneous and traumatic cavernous fistulas were discussed by Varga et al. The normal IOP in traumatic cases is explained by arterial circulatory deficiency. Increased resistance in outflow is attributed to increased episcleral venous pressure. The role of lactic acid concentration in hemorrhagic glaucoma was discussed by Imre et al., explaining also the effect of panretinal photocoagulation.

Kuljača et al. presented an interesting case of secondary glaucoma caused by reactive lymphoid hyperplasia of the conjunctiva and uveal tract, conformed by microscopic findings.

Jerndal illustrated his concept of glaucomatous disease. In this concept congenital glaucoma with recognizable changes of the chamber angle plays an important part (goniodysgenesis). This author favours early surgical treatment.

The features of the chamber angle in glaucoma were studied by Svedbergh et al. They were especially interested in goniodysgenesis and concluded that signs of dysgenesis were more frequently seen in glaucoma patients than in a control group. Pretrabecular membranes were difficult to evaluate.

Finally, Schiødte et al. described their results with panretinal photocoagulation in cases of late stage, complicated glaucoma. They found a combination of panretinal photocoagulation and cyclocryothermia to be successful in a number of cases.

PRESENT AND FUTURE OF COMPUTER ASSISTED PERIMETRY IN GLAUCOMA SELECTED TOPICS

ERIK L. GREVE, TOM J.T.P. VAN DEN BERG
and CHRISTINE T. LANGERHORST

(Amsterdam, The Netherlands)

ABSTRACT

Several possibilities for measurement of defect-intensity (depth) in the assessment phase are described. They are divided into two-zone, three-zone and multi-zone techniques. For threshold measurements, 0.2 log.unit steps (2 dB) have been accepted. For fluctuation analysis repeated measurements are required. Defect intensity can be expressed in relative or in absolute values. Relative intensity values are preferred. Separation of local and general reduction of sensitivity is necessary. The defect volume (sum of local defect intensities) can be calculated and presented with statistical limits. The final solution for such programmes has yet to be found.

Visual fatigue is an important phenomenon in computer assisted perimetry. It can be used for early detection of glaucomatous damage. It may be a troublesome factor in the analysis of fluctuation.

The effect of psychological factors in computer assisted perimetry has been underestimated. It has been shown that a number of patients perform better with psychological support of a trained examiner while the computer takes care of the strategies and the statistics.

The availability of semi-automated procedures in computer assisted perimetry is advocated.

INTRODUCTION

There is a general agreement that Computer Assisted Perimetry (CAP) has advantages over manual perimetry (3, 5, 13). In addition to the increased reproducibility due to standardization of the examination procedures advantages are the possibility for statistical analysis and better print-out.

For glaucoma, CAP is the method of choice in the majority of patients. For a minority a semi-automatic examination may be necessary.

In this review we will discuss a few selected topics. We will not consider screening techniques or different types of instruments. We have written about screening techniques extensively (12, 13). We consider a suprathreshold, threshold-related technique followed by threshold determinations in defects the most efficient. In combination with multiple stimulus presentation this is

1

E.L. Greve, W. Leydhecker & C. Raitta (eds.), Second European Glaucoma Symposium, Helsinki 1984.
© *1985, Dr. W. Junk Publishers, Dordrecht. ISBN 978-94-010-8934-0*

Table 1. Assessment strategies after a suprathreshold, threshold-related detection.

Two zone	= no assessment
Three zone	= normal, relative, maximal
Multi zone	= normal, subdivision relative, max. (L-step size ≥ 0.3)
Threshold	= 0.2 L-steps
Threshold + fluctuation	= double measurements

by far the fastest screening technique. For the detection phase threshold measurements may only be necessary if the screening technique shows a normal result.

ASSESSMENT PHASE

For glaucoma we need to know not only whether there are defects but also what intensity (depth) they have. Several assessment techniques have been developed (Table 1).

A two-zone technique only differentiates between normal and abnormal and is not suitable for glaucoma. A three-zone technique presents data on normal areas, on relative defects and on defects for maximal luminance. Depending on the dynamic L-range of the CAP the intensity of relative defects may be anywhere between 0.0 and 3.0 log.units. Only large intensity changes can be detected with this method.

In manual static threshold-perimetry usually 0.1 log.unit steps are used. Most CAP use 0.2 steps, while some programmes use a 0.6 L-step. The standard deviation of the intensity of relative defects may be in the order of 0.3 or 0.4 log.unit (17). This means that 99% of the answers will be in a range of 1.5 to 2.0 log.unit. Given this large range it is possible to use 0.6 steps to measure the intensity of defects.

Whatever the consideration may be most manufacturers seem to have settled for 0.2 log.unit steps for threshold measurements. A single threshold measurement does not provide information on fluctuation. For decades we have judged progression on single measurements. With clinical experience one could make a fair judgement based on the knowledge that defect intensity can vary considerably.

However, this required a thorough knowledge of the basis of visual function testing and vast experience with visual field examination. Many erroneous judgements have been made. Such judgements can be much more accurate when they are supported by statistical analysis.

For a statistical analysis fluctuation data are required (1, 8, 9, 10, 11, 18). They can simply be acquired by repeating an examination. This, however, is not the most efficient method as the double measurements are really only necessary in some normal areas and in relative defects. The positions where such measurements are made should not be fixed but chosen on the basis of the examination results.

Thus an optimal assessment phase for glaucoma should include threshold

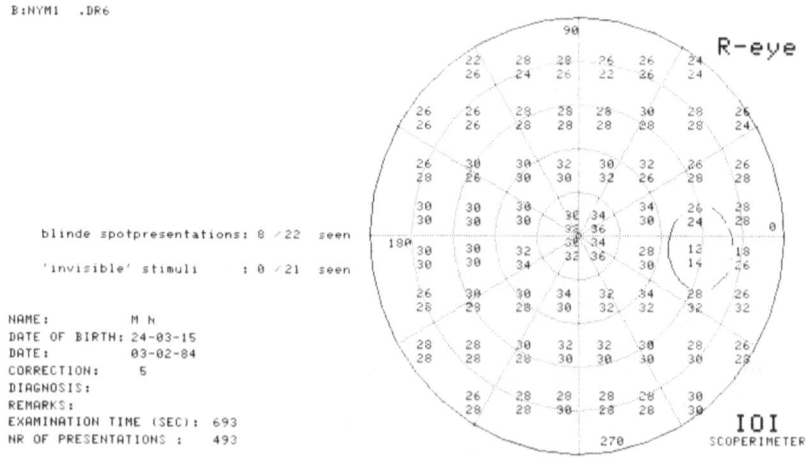

Fig. 1. Double threshold-measurements in a normal subject as performed with the Scoperimeter. In this case as in Fig. 2 the double measurements were performed at all locations.

measurements and data on fluctuation in normal positions and in relative defects. An example of double measurements is given in Figs. 1 & 2.

RELATIVE AND ABSOLUTE INTENSITY

Defect intensity may be expressed as the absolute L-value or as an intensity value relative to normal values (Fig. 3). The latter is comparable to visual acuity values.

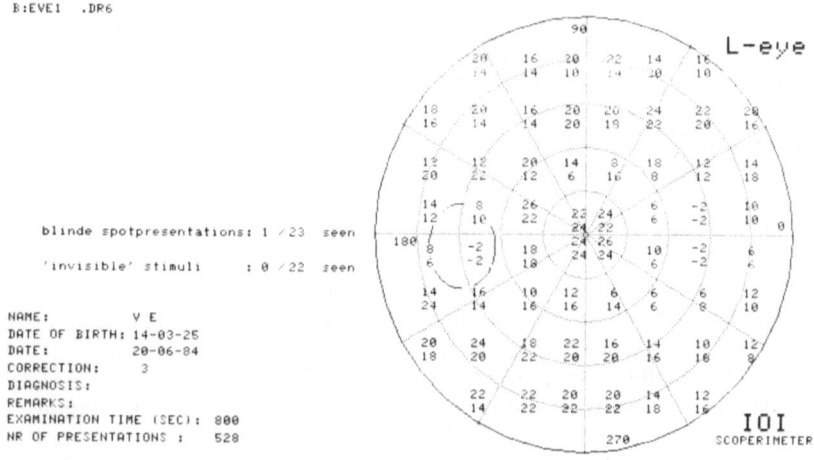

Fig. 2. Double threshold-measurements in a glaucomatous visual field defect as performed with the Scoperimeter.

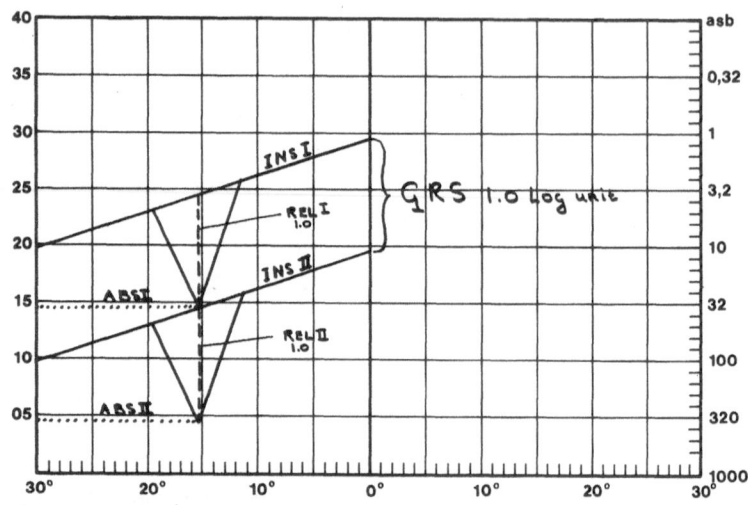

Fig. 3. Absolute and relative intensity of visual field defects. This figure demonstrates two different levels of the individual normal sensitivity (INS I and II). There is a difference of 1.0 log.unit between the two levels of sensitivity or a general reduction of sensitivity (GRS) of 1.0 log.unit in case II. It is clear, however, that the local defect is exactly the same in both cases. The only value that has changed is the general level of sensitivity most probably due to cataract. The relative intensity of the local defect in both cases is 1.0 log.unit, which adequately expresses the fact that no change has occurred in the local (glaucomatous) process.

An absolute value simply presents the threshold luminance. Such presentations do not take in account the normal gradient of sensitivity or the difference between general and local reduction of sensitivity. Absolute values leave much to the personal interpretations of the ophthalmologist. They may even lead to false interpretations. It is logical to use intensity values that are similar at each position. The next step is the determination of general reduction of sensitivity (see also 16). There are often a number of positions which have an equal sensitivity that is better than the sensitivity in other positions. Although their sensitivity may not be normal they still represent normal or near-normal positions as far as glaucoma is concerned, the reduction being caused by a preretinal 'filter', e.g. cataract. The remaining positions with a greater reduction of sensitivity are the 'local' glaucomatous defects. The interpretation of the visual field print-out is greatly facilitated if a relative intensity print-out with separation of general and local reduction of sensitivity is used. Such print-out modes are available for instance in the Octopus, Peritest and Humphrey CAP's.

At this point it may be useful to emphasize that a relative defect is a defect for a certain standard size stimulus with a threshold luminance between normal and maximal. If the maximal luminance is not seen the defect is logically called a defect for maximal luminance and not an absolute defect. The absolute defect on the Goldmann-perimeter is a defect measured with a size V stimulus and maximal luminance or a comparable defect.

4

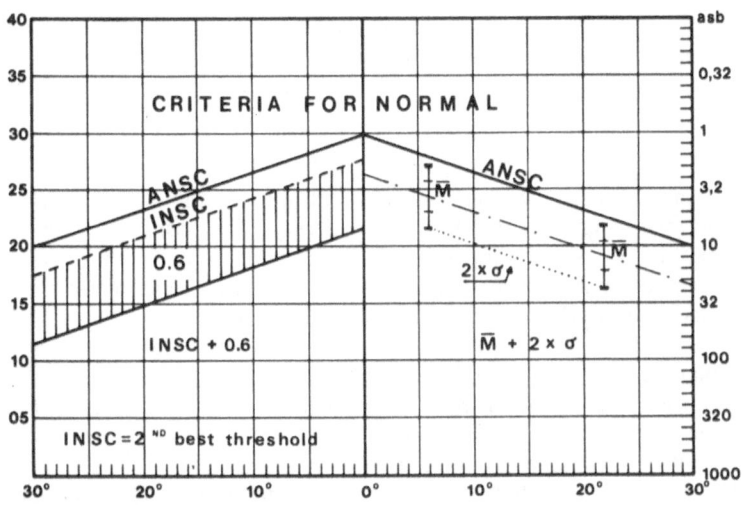

Fig. 4. Criteria for the range of normal sensitivity. Left hand side: the second best threshold is chosen as the INSC: individual normal sensitivity curve. All measurements within this value and 0.6 log.unit higher are considered normal (standard criterion). Right hand side: mean and standard deviation of normal threshold-measurements. The normal range is determined by e.g. 2 × standard deviations of the individual patient.

DEFECT VOLUME

Normal and defect positions can be separated by a set criterion, e.g. normal is any threshold value between the highest sensitivity and 0.6 log.units above it. The criterion is easy to use and has been incorporated in several suprathreshold, threshold related detection strategies (Peritest, Humphrey). A criterion for normal and defect can also be derived from actual fluctuation measurements in normal areas. The limit for normal could be set at mean + 2. standard deviation. (Fig. 4).

Whichever method is used it leads to a separation of normal positions and defect positions. The level of normal sensitivity can be compared with the average interindividual normal sensitivity level. A difference from this average level expressed in log.units is called a general reduction of sensitivity. 'Normal' in the individual case is defined as the best sensitivity. The intensity of defect positions is expressed relative to the individual normal sensitivity.

The defect volume (D.V.) is calculated by adding up the defect intensities at all positions. To this D.V.-value is added a fluctuation value indicating the 99% limits of the D.V. Any significant change should be more than these values (see also 2).

This all seems straightforward and easy. Still, we do not yet have a foolproof programme for the analysis of D.V-change. There are a number of non-statistical factors that influence D.V. and fluctuation. We are not aware of a study that has produced a D.V.-change programme that has been both sensitive and specific in detecting progression or regression.

Further analysis of all factors involved in the variation of D.V. will be

5

necessary. There is no doubt, however, that satisfactory D.V.-change programmes will be available in the not too distant future.

VISUAL FATIGUE

The concept of visual fatigue was first used in perimetry by Enoch (4). He described the phenomenon that the sensitivity of a position in the visual field may deteriorate considerably when tested for an extended period. Or, the threshold value increased after repeated testing. Enoch described this phenomenon for optic nerve disease but not for glaucoma.

Later, Heijl and Drance showed that visual fatigue could also be found in glaucomatous defects (14). We conducted several experiments on visual fatigue in glaucoma. Our main purpose was to detect visual function loss in glaucoma suspects in an earlier stage than hitherto possible. We first used the single position technique as published by Heijl.

The results clearly show a fatigue phenomenon (Fig. 5). While normal areas keep a constant threshold level, in relative defects the threshold level may increase considerably.

Subsequently we tested the fatigue-phenomenon for the whole visual field. Patients with early glaucomatous visual field defects were subjected to repeated automated visual field examination with the Scoperimeter (threshold strategy). It was found that in some patients the visual field defects may enlarge after prolonged tested (20′–30′). (Fig. 6).

This phenomenon, which has several very interesting aspects, may also play a role in fluctuation, and may confuse statistical analysis. If during a visual field examination with a CAP the threshold deteriorates, the values found at the end of the examination may represent a different state of the visual field than the fresh values at the beginning of the examination. It may be fruitful to develop a method that evaluates the influence of fatigue on the visual field results in the individual patient.

PSYCHOLOGICAL FACTORS

There are few reports on the influence of psychological factors in CAP. It should be realized that so far all reports on comparative studies between automatic perimetry and manual perimetry have compared different instruments with different strategies. A study using a similar instrument and strategy does not exist.

We studied psychological phenomena with the Peritest, because this is the only CAP that allows both automatic and semi-automatic presentations. The results of this study are published elsewhere in this volume (15).

Briefly, we examined glaucoma patients twice with the automatic mode and twice with the semi-automatic mode. The main difference between the two examination procedures is the active presence of the examiner during the semi-automatic examination. The examiner can evaluate patient performance, encourage the patient and determine the speed of examination.

6

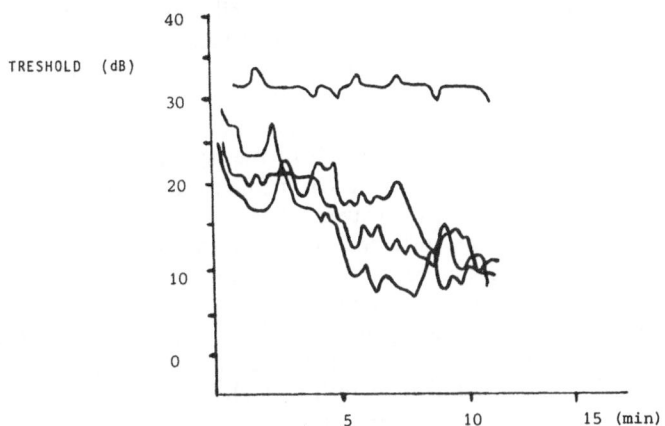

Fig. 5. Local fatigue. The upper curve demonstrates the behaviour of a normal position. The three lower curves show pathological behaviour (= decrease of sensitivity with time).

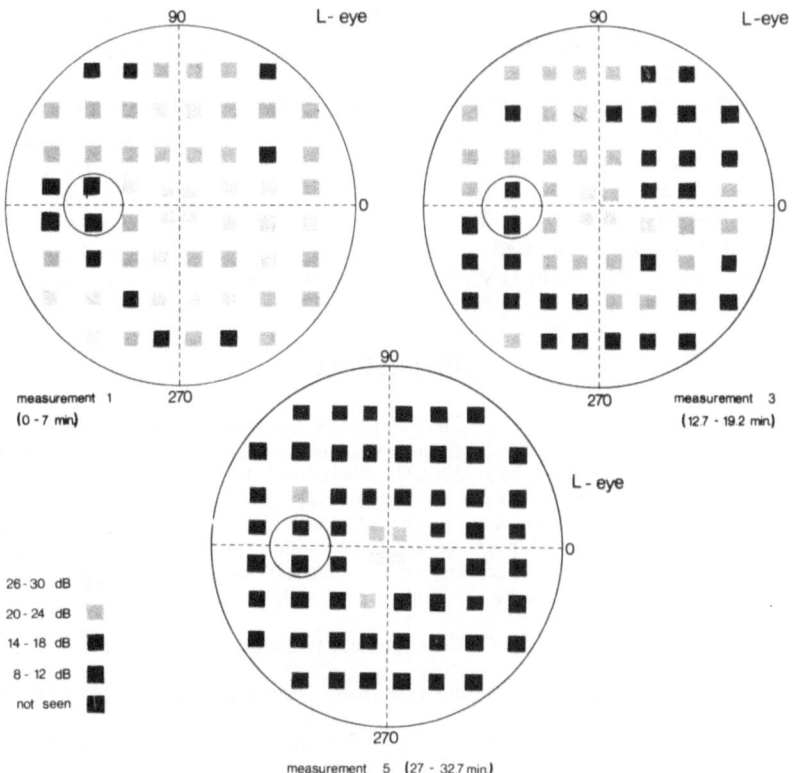

Fig. 6. General fatigue. Three measurements of the same visual field. There is an evident deterioration due to fatigue.

7

The examination strategy was kept basically similar in both procedures. The examination was taped and a psychological evaluation was made after each examination. The psychological score included fixation, reaction and judgement, fatigue, reliability, fear, nervousness, etc.

We found significant differences between the results of automatic and semi-automatic procedures in about half of the patients. Usually the defect volume was smaller in the automatic results. Our second interesting finding was that the average difference between two automatic examinations was almost twice (1.83 x) the difference between two semi-automatic examinations. Similarly, the number of small differences between two examinations was larger in the semi-automatic group.

The somewhat inferior results of atuomatic perimetry were thought to be caused by reaction and judgement problems. Such problems may to a certain extent appear in the false-positive and false-negative score. Other factors were fixation problems. Fatigue and uneasiness were also recorded.

These results do not imply that semi-automatic perimetry is better than automatic perimetry. They do tell us that a number of patients perform better with psychological support. We are afraid that we have been underestimating the role of psychological factors in CAP. It seems we have put an exaggerated trust in the computer. We have forgotten that the computer is only a machine and that this machine also has to deal with 80-year old semi-invalids.

In the past we have advocated flexible CAP's (see also 6, 7), flexible in the sense that they should also be able to operate semi-automatically. Our present study of psychological factors has given us no cause to change our views.

In conclusion, CAP has been greatly improved in the past four years since the first meeting of the European Glaucoma Society in Brighton. Several CAP function well at the clinical level. Further developments, particularly in the field of D.V.-change will make CAP even more exciting.

REFERENCES

1. van den Berg, T.J.T.P., van Spronsen, R., van Veenendaal, W.G. and Greve, E.L. Psychophysics of intensity discrimination in relation to defect volume examination on the Scoperimeter. To be published in Docum. Ophthalmol. Proc. Series.
2. Dannheim, F. Mechanisms for comparing visual fields and their storage in the evaluation of glaucoma. Acta on the 24th Int. Congr. of Ophthalmol., Ed. P. Henkind. Philadelphia, Lippincott. Vol. 1: 654–656 (1983).
3. Drance, S.M. Automatic perimetry: the current state of art. Acta of the 24th Int. Congr. of Ophthalmol., Ed. P. Henkind. Philadelphia, Lippincott. Vol. 1: 160–161 (1983).
4. Enoch, J. Quantitative layer-by-layer perimetry. Invest. Ophthalmol. 17: 1–9–257 (1978).
5. Enoch, J. Perimetry. Today and tomorrow. Docum. Ophthalmol. 55: 307–322 (1983).
6. Etienne, R., Etienne, A. and Sellem, E. Problèmes et solutions de la périmétrie d'aujourd'hui. J. Fr. Ophtal. 6: 179–186 (1983).
7. Etienne, R., Etienne, A. and Sellem, E. Périmétrie moderne: automatique ou manuelle. J. Fr. Ophtal. 6: 927–932 (1983).

8. Flammer, J., Drance, S.M. and Schulzer, M. Covariates of long-term fluctuation of the differential light threshold. Am. Ophthalmol. 102: 880 (1984).
9. Flammer, J., Drance, S.M., Fankhauser, F. and Angustiny, L. Differential light threshold in automated static perimetry. Arch. Ophthalmol. 102: 876 (1984).
10. Flammer, J. and Zulauf, M. The frequency distribution of the deviations in static perimetry. To be published in Docum. Opthalmol. Proc. Series.
11. Gloor, B.P. and Vökt, B.A. Longterm fluctuations versus definite field loss in glaucoma patients. Invest. Ophthal. Vis. Sci. 24: suppl. Arvo: 103 (1983).
12. Greve, E.L. Single and multiple static perimetry in glaucoma: the two phases of visual field examination. Docum. Ophthalmol. 36: 1–355 (1973).
13. Greve, E.L. Performance of Computer Assisted Perimetry. Docum. Ophthalmol. 53: 348–380 (1982).
14. Heijl, A. and Drance, S.M. Deterioration of threshold in glaucoma patients during perimetry. Docum. Ophthalmol. Proc. Series 35: 129–136 (1983).
15. de Jong, D.G.M.M., Greve, E.L., Bakker, D. and van den Berg, T.J.T.P. Psychological factors in computer assisted perimetry; automatic and semi-automatic perimetry. This volume.
16. Krakau, C.E.T. Separation of background and defect in automatic perimetry. Acta Opthalmol. 62: 210–216 (1984).
17. Langerhorst, C.T. Schätzung der Verschiedene Fluktuationsfaktoren bei der Computerperimetrie von Glaukompatienten. Symposium München 1983. To be published.
18. Langerhorst, C.T., van den Berg, T.J.T.P., van Spronsen, R. and Greve, E.L. Results of a fluctuation analysis and defect volume program for automated static threshold perimetry with the Scoperimeter. To be published in Docum. Ophthalmol. Proc. Series.

Authors addresses:
Dr. E.L. Greve
Sint Lucas Hospital
Dept. of Opthalmology
Jan Tooropstraat 164
1061 AE Amsterdam
The Netherlands

Dr T.J.T.P. van den Berg
Eye Clinic of the University of Amsterdam
Academic Medical Center
Meibergdreef 9
1105 AZ Amsterdam
The Netherlands

Dr C.T. Langerhorst
The Netherlands Ophthalmic Research Institute
P.O. Box 6411
Amsterdam, The Netherlands

PSYCHOPHYSICS IN GLAUCOMA. A MODIFIED CONCEPT OF THE DISEASE

JOSEF FLAMMER

(Bern, Switzerland)

Glaucoma is conventionally defined as a disease characterized by high intra-ocular pressure (IOP) leading to excavation of the optic nerve head and progressive visual field loss.

The research work reported has concentrated on two basic questions:

(a) Why does the pressure increase and how can one reduce it?

(b) Why does the increased pressure damage the optic nerve head? Does it damage directly and mechanically or indirectly by reducing circulation.

There are two observations that do not fit this classical pressure theory properly. On the one hand are the so-called low tension glaucomas (glaucomatous damage without elevated IOP) and on the other hand the so-called ocular hypertensives (high IOP without detectable damage in the visual field or optic disc). Some authors postulate, therefore, an individually different sensitivity to pressure. They consider this range as so large that even normal pressure of 10 or 15 may damage some eyes (1). Other research workers no longer consider the elevated IOP as being the only factor producing glaucomatous damage (2); some even consider the elevated IOP just as a symptom and not the cause of this still poorly understood disease (3).

I do not have to emphasize that these different concepts have a major influence on our therapeutic approach and thus have to be considered very carefully.

Based upon the analysis of some psychophysical findings, I will try to present some thoughts about a modified concept of the disease. I would like to emphasize the hypothetical nature of this concept. I am fully aware of the limited character of any hypothesis in a rapidly growing field like glaucoma.

There are several new findings, in psychophysics that have to be built into our concept. One is of special interest. Until recently, we believed that the foveal function is particularly resistant to glaucomatous damage and that it is not affected until very late in the disease process. This opinion was based upon observations with visual acuities and visual fields. The pendulum then swung to the other side and macular changes are now considered to occur at the very beginning and to precede visual field damage. This opinion is based upon observations on color vision and contrast sensitivity. Both are often found to be disturbed in patients with elevated IOP, even in the absence of scotomas (4, 5, 6, 7, 8).

11

E.L. Greve, W. Leydhecker & C. Raitta (eds.), Second European Glaucoma Symposium, Helsinki 1984.
© *1985, Dr. W. Junk Publishers, Dordrecht. ISBN 978-94-010-8934-0*

Actually, color vision changes in glaucoma have been described by many authors since 1883. They were tested very accurately with the Pickford anomaloscope and the 100-hue test. Even if some controversy exists about the nature of the color vision disturbance, there is no doubt that glaucomas have on the average remarkably more color vision changes than normals of the same age. In addition to that, color vision has been shown to have a predictive value for future changes in the visual field. The higher the error in the 100-hue test, the higher is the chance of developing scotomas in the next few years (9).

The interesting fact, however, is that a distinct portion of the patients with irreversible visual field defects has an absolutely normal color sense, whereas other patients with a high error score in the color vision tests have no scotomas in the visual field at all.

This indicates that these two processes are, even though statistically related, at least partially independent. Therefore, none of them is an indispensable precursor of the other.

The findings reported on contrast sensitivity are very similar.

The contrast required to perceive a series of grating targets with different spatial frequencies is on the average higher in glaucomas than in normals (10, 11, 12). This difference is greatest when measured with low spatial frequencies. In a similar way, the sensitivity to flicker modulation is reduced in patients with high IOP. The required contrast for flickering patterns allows a particularly good separation to be made between normals and glaucomas (13). It is also remarkable that chromatic and achromatic activity can be reduced in glaucomas and that these two findings are highly correlated (14).

But how are these foveal functions related to the visual field? We already mentioned the partial independence of scotomas. But this does not mean an independence of the visual field as a whole. Let us briefly recapitulate the perimetric findings in glaucoma. We all know the specific types of scotomas, often beginning paracentrally and showing later the typical shape of a nerve fibre bundle. A well-known manifestation of it is also a nasal step. These typical and specific defects in the visual field are, however, not the only possible changes in the visual field of a patient with high IOP. With the help of good quantitative perimetry we often observe changes such as: diffuse depression of the increment sensitivity, increased short- and long-term fluctuation and fatigue effects (15, 16, 17, 18, 19, 20, 21). Like the changes in color vision and contrast sensitivity, these changes are non-specific but can be observed in patients with high IOP significantly more often than in normals.

Let us examine the fluctuations of the differential light sensitivity briefly.

The short-term fluctuation is known to be increased in relative scotomas as well as in patients with poor cooperation (16). The influence of the latter can be estimated in Octopus perimetry by the rate of false responses in the catch trials. The short-term fluctuation, as well as the so-called homogeneous component of the long-term fluctuation, can, however, be markedly increased in patients with elevated IOP having otherwise still normal visual fields (17).

Another frequent finding is a diffuse depression of the differential light sensitivity (18). This might be due to several shallow scotomas scattered all over or a nearly homogeneous depression of the differential light sensitivity. This diffuse depression can amount to several dB's and is therefore of obvious significance. It has often been overlooked due to the lack of normal confidence values. It is difficult to recognize whether the isopters are constricted (22). It is much easier to give normal values for static perimetry (23). It is, however, self-evident that we find this diffuse damage only in quantitative perimetry.

Fundamental for our present consideration is the question whether all these psychophysical findings are related to each other. Do they represent different sorts of glaucomatous damage or are they possibly an expression of different stages of the disease process?

I strongly believe they are an expression of basically two partly overlapping sorts of glaucomatous damage (Table 1). The first is a diffuse damage

Table 1. Psychophysical changes in glaucoma

Local damage:	— scotomas in the visual field
	— localized increase in scatter
Diffuse damage:	— diffuse depression of the visual field
	— diffuse increase in scatter
	— color vision disturbance
	— decreased contrast sensitivity

comprising more or less the total visual field, including the macula and therefore also including color vision and contrast sensitivity. The second is the presence of localized damages as in the well-known scotomas (24, 25).

This concept is supported by the fact that color vision as well as contrast sensitivity are highly correlated to the diffuse damage observed in perimetry and only weakly to the existence of scotomas (26).

What are the morphological correlates?

This has not yet been answered properly. But our observations indicate that the diffuse damage corresponds to the concentric enlargement of the cup and/or homogeneous pallor of the neuroretinal rim (27) (Table 2).

Nerve fibre counting in histological studies revealed quite diffuse loss in

Table 2. Morphological correlates

Local damage:	— excentric enlargement of the cup
	— notching of the neuroretinal rim
	— disc haemorrhages
	— defects in the nerve fibre layer
	— peripapillary chorioidal atrophy
Diffuse damage:	— concentric enlargement of the cup (decreased area of the neuroretinal rim
	— diffuse pallor of the neuroretinal rim

so-called ocular hypertensives (29). Relatively high visual functions such as color discrimination and contrast sensitivity might be sensitive to such a decrease in the nerve fibre concentration. We, therefore, do not have to postulate additional changes located in the retina.

The increased fluctuation of the differential light threshold can also be explained by a decreased number of nerve fibres. We assume that the brain adapts to a reduced flow of information. On the other hand this adaption increases the scatter, as we know from analogue situations in the technique.

The correlates to the localized defects are eccentric enlargment of the cup and notching of the neuroretinal rim, disc haemorrhages and peripapillary chorioidal atrophy and defects in the nerve fibre layer (30, 31, 32, 33).

What are the pathomechanisms for these two kinds of damage?

There is some evidence that the IOP has a diffuse damaging effect on the axons. This might be a direct mechanical damage that results in a disturbance of the axoplasmic flow and later in a loss of nerve fibers (2, 34). This view is not proven, but is supported by experimental results and the clinical observations of diffuse damage occurring in patients with high IOP but excellent circulation (Fig. 1).

On the other hand, there is some evidence that the local defects are due to a circulation insufficiency, which might lead to a microinfarction of the optic nerve head. This circulation insufficiency can be due to an increased IOP, but it may also be due to other vascular risk factors or circulation problems like postural hypotension (35, 36). The onset of local defects is often sudden as we observe in high tension and low tension glaucomas. I remember an eye physician having IOP in the low twenties and normal visual fields over years. Taking a shower in the morning he noticed the sudden onset of a scotoma. The perimetry done on the same day showed a deep and irreversible nerve fibre bundle defect.

The partial overlap of local and diffuse damage is explained by the assumption that the IOP acts on both mechanisms. In addition, a further circulation insufficiency is more likely to occur in an already mechanically damaged disc.

What are the possible clinical consequences?

1. We should not only check for local defects but also for diffuse damage. This can be done either by the combination of perimetry and a test of foveal function such as contrast sensitivity or color vision or by good quantitative perimetry alone (37). We are developing a new glaucoma program for the Octopus automated perimeter that measures these different possible changes by automated data reduction and permits an easy comparison to normal values and follow up.
2. Having found diffuse damage, we should reduce the IOP. But the finding of a local defect should lead not only to a reduction of the IOP, but also to a search for vascular risk factors, especially if the IOP is only slightly increased. In such cases we might avoid drugs which could reduce the blood supply to the optic nerve head.

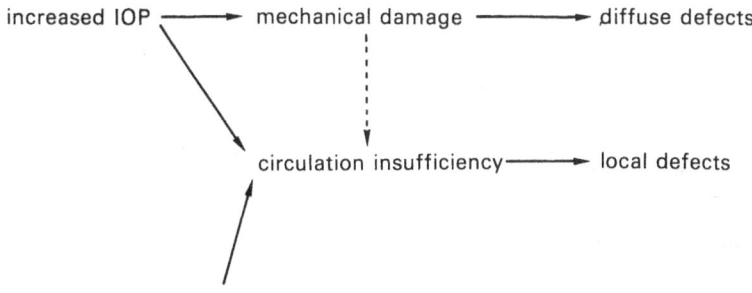

Fig. 1. Schematic depiction of the hypothetical pathomechanisms. An increased IOP may directly cause diffuse damage and, in addition, is one of several risk factors for local, probably ischaemic damage. Furthermore, circulation insufficiency has a higher probability of occurring in an already mechanically damaged optic nerve head.

The crucial question in any glaucoma therapy is not how well it reduces the IOP, but rather, how well it prevents deterioration of the visual function. It is surprising that the drugs we are using are so little studied in this respect (38).

To sum up, I have presented a modified concept of glaucoma which should encompass the different findings currently available. We all realize that we have a long way to go before fully understanding this mysterious disease.

REFERENCES

1. Minckler, D.S. and Spaeth, G.L. Optic nerve damage in glaucoma. Surv. Ophthalmol. 26: 128–148 (1981).
2. Drance, S.M., Sweeney, V.P., Morgan, R.W. and Feldman, F. Studies of factors involved in the production of low tension glaucoma. Arch. Ophthalmol. 89: 457–465 (1973).
3. Krakau, C.E.T. Intraocular pressure elevation – cause or effect in chronic glaucoma? Ophthalmologica, Basel 182: 141–147 (1981).
4. Atkin, A., Wolkstein, M., Bodis-Wollner, I, Anders, M., Kels, B. and Podos, S.M. Interocular comparison of contrast sensitivities in glaucoma patients and suspects. J. Ophthalmol. 64: 858–862 (1980).
5. Poinoosawmy, D., Nagasubramanian, S. and Gloster, J. Colour vision in patients with chronic simple glaucoma and ocular hypertension. Br. J. Ophthalmol. 64: 852–857 (1980).
6. Arden, G.B. and Jacobson, J.J. A simple grating test for contrast sensitivity: preliminary results indicate value in screening for glaucoma. Invest. Ophthalmol. Visual Sci. 17: 23–32 (1978).
7. Motolko, M.A. and Phelps, Ch.D. Contrast sensitivity in asymmetric glaucoma. Int. Ophthalmol. 7: 45–50 (1984).
8. Hyvaerinen, L., Rovamo, J., Laurinen, P., Saarinen, J., Naesaenen, R. Contrast sensitivity in monocular glaucoma. Acta Ophthalmol. 61: 742–750 (1983).
9. Drance, S.M., Lakowski, R., Schulzer, M., Douglas, G.R. Acquired color vision changes in glaucoma. Arch. Ophthalmol. 99: 829–831 (1981).
10. Regan, D., Neima, D. Low-contrast letter charts as a test of visual function. Ophthalmology 90: 1192–1200 (1983).
11. Atkin, A., Bodis-Wollner, I., Wolkstein, M., Moss, A. and Podos, S.M. Abnormalities of central contrast sensitivity in glaucoma. Am. J. Ophthalmol. 88: 205–211 (1979).

15

12. Tyler, Ch.W., Ryu, S. and Stamper, R. The relation between visual sensitivity and intraocular pressure in normal eyes. Invest. Ophthalmol. Vis. Sci. 25: 103–105 (1984).
13. Atkin, A., Bodis-Wollner, I., Podos, S.M., Wolkstein, M., Mylin, L. and Nitzberg, S. Flicker threshold and pattern VEP latency in ocular hypertension and glaucoma. Invest. Ophthalmol. Vis. Sci. 24: 1524–1528 (1983).
14. Adams, A.J., Rodic, R., Husted, R. and Stamper, R. Spectra sensitivity and color discrimination changes in glaucoma and glaucoma-suspect patients. Invest. Ophthalmol. Vis. Sci. 23: 516–524 (1982).
15. Flammer, J., Drance, S.M., Augustiny, L. and Funkhouser, A. Quantification of glaucomatous visual field defects with automated perimetry. Submitted.
16. Flammer, J., Drance, S.M., Fankhauser, F. and Augustiny, L. The differential light threshold in automatic static perimetry. Arch. Ophthalmol. (in press).
17. Flammer, J., Drance, S.M. and Zulauf, M. The short- and long-term fluctuation of the differential light threshold in patients with glaucoma, normal controls and glaucoma suspects. Arch. Ophthalmol. (in press).
18. Stuermer, J., Gloor, B. and Tobler, X. Wie sehen Glaukomgesichtsfelder wirklich aus. Klin. Mbl. Augenheilk. (im Druck).
19. Gloor, B., Stuermer, J. and Voekt, B. Was hat die automatisierte Perimetrie mit dem Octopus fuer neue Kenntnisse ueber glaukomatoese Gesichtsfeldveraenderungen gebracht? Klin. Mbl. Augenheilk. (im Druck).
20. Werner, E.B., Saheb, N. and Thomas, D. Variability of static visual threshold responses in patients with elevated IOPs. Arch. Ophthalmol. 100: 1627–1631 (1982).
21. Heijl, A. and Drance, S.M. Changes in differential threshold in patients with glaucoma during prolonged perimetry. Br. J. Ophthalmol. 67: 512–516 (1983).
22. Chisholm, I.A., Stead, S., Tan, L. and Melenchuk, J.W. Prognostic indicators in ocular hypertension: Can. J. Ophthalmol. 7: 4–8 (1980).
23. Flammer, J. Methoden zur Datenreduktion in der automatischen Perimetrie. In: Neuere Entwicklungen in der Augenheilkunde, H. Merte, ed. (in press).
24. Spaeth, G.L. Low tension glaucoma: its diagnosis and management. Doc. Ophthalmol. Proc. Series 22: 263 (1979).
25. Greve, E.L. and Geijssen, H.C. Comparison of glaucomatous visual field defects in patients with high and low intraocular pressure. Doc. Ophthalmol. Proc. Series 35: 101–105 (1983).
26. Flammer, J. and Drance, S.M. Correlation between colour vision scores and quantitative perimetry in glaucoma suspects. Arch. Ophthalmol. 102, 38–39 (1980).
27. Anctil, J.-L. and Anderson, D.R. Early foveal involvement and generalized depression of the visual field in glaucoma. Arch. Ophthalmol. 102: 363–370 (1984).
28. Balazsi, A.G., Drance, S.M., Schulzer, M. and Douglas, G.R. The area of the neuroretinal rim in glaucoma suspects and early chronic open angle glaucoma: correlation with parameters of visual function. Arch. Ophthalmol. (in press).
29. Quigley, H.A. Histology of human glaucoma optic nerve damage compared to clinical findings in the same eye. In: Krieglstein, G.K. and Leydhecker, W. (eds.): Glaucoma Update II, 83–87, Springer-Verlag 1983.
30. Iwata, K. The earliest finding of primary open-angle glaucoma (POAG) and the mode of progression. In: Krieglstein, G.K. and Leydhecker, W. (eds.): Glaucoma Update II, 133–137, Springer-Verlag 1983.
31. Krakau, C.E.T. Disc haemorrhages – forerunners of chronic glaucoma. In.: Krieglstein, G.K. and Leydhecker, W. (eds.): Glaucoma Update II, 71–76, Springer-Verlag 1983.
32. Anderson, D.R. Correlation of the peripapillary anatomy with the disc damage and field abnormalities in glaucoma. Doc. Ophthalmol. Proc. Series 35: 1–10 (1983).
33. Drance, S.M. Hemorrhage on the disc – a risk factor in glaucoma. In: Krieglstein, G.K. and Leydhecker, W. (eds.): Glaucoma Update II, 77–82, Springer-Verlag 1983.
34. Maumenee, A.E. Causes of optic nerve damage in glaucoma. Ophthalmology 90: 741–752 (1983).

16

35. Goldberg, I., Hollows, F.C., Kass, M.A. and Becker, B. Systematic factors in patients with low-tension glaucoma. Br. J. Ophthalmol. 65: 56–62 (1981).
36. Demailly, P., Cambien, F., Plouin, P.F., Baron, P. and Chevallier, B. Do patients with low tension glaucoma have particular cardiovascular characteristics? Ophthalmologica, Basel 188: 65–75 (1984).
37. Flammer, J., Drance, S.M., Jenni, A. and Bebie, H. JO and STATJO: programs for investigating the visual field with the Octopus automatic perimeter. Can. J. Ophthalmol. 18: 115–117 (1983).
38. Flammer, J. and Drance, S.M. The effect of a number of glaucoma medications on the differential light threshold. Doc. Ophthalmol. Proc. Series 35: 145–148 (1983).

Author's address:
Dr J. Flammer
Augenklinik
Inselspital
CH-3010 Bern
Switzerland

PSYCHOLOGICAL FACTORS IN COMPUTER ASSISTED PERIMETRY; AUTOMATIC AND SEMI-AUTOMATIC PERIMETRY

D.G.M.M. DE JONG, E.L. GREVE and D. BAKKER

(Amsterdam, The Netherlands)

ABSTRACT

The effect of psychological factors on the results of computer assisted perimetry has been underestimated. In order to quantify this effect a group of glaucoma patients was examined twice with a completely automated procedure and twice with a semi-automated procedure on the same instrument, the Peritest. All parameters were similar in both procedures. The examination strategy was also similar. The only difference was the active presence of the examiner during the semi-automated procedure. The examiner judged alertness, fatigue, fixation of the patient and according to his impression determined the speed of examination and provided psychological support.

A psychological score was made during and after the examinations. Defect volumes were calculated for all examinations. In 10 out of 19 cases a significant difference was found between automated and semi-automated procedures. *Intra*-semi-automated defect volume differences were usually larger than *intra*-automated defect volume differences. Thus, variation was less in the semi-automated procedure. The somewhat inferior results of the automated procedure were thought to be mainly caused by reaction and judgement problems of the patients. Other factors involved were fatigue, nervousness and fixation problems.

On the basis of these results and on the general experience with computer assisted visual field examination it is advised to offer the option of a semi-automated procedure in every computer assisted perimeter.

E.L. Greve, W. Leydhecker & C. Raitta (eds.), Second European Glaucoma Symposium, Helsinki 1984.
© 1985, Dr. W. Junk Publishers, Dordrecht. ISBN 978-94-010-8934-0

OPTIC DISC DENSITOMETRIC DATA AND DELAYED VECP IN GLAUCOMA

E. MARRÉ, P. MIERDEL and H.-J. ZENKER

(Dresden, G.D.R.)

ABSTRACT

The colour of the optic disc was quantitatively evaluated by simultaneous photography of the papilla with green and red filters using a stereoscopic fundus camera. The papilla colour is expressed by a numerical index. The colour index data of nasal and temporal areas are compared with the peak delay and rise decrease of VECP occurring when the abrupt stimulus luminance rise (step stimulation) is replaced by a continuously increasing stimulus luminance (ramp stimulation). The results show that pallor of the papilla in early glaucoma (temporal areas) is only conditionally correlated to the VECP data based on the described method.

The colour of the optic disc is considered important for the diagnosis of glaucoma. Since the pallor of the disc is obviously a measure of glaucomatous optic nerve atrophy, it is of interest whether both objective methods, the two-colour densitometry of optic disc and the VECP method, give correlations. This question was investigated in patients with beginning primary open-angle glaucoma (i.e. there were no greater visual field defects apart from small paracentral scotomas or nasal steps) to evaluate the information content of optic disc colour with regard to the functional state of optic nerve system.

METHODS

Optic disc two-colour densitometry (Fig. 1)

Black and white photographs were taken of the disc using a modified stereoscopic fundus camera which contained a green filter in one optical path and a red filter in the other. For calibration several neutral density filters were photographed on the same strip of the film. Densities derived from areas of the temporal and nasal rim of the disc were measured from the simultaneously taken red and green partial images of the stereophotographs by a rapid photometer. The colour of these areas was expressed as a numerical index (colour index) which is based on simple analysis of the optical densities of the two different light components (red and green) within the corresponding colour space (1).

19

E.L. Greve, W. Leydhecker & C. Raitta (eds.), Second European Glaucoma Symposium, Helsinki 1984.
© *1985, Dr. W. Junk Publishers, Dordrecht. ISBN 978-94-010-8934-0*

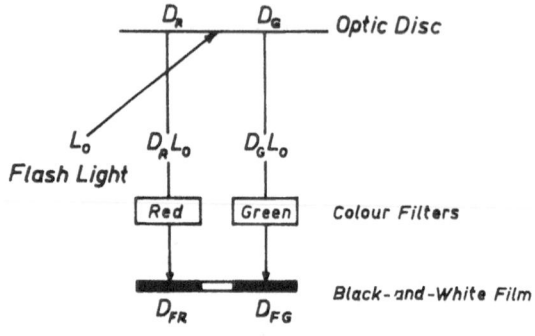

$$D_{FR}, D_{FG} \quad \text{— By Means of Calibration} \longrightarrow D_R, D_G$$

$$\boxed{\text{COLOUR INDEX} \quad D_R/D_G}$$

D_R, D_G Density of Optic Disc in Red or Green Light

D_{FR}, D_{FG} Film Density of Red or Green Partial Images

Fig. 1. Principle of the two-colour densitometry method.

VECP-method (Fig. 2)

The visual evoked cortical potentials were recorded bipolarly from the Area striata. As a measure of the transmission capacity of optical nerve system served the wave form alteration of the on-VECP in response to an abrupt linear increase of luminance (ramp stimulus), as compared to luminance step stimulation. The parameters of the wave of which the normal peak latency is of the order of magnitude of 90 ms were used (delay of peak latency and decrease of wave rise). A special stimulator (low voltage lamps, electromagnetic shutter, slow speed shutter resp.) produces a $5°$ stimulus centred in a $20°$-background light and with a luminance of about 10,000 cd/m². The stimulus is superimposed on a permanently visible light spot of the same colour and size as the stimulus, but near threshold intensity. The stimulus light is mechanically modulated to generate a defined temporal luminance rise. The rise time, approximately linearly sloped, amounts to 200 ms (ramp stimulation). A terminal value of about 80,000 cd/m² was used. The rise time of the step stimuli was below 10 ms. Both the step and the ramp stimuli had a total duration of 500 ms. White or blue stimuli with a white or yellow background illumination were used (Fig. 1).

RESULTS (TABLE 1)

The colour index of examined glaucomatous eyes showed a significant difference with normals only in temporal rim data. The correlation coefficient

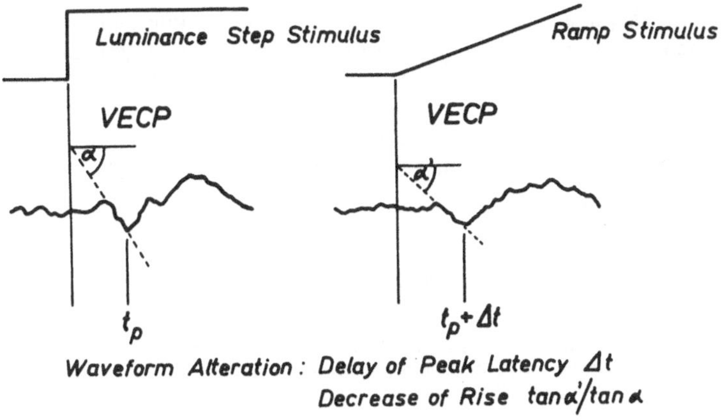

Fig. 2. Delayed VECP method.

between the temporal colour index and VECP wave alteration was calculated to 0.19 (white stimuli), but it is not significant. The correlation between the colour index of selected rim parts, corresponding to visual field defects and VECP data was no better and also not significant ($r = 0.22$).

The significant increase of VECP delay and decrease of wave rise at white stimulation in glaucoma patients is noteworthy. At blue stimulation the difference is only significant for a level of confidence of 0.90 in peak delay.

DISCUSSION

The small number of analysed glaucomatous eyes makes it difficult to draw exact conclusions. A problem is how to sufficiently dilate the pupils of glaucoma patients (above 5.5 mm) so as to make possible an accurate photography of the optic disc. Of 26 patients the dilation succeeded in only 12 cases.

Table 1. Means of densitometric data (colour index) and VECP data in normals and glaucoma patients.

	Normals	Glaucoma patients	Significance of difference (95%)
Colour index			
Temporal	2.09	1.70	yes
Nasal	2.17	2.00	no
VECP Peak delay			
White stim.	21 ms	37 ms	yes
Blue stim.	22 ms	31 ms	no
VECP tan α'/tan α			
White stim.	0.72	0.54	yes
Blue stim.	0.65	0.63	no

The relative large standard deviation of the colour index in normals is an indication of its small informative value. Nevertheless a significant decrease of temporal colour index in the examined eyes with initial stages of glaucoma could be found. The VECP data in these patients refer to manifest functional deficiencies of the optic nerve. But the results show that colour (pallor) of the papilla is only conditionally correlated to the VECP data based on the described method.

REFERENCE

1.   Zenker, H.-J., Mierdel, P. and Marré, E. Quantitative evaluation of pallor-disc ratio and colour of the optic disc by a photographic method. Graefes Arch. Clin. Exp. Ophthalm. 220: 184 (1983).

Author's address:
Dr P. Mierdel
Medizinische Akademie Dresden
Augenklinik
Fetscherstr. 74
G.D.R. 8019 Dresden

CORRELATION OR NON-CORRELATION BETWEEN GLAUCOMATOUS FIELD LOSS AS DETERMINED BY AUTOMATED PERIMETRY AND CHANGES IN THE SURFACE OF THE OPTIC DISC?

S.A. DIMITRAKOS, U. FEY, B. GLOOR and P. JÄGGI

(Basle, Switzerland)

ABSTRACT

The development of field loss as revealed by Octopus perimetry in one eye selected at random in each of 35 patients who had clearly-established glaucoma is shown. The observation period was up to 5 years. In this time half of the fields of the eyes became worse, the other half became better.

From these 35 patients, there were 23 eyes which could be followed by fundus photography and planimetry of the optic disc. Seven of these eyes showed an increase of surface of neuroretinal rim, 18 a decrease. The change of surface is only in two eyes clearly outside the error of measurement.

There is no clear or linear correlation between (1) loss and cup/disc ratio or surface of the rim; (2) change of field loss and change of surface of the rim. This may be explained by the fact that considerable short- and long-term fluctuations in the glaucomatous fields overshadow what was going on at the neuroretinal rim, but also that an enlargement of the cup is not the only parameter which can tell what happens to the nerve fibers in the optic disc.

INTRODUCTION

Automated static threshold perimetry, as performed with the Octopus perimeter, exposed how difficult the assessment of progress of glaucomatous field damage may be (11, 12). This became easy to understand when, with semi-automated perimetry (15) and with automated perimetry, it could be demonstrated that short- and long-term fluctuation of differential light sensitivity threshold are a common feature in fields of patients with glaucoma (8, 9, 10, 11, 12, 19, 28). Betz et al. (4, 5) and many others (1, 6, 7, 14, 16, 17, 20, 24, 25, 27, 29) have presented methods for measuring the neuroretinal rim of the optic disc and have found reasonable correlations with the changes in the visual field of glaucoma patients as revealed by perimetry with the Goldmann apparatus (4, 5) and the Octopus (1, 7). Therefore, it became quite an obvious next step to combine measurements of the surface of the optic disc, especially of the neuroretinal rim, with investigations of the visual field with automated static perimetry not only to evaluate the actual stage but also the course of the disease. Preliminary results of this undertaking were

23

E.L. Greve, W. Leydhecker & C. Raitta (eds.), Second European Glaucoma Symposium, Helsinki 1984.
© *1985, Dr. W. Junk Publishers, Dordrecht. ISBN 978-94-010-8934-0*

quite puzzling (14), and what we are going to present in this paper will generate at least as many problems as it solves.

This investigation has two parts: In the first part, our follow-up data of Octopus fields of our glaucoma patients presented earlier (11) are brought up-to-date. They form the back-ground against which the need for better criteria to evaluate the course of the disease is made obvious.

In the second part, the results of the planimetric measurements of the neuroretinal rim of the optic disc over approximately the same period of time are presented and correlated to the changes in the visual field as revealed by Octopus perimetry.

MATERIALS AND METHODS

Development of fields of glaucoma patients as revealed by Octopus perimetry

Among the 126 patients with ocular hypertension and/or glaucoma who could be followed during at least 3 years, only 35 patients were chosen, of whom the diagnosis of glaucoma appeared absolutely justified for further evaluations. There were 16 women and 19 men, 37 to 84 years old; their glaucoma had been known for 4 to 27 years. These patients had to satisfy the following criteria: open angle, intraocular pressure untreated ≥ 25 mm Hg or cup/disc-ratio ≥ 0.8 and visual field defects of various extent. All the patients were under topical glaucoma therapy, and 10 of them had had trabeculectomy before the study began.

For further computations only one eye of each patient was chosen at random. In these eyes, the visual acuity at the most recent examination ranged from 0.4 to 1.0 (mean 0.81 ± 0.18). The cup/disc ratio was estimated by means of repeated biomicroscopy and/or color photography. The readings from each eye were averaged. Visual fields were recorded by means of auto-mated perimetry with Octopus programs 31 and 33 and evaluated with program delta 'series' and program delta 'change' (3). All patients had at least 4 recordings, and 23 patients had 6 consecutive ones. The observation period was 2 to 3 years for 5 patients, 3 to 4 years for 5 patients, 4 to 5 years for 9 patients, and 5 to 6 years for 16 patients.

Planimetric measurements of the neuroretinal rim of the optic disc

In 26 eyes of the 35 aforementioned patients, stereo photographs were available for follow-up periods of 1 to 5 years (mean 2.8 years). The stereo photographs were made with a Zeiss fundus camera at a magnification of 2.5 times. The slides were projected on a white paper. The magnification due to projection was 22 times, resulting in a final magnification of 55 times. A line drawing of the projected picture was made, delineating the margin of the optic disc and the inner margin of the neuroretinal rim or the excavation and comparing this two-dimensional figure with the stereoscopic appearance all the time. For discrimination between the neuroretinal rim and excavations, the criteria of Betz et al. (4, 5) were applied. Each disc was drawn three times

24

independently, and each drawing was measured by planimetry. The surface of the whole optic disc, of the excavation, and of the neuroretinal rim are expressed in units originating from the magnification of the projected slide and, after conversion in mm^2 (1 unit = 0.03 mm^2).

The error of measurement due to planimetry of the drawn surface is < 1%, and the error in the estimation of the border-line between the neuro-retinal rim and the excavation is 6%. The main source of error is unsharp focussing of the optic disc on the plane of the film. The magnification factor originating from ametropia could purposely be neglected, because our aim was not to distinguish between normal and pathological findings, but to correlate *change* of the surface of the rim with *change* of the visual field.

RESULTS

Development of fields of glaucoma patients as revealed by Octopus perimetry

The total loss as revealed by program delta 'series' ranged from 12 to 1599 dB (note that the total sensitivity in the 30° field is around 2000 dB [≈ 70 × 29!]). If the fields examined in the first half of the follow-up period are compared with the fields checked in the second half of the follow-up period, the fields of 18 eyes changed for the worse (1 ± 23 dB to 699 ± 72 dB) and 17 eyes changed for the better (7 ± 45 dB to 793 ± 123 dB).

In Fig. 1 the total loss of sensitivity found at the first examination of the field is taken as a starting point. The change of total loss with regard to this base is depicted. Some of the field were quite stable, but there are some peculiar follow-ups, e.g. no. 1: From the first to the second examination (14 months later) this field showed considerable gain of sensitivity and then stayed stable for another $3\frac{1}{2}$ years. Field no. 2 showed an amelioration from the first to the second examination, then stayed stable for about 2 years, showed at that time another amelioration and finally remained stable for another 3 years on this level. At each full year of follow-up, sample section is made from the plots (upper half of Fig. 1), showing that the distributions of amelioration and deterioration remain almost symmetrical even over a period of 5 years.

In Fig. 2 the relation between the mean of total loss (y-axis) and cup/disc ratio of the 35 eyes is shown. The correlation coefficient of r = 0.352 shows that there is, if at all, only a weak, or probably non-linear correlation between cup/disc ratio and loss of differential light sensitivity in the 30° field.

Planimetric measurements of the neuroretinal rim of the optic disc

In Table 1 the change of the surface of the rim is shown. The error of measurement is used for classification, one-δ being 3.7 u (0.111 mm^2). Seven of the surfaces increased, but five of them are in the one-δ group, and 18 decreased, but 10 of them are in the one-δ group. The overall tendency is toward decrease, but only in two cases did this tendency show up to be outside error of measurement with a 99.77% probability.

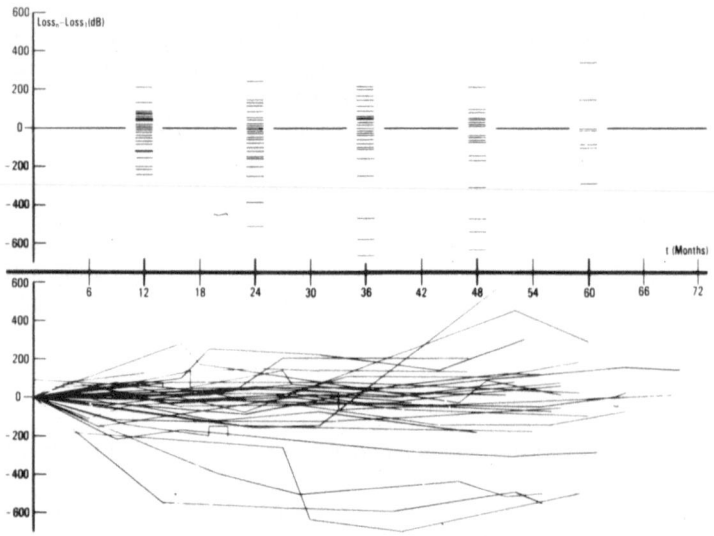

Fig. 1. Development of the visual field as revealed by Octopus perimetry (programs 31 and 33) over 1 to 5 years in 35 eyes with chronic simple glaucoma.

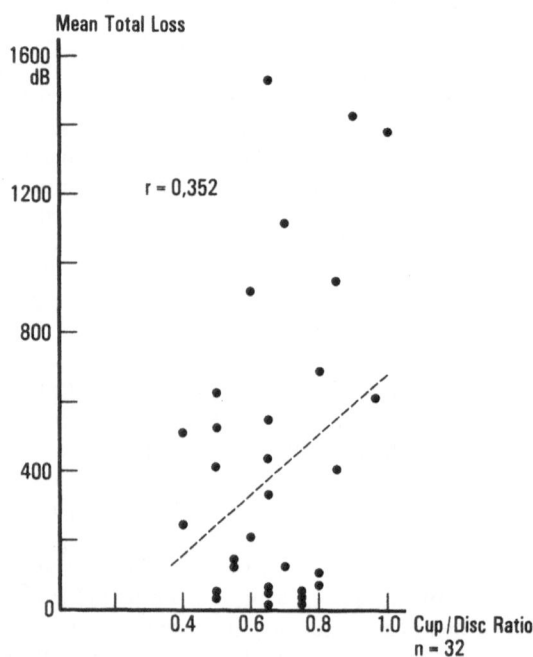

Fig. 2. Correlation between mean field loss and cup/disc-ratio in 35 eyes with chronic simple glaucoma.

Table 1. Changes of the neuroretinal rim. 1 u = 0.03 mm²; 1 = 3.7 u

	0 – 3.7 u	3.71 – 7.41 u	7.41 – 11.1 u	> 11.1 u
+ Increase of surface	5	1	1	
— Decrease of surface	10	6		2

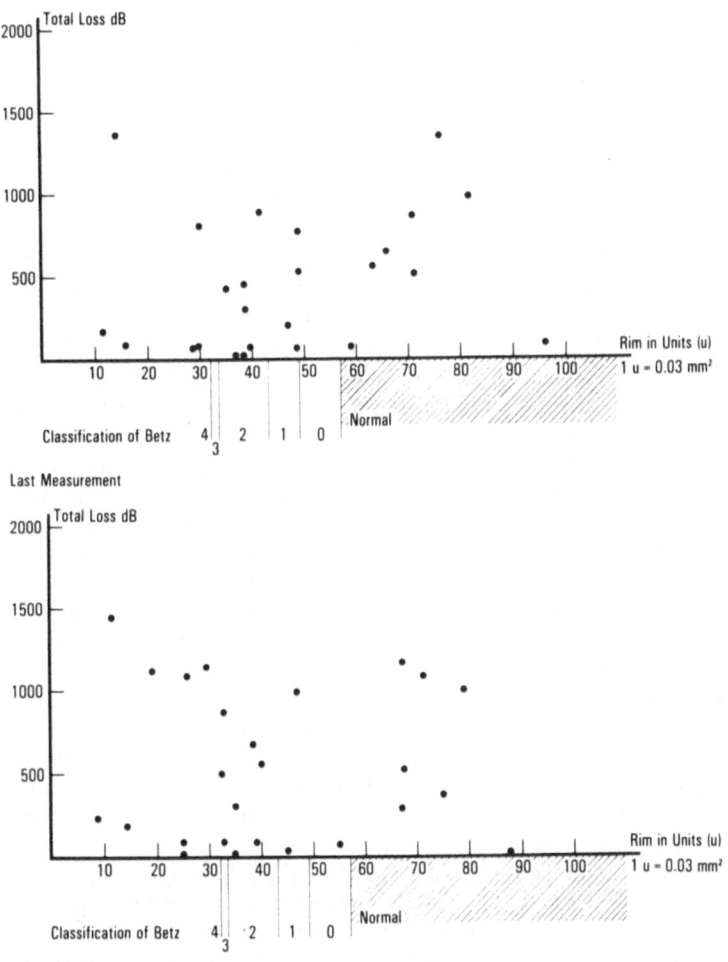

Fig. 3. Correlation between total loss and surface of the rim at the time of the first measurement (a, top), and of the last measurement (b, bottom).

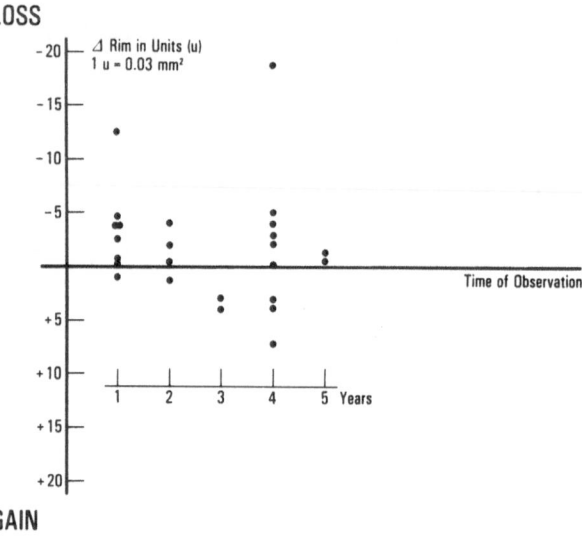

Fig. 4. Correlation between change of rim and time period of follow-up observation.

In Figs. 3a & b, the relation between total loss and surface of the rim of the first (3a) and of the last measurements (3b) is shown. No linear correlation exists. We have to accept that so-called normal rims can be accompanied by the considerable field loss. In Fig. 4 the change in the surface of the rim is correlated to the time period of follow-up. There is no clear trend which would show that, in a time period of up to 5 years, the surface of the rim would decrease with time.

In Fig. 5 the change of sensitivity and of the rim in surface units is depicted (+ sign on the y-axis means loss of sensitivity, − sign on the y-axis means gain of sensitivity; − sign on the x-axis means diminution of the surface of the rim, + sign on the x-axis means gain of the surface of the rim). The ± one-δ area of measurement-error of the surface of rim is also shown, and as a range for long-term fluctuations ± 300 dB are somewhat arbitrarily assumed (see 3, 8, 9, 10, 12). There is a tendency toward loss of the surface of the rim and of the field, but note that, in some cases with this decrease of surface of the rim, an increase of sensitivity is also possible; this means that the surface of the rim and field changes can progress in opposite directions.

In 5 eyes the decrease of the surface of the rim was more pronounced in one quadrant than in the others, but also in these cases no clear correlation between sectoral decrease of surface and field loss in the corresponding quadrant could be found.

These facts may be further illustrated by the following examples:

S.F. (Table 2) is a 67-year-old patient with a history of glaucoma for 14 years. After maximum medicamentous therapy, he had a trabeculectomy in December 1982 and revision of this trabeculectomy in March 1983 on the right eye; ever since, the tension was controlled.

Planimetry of disc and Octopus field examination both show an aggravation

28

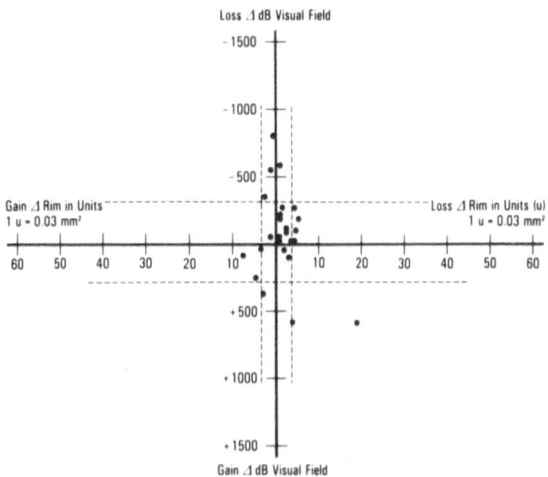

Fig. 5. Correlation between change of sensitivity and change of surface of the rim.

Table 2. Patient no. 1. S.F. 67y chronic open-angle glaucoma RE.

	Surface (mm²)	Rim (u)	Excavation %	Total loss dB
1979	1.41	38.0	45.3	296
1983	0.98	32.7	63.7	499
Δ	− 0.43	− 5.3	+ 18.4	− 203

of the disease; we seem to have good correlation between these two parameters.

U.E. (Table 3) is a 59-year-old woman, whom we have known as having
glaucoma for 11 years. Already at the first examination, the disc of her
right eye was almost totally excavated. First she was treated with medication:
then followed a trabeculectomy in 1967. The further course of her disease
showed repeated peaks of intraocular pressure even with maximum medication.
In January 1984 a lasertrabeculoplasty was made (180°, nasally). Note on
the table that, in our observation period, both the disc and the visual fields
remained almost unchanged. Actually you would expect a much greater loss
of sensitivity with such a small rim.

Table 3. Patient no. 2. U.E. 59y chronic open-angle glaucoma RE

	Surface (mm²)	Rim (u)	Excavation %	Total loss dB
1982	0.47	15.7	76.3	90
1983	0.44	14.7	78.2	159
Δ	+ 0.03	+ 1.0	+ 1.9	− 69

T.V. (Table 4) is a 51-year-old male patient who had glaucoma for 4 years
with initial pressure of 14 mm Hg. The pressure is controlled with maximum

Table 4. T.V. 52y chronic open-angle glaucoma LE

	Surface (mm²)	Rim (u)	Excavation %	Total loss dB
1979	2.37	79.0	8.5	916
1983	2.25	57.0	8.9	369
Δ	− 0.12	− 4.0	+ 0.4	+ 547

glaucoma therapy. Note that the rim is of normal extent; there is almost no excavation but, nontheless, visual fields exhibit a quite extensive field loss.

DISCUSSION

If the border of the optic disc were a circle and if excavation were to progress evenly in each part of the disc, determination of the cup/disc ratio could theoretically be as good a parameter as the measurement of the surface of the rim for evaluating progressing excavation. However, because the optic nerve head border is not a perfect circle and because excavation does not progress evenly in different sectors of the disc (4, 5, 6, 7, 18, 20; 23, 24, 25, 26, 27, 29), measurement of the surface of the neuroretinal rim seems to be a much better tool for evaluating these changes than observation of the cup/disc ratio (1, 4, 5, 6, 7, 14, 18, 20, 23, 24, 25, 27, 29). There is also no doubt that automated static determination of differential light sensitivity thresholds is a better tool than kinetic and static hand perimetry in the evaluation of what is going on in the visual field of glaucoma patients. Nevertheless, to answer clearly the question asked in the title − is there a correlation between glaucomatous field loss as determined by automated perimetry and changes in the surface of the optic disc?− we must say that no linear or simple correlation between field loss and decrease of surface of the neuroretinal rim could be found in our patients during a mean observation period of 2.8 years.

However, this can be explained quite easily, at least to a certain extent, just by what was found by automated static perimetry earlier: Increase of scatter or short- and long-term fluctuation is strongly correlated to increase of loss of differential light sensitivity threshold, as long as no absolute scotoma has developed (8, 9, 10, 12, 13, 28). Long-term fluctuations may reach up to 600 dB, and this would be about 30% of the whole sensitivity − to use this mathematical incorrect expression just once, because measurement of sensitivity in dB is a logarithmic scale. With respect to long-term fluctuations, the error of measurement of the surface of he rim in the range of 6% is relatively small.

In our figures the direct measurements of the surface of the rim are shown, by which the factor of magnification originating from ametropia or length of the globe was not considered. Even if this factor reaches 10% for a + 12 diopter hypermetropic eye and 24% for a − 15 diopter eye, it is unimportant as long as we are looking for changes and as long as this change is not larger than 15%, which is the case in our last group in table 1. In this extreme case of a − 15 diopter myope, the magnification error would be 15% of 24%,

30

which is about 4% and therefore still smaller than the error of measurement. But for longer follow-ups when larger changes of the surface or the rim have to be expected, magnification would become important, and we are going to consider these facts in the future. Nevertheless, the largest errors are introduced if the disc is not sharply focussed on the plane of the film of the camera (see also 21 and 22).

Because long-term fluctuations in static perimetry may, as mentioned before, reach 600 dB in the 30° field, a gain of sensitivity is not surprising, even if the surface of the rim shows a tendency to diminish. Fluctuations outweigh the error of measurement of the surface of the rim. Therefore we would consider loss of the surface of the rim as being a more reliable indication of true change for the worse in the overall situation of a given glaucoma patient. And, considering both parameters together, we are certainly coming closer to the truth.

That glaucomatous field loss develops from zero in a normal looking disc with a cup/disc ratio of 0.2 to 0.4 or a rim surface of 84 to 90% to blindness in a disc with no detectable rim is clear to everybody. But to elucidate the events and type of correlations – these correlations are certainly not linear – between field changes and disc changes between these two extremes is more difficult and has only begun. Different types of transitional damages, the distribution of definitely lost nerve fibers, and the organization in overlapping receptive fields of the retina may not only be responsible for the scatter in differential light sensitivity threshold, the so-called short- and long-term fluctuations, but may also be the reason that a relatively simple retinal function, with differential light sensitivity really is, can in extreme cases remain intact until 65% of the surface of the rim or of the nerve fibers (16), respectively, corresponding to a cup/disc ratio of 80%, is lost. On the other hand, if a cup/disc ratio of 0.4 is present and therefore the surface of the rim still comprises 84% of the full-sized disc, considerable field loss can be revealed by automated static perimetry. Then the question arises whether the neuroretinal rim, as measured by planimetry, may be at least in some cases also a very questionable parameter for evaluating what is going on in the nerve fibers of the optic nerve head, perhaps e.g. we are sometimes measuring a variable amount of glial tissue instead of nerve fibers. There is again some need to evaluate the rim three-dimensionally, even if Betz et al. abandoned stereometry of the cup because they found no advantages over planimetry.

REFERENCES

1. Balaszi, A.G., Drance, S.M., Schulzer, M. and Douglas, G.R. The area of the neuro-retinal rim in glaucoma suspects and early chronic open-angle glaucoma: correlation with parameters of visual function. Arch. ophthal. (Chicago) (in press).
2. Balaszi, A.G., Roorman, J., Drance, S.M., Schulzer, M. and Douglas, G.R. The effect of age on the nerve fibre population of the human optic nerve.
3. Bebie, H. and Fankhauser, F. Program Delta. Manual for the use of, INTERZEAG November (1981).
4. Betz, Ph., Camps, Fr., Collingnon-Brach, C. and Weekers, R. Photographic stéréoscopique et photogrammétrie de l'excavation physiologique de la papille. J. Fr. Ophthalmol. 4 (3): 193–203 (1981).

5. Betz, Ph., Camps, F., Collingnon-Brach, J., Lavergne, G. and Weekers, R. Biometric study of the disc cup in open-angle glaucoma. Graefe's Arch. Clin. Exp. Ophthalmol. 218: 70–74 (1982).
6. Caprioli, J., Spaeth, G.L., Moster, M.R. and Lebowitz, H. Quantitative determination of glaucomatous optic nerve changes. Supp. to Invest. Ophthalmol. & Vis. Sc. 25 (3): 98 (1984).
7. Drance, S.M. and Balaszi, G. Die neuroretinale Randzone beim frühen Glaukom. Klin. Mbl. Augenheilk. 184: 271–273 (1984).
8. Flammer, J., Drance, S.M. and Schulzer, M. The estimation and testing of the components of long-term fluctuation of the differential light threshold. Docum. Ophthalmol. Proc. Series 35: 383–389 (1983).
9. Flammer, J., Drance, S.M. and Zulauf, M. The short- and long-term fluctuation of the differential light threshold in patients with glaucoma, normal controls & glaucoma suspects. Arch. Ophthalmol. (in print).
10. Flammer, J., Drance, S.M., Fankhauser, F. and Augustiny, L. The differential light threshold in automated static perimetry. Arch. Ophthalmol. (in print).
11. Gloor, B. Die Computerperimetrie in der langfristigen Beurteilung des Glaukoms. Krieglstein, G.K., Leydhecker, W. Medikamentöse Glaukomtherapie. J.F. Bergmann Verlag, München 59–72 (1982).
12. Gloor, B.P. and Vökt, B.A. Long-term fluctuations versus definite field loss in glaucoma patients. Suppl. to Invest. Ophthalmol. & Vis. Sci. 24 (3): 103 (1983).
13. Gloor, B., Stürmer, J. and Vökt, B. Was hat die automatisierte Perimetrie mit dem Octopus für neue Kenntnisse über glaukomatöse Gesichtsfeldveränderungen gebracht? Klin. Mbl. Augenheilk. (1984).
14. Gloor, B., Jäggi, P. and Stürmer, J. Wo steht die Perimetrie im Verlaufe des Glaukoms? Merté, H.J. und Mertz, M. Neuere Entwicklungen in der Ophthalmologie. (in print).
15. Hart, W.M. and Becker, B. The onset and evolution of glaucomatous visual field defects. Am. Acad. Ophthalmol. 89 (3): 268–279 (1982).
16. Hitchings, R.A., Brown, D.B. and Anderton, S.A. Glaucoma screenings by means of an optic disc grid. Br. J. Ophthalmol. 67 (6): 352–355 (1983).
17. Hitchings, R.A., Genio, C., Anderton, S. and Clark, P. An optic disc grid: its evaluation in reproducibility studies on the cup/disc-ratio. Br. J. Ophthalmol. 67 (6): 356–361 (1983).
18. Holmin, C. Optic disc evaluation versus the visual field in chronic simple glaucoma. Acta Ophthalmol. 60: 275–283 (1982).
19. Langerhorst, C.T., van den Berg, T.J.T.P. and Greve, E.L. Schätzung der verschiedenen Fluktuationsfaktoren bei der Computerperimetrie von Glaukompatienten. Neuere Entwicklungen in der Ophthalmologie, ed. Merté, H.J. und Mertz, M. Beihefte Klin. Mbl. Augenheilk. (in print).
20. Lewis, R.A., Hayreh, S.S. and Phelps, Ch.D. Optic disc and visual field correlations in primary open-angle and low-tension glaucoma. Am. J. Ophthalmol. 96: 148–152 (1983).
21. Lotmar, W. Rapid detection of changes in the optic disc: stereochronoscopy. Int. Ophthal. 2, 3: 169–174 (1980).
22. Lotmar, W. Dependence of magnification upon the camera-to-eye-distance in the Zeiss fundus camera. Acta Ophthalmol. 62: 131–134 (1984).
23. Motolko, M. and Drance, S.M. Features of the optic disc in preglaucomatous eyes. Arch. Ophthalmol. 99: 1992 (1981).
24. Pederson, J.E. and Anderson, D.R. The mode of progressive disc cupping in ocular hypertension and glaucoma. Arch. Ophthalmol. 98: 490 (1980).
25. Pdereson, J.E. and Herschler, J. Reversal of glaucomatous cupping in adults. Arch. Ophthalmol. 100: 426 (1982).
26. Quigley, H.A. Addicks, E.M. and Green, R.W. Optic nerve damage in human glaucoma. III Quantitative correlation of nerve fiber loss and visual field defect in glaucoma, ischaemic neuropathy, papilledema and toxic neuropathy. Arch. Ophthalmol. 100 (1982).
27. Sommer, A., Pollack, I. and Maumenee, A.E. Optic disc parameters and onset of

glaucomatous field loss: I. Methods and progressive changes in disc morphology. Arch. Ophthalmol. 97: 1444 (1979).

28. Stürmer, J., Gloor, B. and Tobler, H.J. Wie sehen Glaukomgesichtsfelder wirklich aus? Klin. Mbl. Augenheilk. (1984).

29. Takamoto, T. and Schwartz, B. Quantification of cup shape in normals, ocular hypertension and glaucomas. Suppl. to Investigative Ophthalmol. & Visual Science. 25 (3): 97 Arvo (1984).

30. Werner, E.B. and Drance, S.M. Increased scatter of responses as a precursor of visual field changes in glaucoma. (In print).

Author's address:
Prof. B. Gloor
Univ.-Augenklinik
Augenspital
Mittlere Strasse 91
CH-4056 Basle
Switzerland

COMPUTERIZED ANALYSIS OF VISUAL FIELDS

C.E.T. KRAKAU and CATHARINA HOLMIN
(Lund, Sweden)

ABSTRACT

A system for computerized analysis of visual field records (COMPETER) is described. The salient features of the field, such as localization and depth of defects, are expressed in a condensed form by a small number of parameters. The system is self-educating since it starts from complete ignorance and becomes an expert system by analysing and memorizing a great number of fields.

The efficiency of the system is assessed by making it carry out a comparison between glaucomatous disc changes and the visual field analysis. 'Saucerization' was associated with a general reduction of sensitivity, whereas 'notch' meant a characteristic pattern with local sensitivity reduction.

INTRODUCTION

The visual fields recorded by computerized devices provide the result in numeric form, well suited for further automatic processing. In fact, the evaluation of the perimetry results has been improved in several ways by making the computer do some numerical work on the crude threshold values. It even seems likely that the whole interpretation of the field test might be entrusted to the computer. A first step for this purpose was taken with the design of a system capable of suggesting diagnoses on the basis of its own experience. In the present pilot study it is demonstrated how this system works when applied to a specific problem, i.e. evaluation of the connection between visual field results in a glaucoma material and the evaluation of changes in the optic disc.

From the appearance of the disc it is possible to decide correctly the presence or absence of visual field defects in a high percentage, provided both disc and visual field are studied with appropriate techniques. To no small extent the size of the field defect was also correlated to the severity of the disc changes (1). The fact that structural defects of the papilla are mapped onto the visual field as scotomata etc. makes it likely that a detailed analysis might reveal more specific disc-field correlations.

35

E.L. Greve, W. Leydhecker & C. Raitta (eds.), Second European Glaucoma Symposium, Helsinki 1984.
© *1985, Dr. W. Junk Publishers, Dordrecht. ISBN 978-94-010-8934-0*

DISC CODE

The upper and lower half of the disc were judged separately and the following classification code was used: normal (A), saucerization (B), narrow regular rim (C), incomplete notch (D), complete notch (E), more extensive excavation reaching the disc margin (F), (1) (Fig. 1). Saucerization denotes a shallow excavation with a configurational cup larger than the colour cup. On plain photographs this is recognized by the course of the vessels, which are often angulated at the border, and a smooth bend over the papilla, the border of which also appears abnormally distinct.

FIELD PARAMETERS

The information about the field is the set of threshold values for all points tested. This has to be condensed into a smaller number of parameter values in order to be manageable. The choice of parameters is in the first place a result of educated guesses. The following set is tentative; experience will indicate where improvements are possible.

1. Threshold values of point groups. The mean threshold value for the points of each quadrant arc in the circles at 5, 10, 15, and 20 degrees of excentricity — 16 arc values altogether — were calculated. The threshold values at each point can take one of 16 values. To simplify handling we permit each arc mean to be only one digit (0—9). The mean is thus divided by 1.6 and the decimals are disregarded. The numbers denote the relative sensitivity of the quadrant arcs and constitute the main part of the field code.

2. The number of *defect points* and *very defect points*. The number of points whose threshold is more than 2 steps below the maximal in each excentricity circle are counted and denoted *defect* or *very defect*. Points whose value lie more than 4 steps below the maximal are the very defect points. The total number of defect and very defect points of all circles is divided by 4. The decimals are disregarded. Since all values above 9 are denoted 9, we have single figures related to defect and very defect points.

Codes from different fields are accepted as similar if the difference between two codes is higher than one at none of the 18 codes numbers. The choice of one is of course arbitrary and chosen to reduce the number of different sets of code.

PROCEDURE

The system which has to take care of and process the visual field results and disc estimates is completely ignorant initially, but as it stores this information it becomes gradually more and more 'educated' (Fig. 2). From the field result (as a rule stored on 'flexible disc') the computer calculates the field code set. The computer asks for the optic disc code. Various situations are now possible.

36

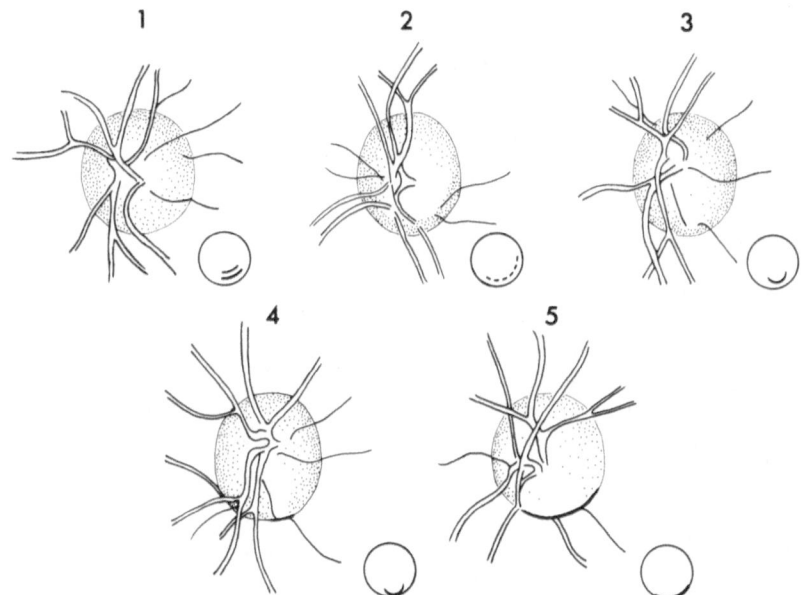

Fig. 1. Skeleton drawings of the signs used in the classification of the discs. 1) Saucerization (B), 2) Narrow rim (C), 3) Incomplete notch (D), 4) Complete notch (E), 5) Extensive loss of tissue reaching the disc margain (F). The sign referred to is located in the lower half of the disc.

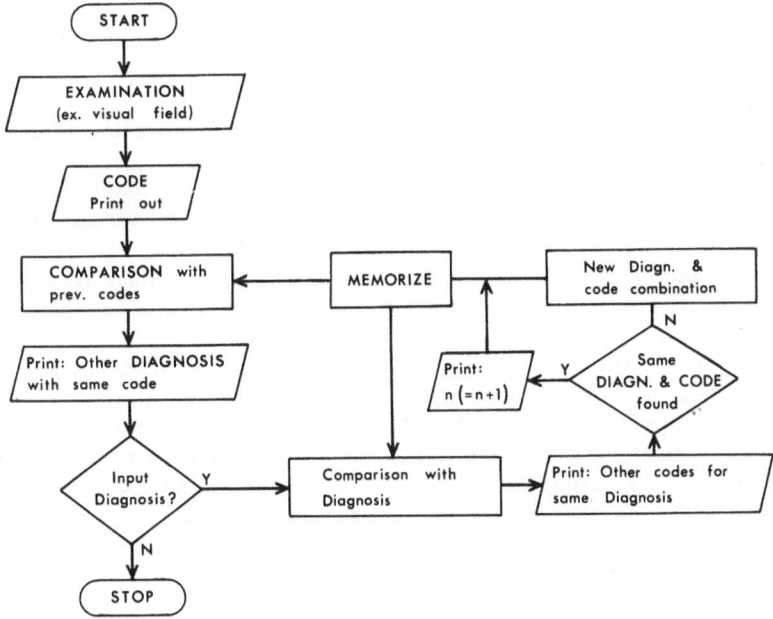

Fig. 2. Flow diagram, showing learning and diagnosis-suggesting process. 'Diagnosis' = disc code.

```
A  REC.NR   89
   SIN
     37   36   34   37   57   63   62   60   49   56   61   44   20   20   22   22

   ARC 5,10,15,20                                              DEF.& V.DEF PKT,-,N
     7   7   7   7   7   7   7   7   6   7   7   5   6   6   6   6 : 5   1
   DIAGNOS:NN......
   IDENT.CODE - DIAGNOS:AA......                      16
   IDENT.CODE - DIAGNOS:BB......                       3
   IDENT.CODE - DIAGNOS:FF......                       1
   IDENT.CODE - DIAGNOS:DD......                       1

B  REC.NR   521
   DX
     17   21   11   17   27   33   23   27   33   27   33   27   16   6   16   6

   ARC 5,10,15,20                                              DEF.& V.DEF PKT,-,N
     3   4   2   3   3   4   2   3   4   3   4   3   5   1   5   1 : 0   9
   DIAGNOS:AE......
   ID.DIAGN.-DIFF.CODE
     4   0   6   6   2   4   6   6   3   3   6   5   5   1   5   5 : 3   5 : 1
   ID.DIAGN.-DIFF.CODE
     2   1   6   6   1   0   5   6   4   3   5   5   0   5   5   2 : 4   7 : 1
   ID.DIAGN.-DIFF.CODE
     1   0   5   5   3   5   5   5   4   4   5   3   3   4   4   4 : 6   2 : 1
   ID.DIAGN.-DIFF.CODE
     0   0   0   3   1   0   1   5   1   0   2   4   4   0   0   5 : 1   9 : 1
   ID.DIAGN.-DIFF.CODE
     2   0   6   6   0   0   6   0   0   6   4   0   1   5   3 : 2   8 : 2
   IDENT.CODE - DIAGNOS:CE......                       1
   ID.DIAGN.-DIFF.CODE
     4   0   6   7   0   3   6   3   4   6   6   5   3   5   6 : 3   5 : 1
   ID.DIAGN.-DIFF.CODE
     3   0   6   6   0   0   6   6   0   0   5   4   5   0   5   4 : 3   7 : 1
   ID.DIAGN.-DIFF.CODE
     1   1   6   6   0   0   6   6   3   0   6   4   0   5   5   5 : 2   7 : 1
   ID.DIAGN.-DIFF.CODE
     0   0   6   6   2   3   6   6   5   5   6   5   5   5   6   5 : 3   4 : 1
```

Fig. 3. Suggested diagnoses for given field code. NN = diagnosis unknown, AE = upper part of the disc normal; notch in the lower part. Various field codes with the same disc diagnosis printed out.

1. Neither disc nor field codes have previously been encountered by the computer.
2. The computer may have encountered the same disc code before, but not the field code. The various field codes with the same disc code are printed out.
3. The same field code but not disc code has occurred earlier. These disc codes are printed out. All three combinations 1–3 are new and therefore stored in the memory.
4. The same codes for both field and disc have occurred earlier. The number of occurrences of this combination is updated by one.

The survey printed out (Fig. 3) at each consultation of the system contains frequency figures which makes it possible to obtain the set of conditional probabilities for all disc codes associated with a specific field code and also the set of all field codes associated with a specific disc code.

MATERIAL

From the group of patients followed at the glaucoma care unit, Lund, a sub-group of 140 eyes were chosen for the comparison of field with disc changes.

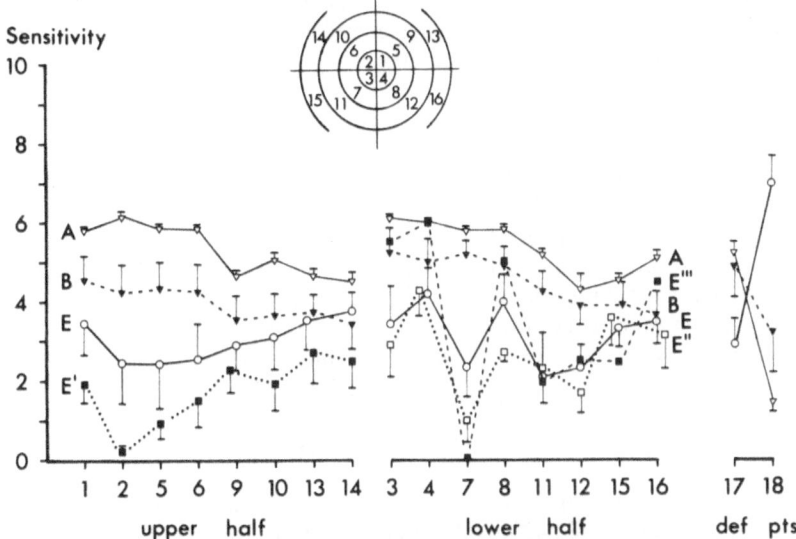

Fig. 4. Profiles for Normal (AA), Saucerized (BB) and Notched discs (EE, E′, E″, E‴).
Top part: sectors of the visual field enumerated. Bottom part: abscissa axis = Sector
number, ordinate axis = Sensitivity mean value

All patients had at least one eye with glaucomatous field defects according
to the definition used in the previous papers (2). Fundus photographs of
acceptable quality and reliable field tests obtained with the automatic device
Competer were available in all cases.

RESULTS AND DISCUSSION

In Fig. 4 the mean values are drawn of the field codes for the following disc
codes: normal (AA), saucer (BB), notch (EE).
  The disc changes range from normal to the most advanced destruction of
the disc. There is a parallel decrease of the threshold level.
A: The discs assessed as normal (AA) were in fact without field defects to a
  high extent. In 12 out of 66 cases there were parameter values 2 steps
  below (or more) the thresholds of the main group.
B: In the discs considered 'saucerized' there were fields with a general
  sensitivity reduction in all areas compared to the normals.
E: Discs with 'notch' had without exception a lower sensitivity. Notches at
  the inferior pole of the disc were connected with lowered sensitivity
  preferentially in the 5 degree upper nasal arc, whereas the upper notch
  showed a lowered sensitivity in the inferior 10–15 degree nasal arc. E′,
  E″ and E‴ in Fig. 4 refer to groups with different upper and lower codes.
  They were included to demonstrate the similarity of the E-profiles.

The disc diagnoses 'narrow rim' and 'incomplete notch' were the least distinctly discernible codes, showing considerable overlapping with other evaluations. The boundaries between the groups of the optic disc classification are by no means clear. Improved technique for inspection could no doubt make the disc diagnosis more reliable. The set of visual field parameters is tentative, but the system itself gives indications for optimizing the set. But in spite of every improvement at both ends a perfect disc-field correspondence can hardly be achieved, since the variability from one field test to another introduces an inevitable blurring of the disc-field relations.

Saucerization represents a diffuse consumption of disc tissue, and accordingly this evaluation is connected with a general reduction of the sensitivity level. On the other hand, the distinct substance defects constituting notches also have more specific dips in the profile of the field code.

ACKNOWLEDGEMENTS

This work was supported by grants from the Swedish Medical Research Council (project No B84-4X-5202-7C) and H. and L. Nilsson's Foundation.
Fig. 1 is reproduced with kind permission from Acta Ophthalmol.

REFERENCES

1. Holmin, C. Optic disc evaluation versus the visual field in chronic glaucoma. Acta Ophthalmol (Copenh.) 60: 275 (1982).
2. Holmin, C. and Krakau, C.E.T. Regression analysis of the central visual field in chronic glaucoma cases. Acta Ophthalmol (Copenh.) 60: 267 (1982).

Authors' address:
Dept. of Experimental Ophthalmology
University Eye Clinic
S-221 85 Lund
Sweden

THE VISUAL FIELD QUANTIFICATION ISSUE

R. ETIENNE and E. SELLEM

(Lyon, France)

ABSTRACT

It is always difficult to compare visual fields of glaucoma patients, in order to evaluate the progression of the disease. Modern perimetry offers a solution to this problem in replacing the cartographic reading by a number evaluating a 'deficit ratio'. This quantification in percentage of visual field destroyed is very simple to perform if the results of examination are expressed in classes of Log. L. U.

At the time of the kinetic perimetry, the visual fields chart had the appearance of a topographical map. As the resulting area, the isopter was not in any way geometric, its surface was barely measurable. This calculation was made all the more difficult due to enclosed patches of non vision, scotomas, which further reduced the total area. The first, in 1897, Groenow (8) noticed that it was difficult to compare successive visual fields of a glaucomatous patient.

An ophthalmologist, whose name is now forgotten, proposed to define the areas of vision and the scotomas and to weight them. However, this method did not prove to be a practical one. Nonetheless, it is worthy to note that a useful notion was introduced: the scotomatous mass.

More recently, Ben Esterman (1967–1968) (3) made a praiseworthy quantification attempt, concerning the Bjerrum's campimetry and H. Goldmann's kinetic perimetry, the importance of which concerns us regarding the central visual field.

When Friedmann's visual field analyser was developed and the visual fields chart took on the appearance of an abstract painting, i.e. a page plotted with values of luminance of differential threshold, things began to simplify. Based on the numeric representation of these findings, Ph. Demailly and Papoz (1) were able to make known a calculation of 'visual capacity' either for the total area of the visual field, or for five (5) concentric zones. C. Holmin and C.E.T. Krakau (9) used in a similar manner the data furnished by the 'Competer' and, just as is the case with visual capacity, the 'performance' diminishes with the accentuation of the perimetric damage.

The printout of the visual fields takes on a different appearance with the Peritest and the grouping of classified responses (Fig. 1). Thus, when using

41

E.L. Greve, W. Leydhecker & C. Raitta (eds.), Second European Glaucoma Symposium, Helsinki 1984.
© *1985, Dr. W. Junk Publishers, Dordrecht. ISBN 978-94-010-8934-0*

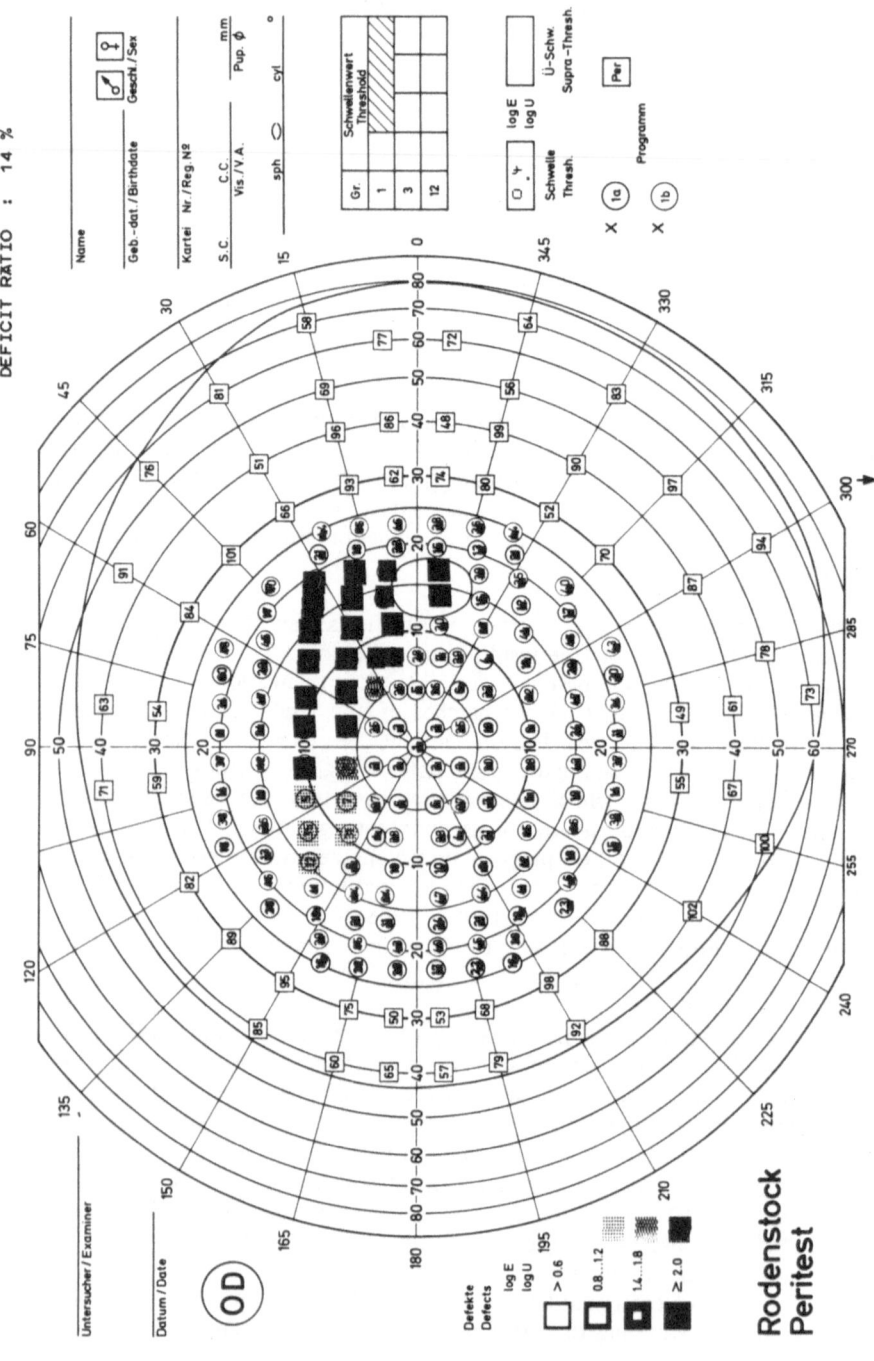

Fig. 1. Deficit ratio (D.R.) in a case of glaucomatous scotoma. d = 63. Peritest: program 1a + 1b. D = 447. The differential threshold is: 0.4 Log. U.L. D.R. = d/D × 100 = 14%.

Table 1. Advantages and disadvantages of the two strategies of the Peritest

Automatic strategy	Our opinion		Semi-automatic strategy
No human relation	BAD	GOOD	Human relation
Possible unexperimented operator	GOOD?!	BAD?!	Operator having to be experimented
Theoretical uniformity and reproducibility	GOOD	BAD?	Operator's influence, in fact more beneficial than troublesome
Longer duration of the test	BAD	GOOD	Shorter duration of the test
Unjustified variations of the individual threshold	BAD	GOOD	No unjustified variations of the individual threshold, determined by the operator
No multiple stimuli	BAD	GOOD	Multiple stimuli are possible
No located study	BAD	GOOD	Located study is possible

this instrument, nothing is easier than to numerically evalute the central 25° of the visual field (Table 1, Fig. 2).

Indeed:
— The number of points examined remains invariable in each program (1a or 1b or the central 10°).
— The position is distributed in a relatively homogeneous fashion.
— The deficits are groups and classified according to their depth. We no longer have the dispersion of all the values of the differential threshold, as it is given up by the visual field analyser. The grouping of the classes allows for the use of symbols.

Using this apparatus, E. Greve and D. Bakker (6) employed a defect volume which, it seems, is more difficult to calculate than our deficit ratio (D.R.), in which instance we only take into consideration the reduction of localized sensitivity, while the value of the differentiation threshold was already calculated before the test.

The value 1 is given to deficits within class I (i.e. the points seen at the value of the differential threshold increased by U.L. Log. 0.8 to 1.2), the value 2 to those of class II (threshold + U.L. Log. 1.4 to 1.8) and 3 to those of class III (threshold + U.L. Log. > 2).

These *bad scores* are added up (= d). The deficit ratio (D.R.) is the percentage of the actual deficit (d) in relationship to the total theoretical deficit (D) of the selected program.

Introducing a percentage allows a comparison between visual fields resulting from different programs (e.g. 1a, 1a + 10° or 1a and 1b).

The deficit ratio of a pathological visual field is thus:

$$D.R. = \frac{d}{D} \times 100$$

The program 1a consists of a test of 78 points: if all were seen, the deficit would be zero; if none were seen, the deficit would be evaluated as 234 − 3, therefore 231, since the blind spot is also measured (thus a class III response).

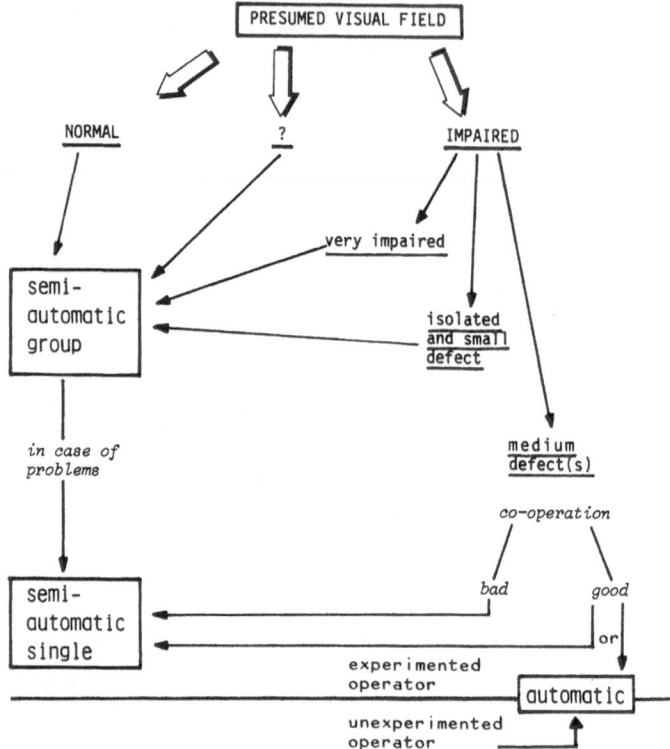

Fig. 2. Choice of strategy with the Peritest.

Using the program 1a + 1b, we similarly have:

$$D = 3 \times 151(-6) = 447$$

The deficit ratio is thus:

$$\frac{d}{447} \times 100$$

Given that the dispersion of points is not homogeneous within the 25° due to the fact that the distribution is the double within the 10° sector, it becomes imperative to run not only the 1a program but also 1a + 10° and to calculate the D.R. of this central zone, which is the most important functional one:

$$D.R. (10°) = \frac{d}{117} \times 100$$

The deficit ratio (Table 3), is thus the inverse of the visual capacity or of the Swedish performance. It appears that the patient is more sensitive to a partial loss of vision as opposed to a percentage maintained: for example, 'You have lost 25 per cent of your visual capital' sounds very clear for the patient.

Table 2. Calculating the RD according to the different programs

Programme	D (25°)	RD (25°)	D (10°)	RD (10°)
1a	231	$d_{1a}/2.31$	66	$d_{10°}/0.66$
1a + 1b	447	$d_{1a+1b}/4.47$	117	$d_{10°}/1.17$
1a + 10°	231	$d_{1a}/2.31$	117	$d_{10°}/1.17$

Furthermore, in addition to the deficit ratio, the value of the differential threshold is known. It is dependent upon:
— The transparency of the environment.
— The central, pericentral and peripheric retinal sensitivity.
— To a lesser degree, the size of the pupil.

Thus, with two results, that of the differential threshold and of the deficit ratio, a change in the state of a glaucomatous patient can be evaluated at visual field check-up. If the threshold remains constant and the deficit ratio increases, the glaucoma advances. If the deficit ratio remains constant but the value of the threshold increases, a beginning cataract, for example, could be diagnosed.

The only problem, not the least of which and one which is relevant to all patients, is to increase to a certain extent the number of perimetric examinations so as to have an idea of the intra-individual fluctuation of the response. Despite today's ongoing technological revolution, we must bear in mind that the exploration of the visual field will always remain a psychophysiological test.

REFERENCES

1. Demailly, Ph. and Papoz, L. Long term study of visual capability in relation to intraocular pressure in Chronic Open Angle Glaucoma. Doc. Ophth. Proc. 14: 331–335 (1977).
2. Esterman, B. Grid for scoring visual fields tangent screen. I. Arch. Ophthal. 77: 780–786 (1967).
3. Esterman, B. Grid for scoring visual fields. II. Perimeter Arch. Ophthal. 79: 400–406 (1968).
4. Etienne, R. and Sellem, E. Problèmes et solutions de la Périmétrie d'aujourd'hui. J. Fr. Ophtal. 6: 179–186 (1983).
5. Etienne, R., Etienne, A. and Sellem, E. Périmétrie moderne: automatique ou manuelle? J. Fr. Ophtal. (in press).
6. Greve, E. and Bakker, D. Personal Communication (1982).
7. Greve, E. Peritest. Doc. Ophthalmol. Proc. 22: 71–74 (1980).
8. Groenow. Veber die Berechnung der Erwebsfahigkeit bei Sehstorgen Deutsch Med. Ztg. (1897).
9. Holmin, C. and Krakau, C.E.T. Visual field decay in normal subjects and in cases of chronic glaucoma. A.V. Greefe's Arch. Klin. Ophthalmol. 213: 291–298 (1980).
10. Lavergne, G. L'analyse quantitative des déficits du champ visuel. J. Fr. Ophtalmol. 6 (11): 933–939 (1983).
11. Leydhecker, W. Perimetry update. Ann. Ophthalmol. 15: 511–543 (1983).

Authors' address:
31 Rue Ferrandière
69002 Lyon
France

COMPUTERIZED LOCATION OF FLUCTUATION AND CHANGES IN GLAUCOMATOUS VISUAL FIELDS

M. MERTZ and U. ZIRKEL
(Munich, F.R.G.)

ABSTRACT

With the aid of image analysis strategies fluctuations and changes are located and identified in follow-up measurements of the visual field using data gained by Octopus static perimetry. After performing rational spline interpolation on the single examination data sets the local variations of sensitivity are calculated and displayed on the television screen of the Kontron image analysis system IBAS/IPS, the standard deviations being converted to grey scale levels. By a superposition of isopters derived from the starting field the site of the variations referring to visual field details such as existing or presumed scotomas can be recognized easily.

INTRODUCTION

The main task of computer perimetry in glaucoma seems to be to give information about the existence and progress of defects in the visual field. Very often, this information is hidden by normal and pathologically increased fluctuations of the values. On the other hand, increasing fluctuations are discussed to be an early indication to a beginning glaucomatous nerve fiber degeneration (1, 2, 4). In this paper, a new method is shown to detect, locate and quantify visual field changes of any kind, such as short- and long-term fluctuations, and real deteriorations as well as possible improvements. This method may be suggested as a visualization of a statistical Delta program.

THE METHOD

The procedure is based on visual field data processing methods already published (5, 6, 7, 8, 9), giving the opportunity to display visual fields in forms of either grey scale charts, isopters or three dimensional pictures. Compared to the well known Octopus Delta program which gives an overall statistical analysis it is seen as an additional tool to determine the site of detectable visual field variations.

47

E.L. Greve, W. Leydhecker & C. Raitta (eds.), Second European Glaucoma Symposium, Helsinki 1984.
© *1985, Dr. W. Junk Publishers, Dordrecht. ISBN 978-94-010-8934-0*

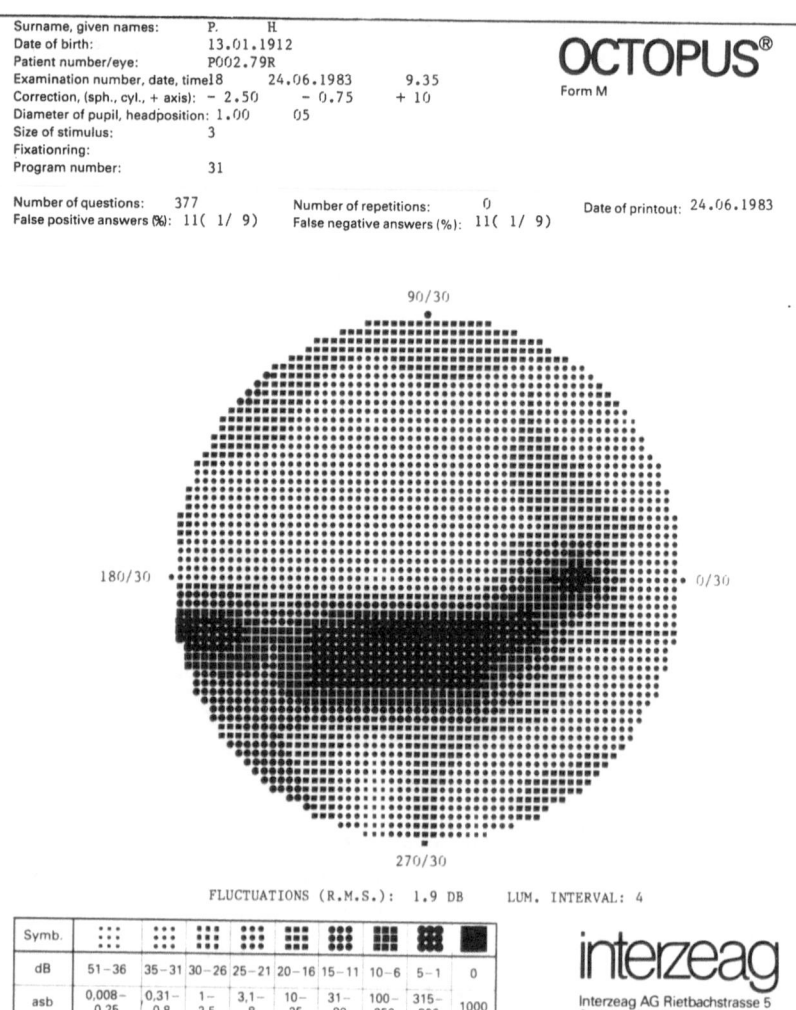

Surname, given names: P.   H
Date of birth: 13.01.1912
Patient number/eye: P002.79R
Examination number, date, time18   24.06.1983   9.35
Correction, (sph., cyl., + axis): − 2.50   − 0.75   + 10
Diameter of pupil, headposition: 1.00   05
Size of stimulus: 3
Fixationring:
Program number: 31

Number of questions: 377
False positive answers (%): 11(1/ 9)

Number of repetitions: 0
False negative answers (%): 11(1/ 9)

Date of printout: 24.06.1983

OCTOPUS®
Form M

90/30

180/30

0/30

270/30

FLUCTUATIONS (R.M.S.): 1.9 DB   LUM. INTERVAL: 4

Symb.	⋮⋮⋮	⋮⋮⋮	⦂⦂⦂	⦂⦂⦂	▦	▦	▩	▩	■
dB	51 − 36	35 − 31	30 − 26	25 − 21	20 − 16	15 − 11	10 − 6	5 − 1	0
asb	0,008 − 0,25	0,31 − 0,8	1 − 2,5	3,1 − 8	10 − 25	31 − 80	100 − 250	315 − 800	1000

1 asb = 0,318 cd/m²

interzeag

Interzeag AG Rietbachstrasse 5
CH-8952 Schlieren Switzerland

Fig. 1. Central 30° visual field, right eye, of a 67-year-old male glaucoma patient. Octopus program 31. Note the typical Bjerrum scotoma.

All data handling, calculations and displaying are done in the fast television image analysis system IBAS/IPS (Kontron) using both routines commercially available and software developed in our laboratory. Like every image analysis procedure the method can be explained best with the aid of pictures. These are taken from a glaucoma case report concerning follow-up investigations over three years.

CASE REPORT AND METHODOLOGICAL DETAILS

The visual field of the right eye of a 67-year-old male patient showed a typical Bjerrum scotoma (Fig. 1). In a three year follow-up, investigated with the original Octopus Delta program, some different short-term fluctuations were recognized, and long-term changes occurred too, the location of which are given roughly in the tables (Fig. 2). As shown, the overall fluctuation is noticed, and the figures describing the amount of changes (e.g. mean loss and mean sensitivity) are given referring to quadrants and excentricities. We are interested in a more distinct local evaluation, or at least in a better visualization of what is going on and *where* the changes take place. For this purpose, the values of the central visual field examinations (Octopus program No. 31) were used to calculate continuous grey scale charts with the aid of a non linear, rational spine interpolation algorithm (Fig. 3).

By this means, a picture can be produced on a television screen looking very similar to an origianal Octopus printout, but being composed to thousands of picture points (called 'pixels'), all having a defined grey value and location (there are more than 5000 pixels in one line). In order to facilitate the interpretation, isopters of any desired step width can be calculated at a second. In the case shown here, 5-dB-steps were chosen and superimposed on the picture as indicated on top of it (Fig. 4). Due to the very high storage capacity of our computer, several entire pictures of this kind (without isopters, naturally) can be taken into its memory, and a point-to-point statistical analysis can be performed subsequently.

As a result, we can obtain a picture which shows up the topological distribution of the changes in this individual field over the three years time investigated (Fig. 5). It is composed of the integer values of the standard deviation at each picture point. Thus, the white spots represent areas with severe changes (up to 6 dB), while the black spots represent areas with very stable sensitivity.

To faciliate interpretation, we have again cut the continuous shaded picture into defined dB-grey scale planes (Fig. 6). One can now conjecture that the greatest degree of change is located in the region of the Bjerrum scotoma. To prove this more exactly, we took the isopters from the original field (Fig. 4) and put them into the fluctuation picture. And this is the final step in our procedure (Fig. 7).

RESULTS

(1) The greatest variations took place at the lower margin of the Bjerrum scotoma.

(2) There is another maximum located between the blind spot and the center.

(3) A third region of marked variation is seen at the edge of the tested area at 5 o'clock.

P. H.
13.01.1912
P002.79R OD
(03,07,10,16,18)

PROGRAM DELTA V 2.0
MODE : SERIES

3

31 33

	EX1	EX2	EX3	EX4	EX5	SUMMARY
DATE OF EXAM : DAY	07.01	27.05	07.04	25.11	24.06	
YEAR	1980	1980	1981	1982	1983	
PROGRAM / EXAMINATION	31/03	33/07	31/10	31/16	31/18	
TOTAL LOSS (WHOLE FIELD)	229	193	307	425	300	290 ± 39
MEAN LOSS (PER TEST LOC)						
WHOLE FIELD	3.3	2.8	4.5	6.2	4.3	4.2 ± 0.6
QUADRANT UPPER NASAL	0.0	0.0	2.1	1.6	0.0	0.7 ± 0.5
LOWER NASAL	8.8	8.5	13.1	13.7	12.2	11.2 ± 1.1
UPPER TEMP.	0.5	0.0	0.0	0.9	0.8	0.4 ± 0.2
LOWER TEMP.	6.0	3.2	4.7	10.3	5.6	6.0 ± 1.2
ECCENTRICITY 0 - 10	9.7	8.9	9.6	11.2	9.7	9.8 ± 0.4
10 - 20	4.1	2.7	5.6	7.0	6.5	5.2 ± 0.8
20 - 30	1.2	1.4	2.4	4.3	1.6	2.2 ± 0.6
MEAN SENSITIVITY						
WHOLE FIELD (N: 24.0)	19.7	*	17.9	16.4	18.6	* ± *
QUAD.UPP.NAS.(N: 23.0)	23.3	*	19.3	19.4	22.2	* ± *
LOW.NAS.(N: 24.0)	14.4	*	10.4	9.8	11.4	* ± *
UPP.TMP.(N: 23.3)	21.2	*	21.5	19.8	21.3	* ± *
LOW.TMP.(N: 24.7)	17.2	*	17.9	13.8	17.6	* ± *
ECC. 0 - 10 (N: 27.2)	16.7	*	15.9	15.1	16.6	* ± *
10 - 20 (N: 24.8)	19.7	*	18.1	16.2	17.4	* ± *
20 - 30 (N: 22.6)	20.6	*	18.2	16.9	19.8	* ± *
NO. OF DISTURBED POINTS	17	15	26	36	20	23 ± 4
R.M.S. FLUCTUATION	2.3	*	2.8	0.8	1.9	2.0
TOTAL FLUCTUATION						3.0

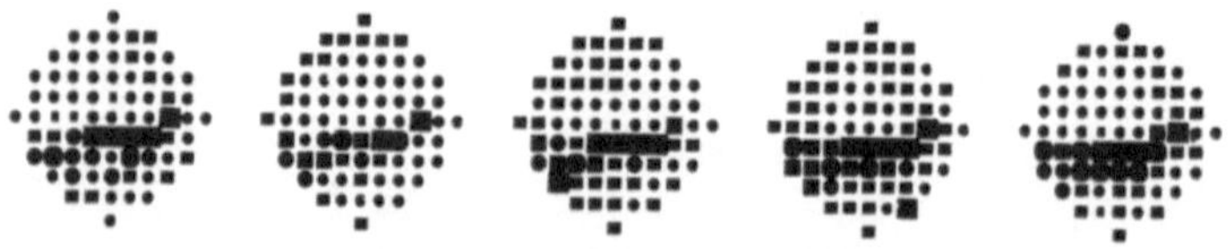

Fig. 2. Statistical Delta investigation in the same eye over a more than 3 year follow-up period. Note the excellent statistics, but more or less poor information about the locations, which can be extracted only by a rather tedious comparison of figures.

(4) The upper quadrants seem to be considerably calm. The standard deviation is mostly about 2 dB, with the exception of only one small paracentral area (superior to the fixation point) which reaches 4 dB.

Rational splines

$g_1 = 1 - t$ $\qquad\qquad g_2 = t$

$$t = \frac{x - x_k}{\Delta x}$$

$$g_3 = \frac{(1-t)^3}{p_t + 1} \qquad\qquad g_4 = \frac{t^3}{p(1-t) + 1}$$

Free parameter: p

Limit: $p \to \infty$ Linear interpolation

$\qquad\quad p = 0$ cubic splines

The function has to fit in every $x_i y_k$

The function has to be two times differentiable $\Rightarrow$ destination of the coefficients a_{ki}

Fig. 3. The system of equations used for the non linear interpolation between the measured points.

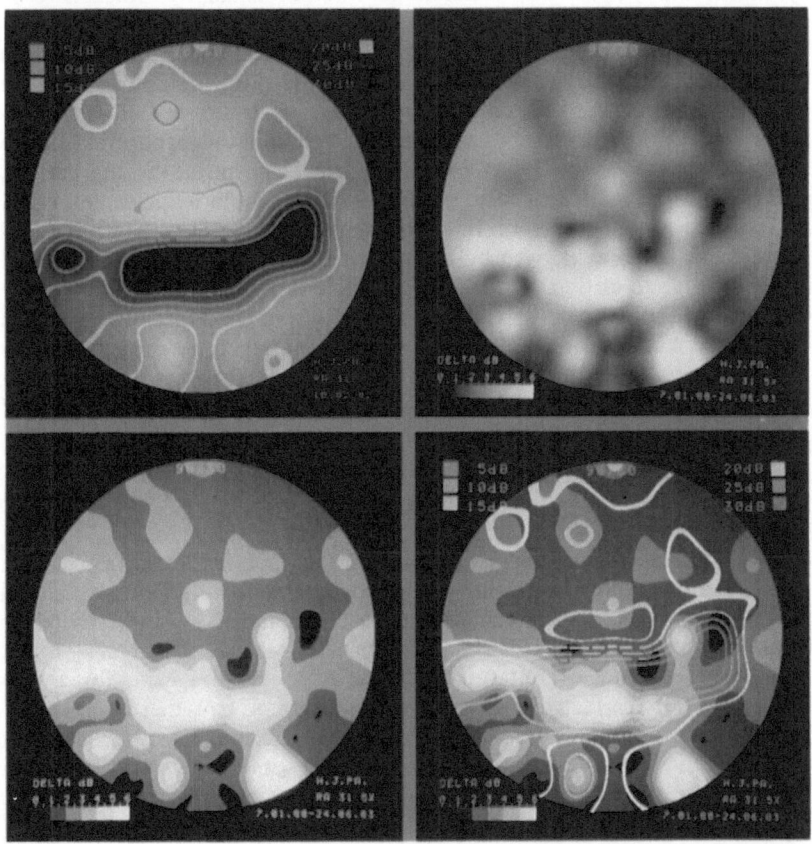

Fig. 4. (upper left). Interpolated, continuous shaded picture of the same visual field, as taken from the television screen photographically. Note the superimposed 'isopters' calculated from these data and giving additional information about the values of sensitivity.

Fig. 5. (upper right). Total variability in the visual field during the 3 year follow-up period, the picture composed of the standard deviation in every point (pixel).

Fig. 6. (lower left). For better orientation, the picture is cut into decible planes. Note dB-scale at the left lower corner.

Fig. 7. (lower right). Superimposed isopters (derived electronically from Fig. 4) reveal the sites of variation maxima (see text).

DISCUSSION

(1) The fact that the maximum of variability is seen at the lower margin (and not beneath the center!) can be interpreted in such way that the deterioration of this visual field did not move towards the fixation point, but was speading to areas neighbouring the scotoma in a peripheral direction. This may have its cause in the special situation of the concerned nerve fiber layers in this eye, and, moreover, may have some prognostic importance too, concerning the indication for a filtrating operation and its probable risk.

(2) On the contrary, the location of the second maximum of variations – between the blind spot and the fixation point – might let us expect a growing danger for the fixation point. On the other hand, it may be created by chance only, as a result of horizontal fixation instability. This has to be proven by further investigations.

(3) The third maximum (at the lower edge of the visual field measured) seemed to correspond neither to the patient's individual field nor to general experience in glaucoma. Therefore, we looked up to the six Octopus examination sheets the calculation was based on, and could recognize that in one examination the testing point concerned had been missed by the patient, giving the value 0. In this way, misinterpretation could be prevented easily by a guided look to the data. In contrast, if you would have had the global statistical data only, as given by the known Delta programs, you would not have been able to distinguish those three different changes so easily.

(4) Concerning the considerable low variations in the upper two quadrants one may assume that the existing Bjerrum scotoma may be caused more by a local nerve fiber degeneration (wherever sited) than by a generalizing process. This may be of importance in the recent discussion of the value of diffuse and local acting factors of disturbance in the glaucomatous eye.

CONCLUSION

A computerized evaluation method for an easy location, identification and quantification of changes in the visual field feasable for any follow-up period has been demonstrated. It enables one to check rapidly whether there are big variations and towards which region the deterioration will probably move. On the other hand, overinterpretation has to be avoided carefully, always being aware of the fact that all calculations are based on rather few measurements. But, if it holds true that the different kinds of fluctuations, their detection and their definition versus real changes are of some importance for the prognosis of the glaucomatous visual field decay, we hope to have made some contribution to the solution of this problem.

REFERENCES

1. Flammer, J. Methoden zur Datenreduktion in der automatischen Perimetrie. Neuere Entwicklungen in der Ophthalmologie. München, 28.–31.10.1983. Bücherei des Augenarztes, Enke (in press).

2. Gloor, B., Jäggi, P., Stürmer, J. Wo steht die Perimetrie im Verlauf des Glaukoms? Neuere Entwicklungen in der Ophthalmologie. München, 28.–31.10.1983. Bücherei des Augenarztes, Enke (in press).
3. Gramer, E. Computerperimetrie bei Glaukom. In: Programmgesteuerte Perimetrie. Hrsg.: W. Leydhecker und G.K. Krieglstein. Kaden Verlag, 99 (1982).
4. Langerhorst, C.T., van den Berg, T.J.T.P. und Greve, E.L. Schätzung der verschiedenen Fluktuationsfaktoren bei der Computerperimetrie von Glaukompatienten. Neuerer Entwicklungen in der Ophthalmologie. München, 28.–31.10.1983. Bücherei des Augenartzes, Enke (in press).
5. Mertz, M. and Schultes, N. Greyscale and isopters. First Internat. Meeting on Automated Perimetry System Octopus. Zürich, 6.–7.4.1979.
6. Mertz, M. Die Rolle des Arztes bei der Computerperimetrie. In: G.K. Krieglstein, W. Leydhecker (Hrsg.): Programmgesteuerte Perimetrie. Heidelberg: Kaden: 15 (1982).
7. Mertz, M. Retinale Ortsbestimmung rasterperimetrisch nachgewiesener Skotome. Neuere Entwicklungen in der Ophthalmologie. München, 28.–31.10.1983. Bücherei des Augenarztes, Enke (in press).
8. Mertz, M. Three dimensional visual field analysis, its history and present state. University of California, San Francisco, Dec. 12, 1983.
9. Weber, B. and Spahr, J. Zur Automatisierung der Perimetrie; Darstellungsmethoden perimetrischer Untersuchungsergebnisse. Acta Ophthalmol. 54: 349 (1976).

Author's address:
Prof. Dr M. Mertz
Dipl.-Phys. U. Zirkel
Augenklinik rechts der Isar
    der Technischen Universität München
Ismaninger Str. 22
D-8000 München 80
F.R.G.

THE HUMPHREY FIELD ANALYZER: CONCEPTS AND CLINICAL RESULTS

ANDERS HEIJL

(Malmö, Sweden)

ABSTRACT

The technical data, test strategies and printout modes of the new Humphrey Field Analyzer are briefly described. Clinical experiences, main advantages and shortcomings are reported.

INTRODUCTION

The concepts behind the new Humphrey Field Analyzer (HFA) are to provide a fully automatic computerized perimeter with:
1. A projection system.
2. Precise threshold strategies.
3. Time-effective supraliminal testing strategies related to the individual sensitivity of the tested field.
4. Flexible custom tests.
5. Space-adaptive screening.
6. Specific glaucoma and neuro patterns.
7. Floppy disc system for storing fields, enabling follow-up examinations using data from prior tests and statistical analysis of test results.
8. Standard Goldmann stimuli and background.

HARDWARE

The most important technical specifications of the HFA (Fig. 1) are shown in Table 1.

SOFTWARE

The HFA has a number of different test strategies and point patterns.

55

E.L. Greve, W. Leydhecker & C. Raitta (eds.), Second European Glaucoma Symposium, Helsinki 1984.
© 1985, Dr. W. Junk Publishers, Dordrecht. ISBN 978-94-010-8934-0

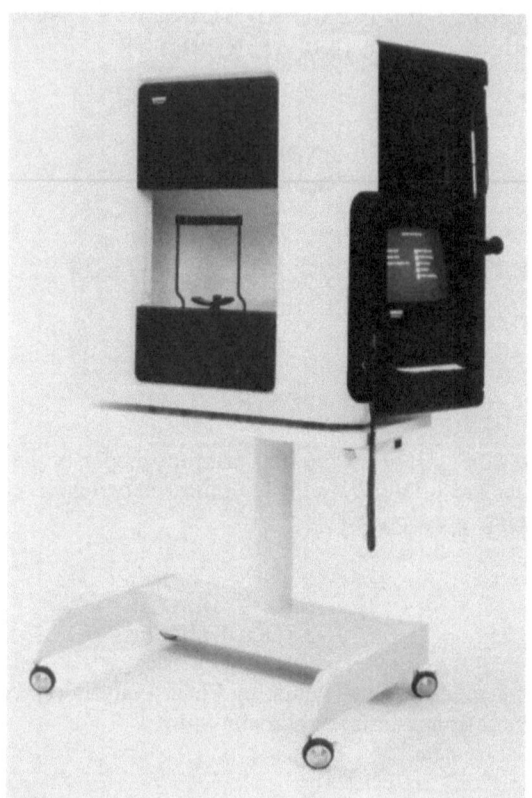

Fig. 1. The Humphrey Field Analyzer.

Table 1. Some technical specifications of the HFA

Stimulus presentation	Static
Stimulus duration	0.2 sec
Stimulus source	Incandescent lamp, projection system
Stimulus intensities	0.08–10,000 asb (neutral density filters + filter wedge)
Stimulus intensity range	5.1 l.u.
Stimulus size	Goldmann V–I
Stimulus colours	White, blue, red, green
Background	Hemisphere, 330 mm radius
Background luminance	31.5 asb
Computer	Intel 8088 processor, 64 kbytes RAM + 64 kbytes ROM
Input unit	CRT (cathode ray tube)/lightpen system
Output unit	Impact printer + CRT
Disc system	Two 5.25″ floppy disc drives (2 × 400 kbytes)
Fixation monitoring	Blind spot type + telescope

Test strategies

There are three different types of test strategies:
1. Threshold strategies;

2. Supraliminal screening strategies; and
3. Space-adaptive screening strategy.

1. Threshold strategies. The basic thresholding strategy (Full Threshold) starts by determining the threshold in four primary points. The stimuli are initially presented at supposedly supraliminal intensity levels, and the intensities are decreased in 4 dB steps until the stimulus is no longer perceived. The test process then reverses and moves in 2 dB steps until the stimulus is seen again. This procedure is performed twice at each primary point. The results at these four points are then used to determine the starting levels of the test process in neighbouring secondary points. In these, the same logic is used as in the primary points, but the threshold is measured once. If at this stage the measured threshold is within 4 dB of the expected (the threshold of the neighbouring point from which the starting level was determined plus correction for location) the test is finished, otherwise the threshold is measured again. The measured thresholds in secondary points are used to determine starting levels for tertiary points and so forth. This approach saves time by taking advantage of the a priori knowledge that threshold values of neighbouring points normally are similar.

If previous threshold data from the same eye are available from disk, two other threshold technique may be used:

a. In the Full Threshold from prior Data strategy, the most recent test results from the same eye are used to determine the initial intensity levels used for the threshold bracketing at each test point.

b. The Fast Threshold Strategy is a different logic where each point is tested with a stimulus 2 dB brighter than the stored value from an earlier test. If this stimulus level is seen, no attempt is made to determine the threshold. Only points missed twice at this level are subjected to threshold determination. This strategy, can be regarded as an individually tailored, slightly supraliminal screening, the objective of which is to see whether the field has deteriorated since the previous examination.

2. Supraliminal screening strategies. The HFA has four different screening test strategies. Three of these are threshold-related, supraliminal tests where the stimulus intensities used are based on actual threshold determinations in four primary points. The target intensity is corrected for eccentricity and presented 6 dB above the expected threshold. Missed points are retested. In the Supra Threshold Strategy the points are classifed into two categories, seen and not seen; in the Three Zone Strategy all points missed twice are tested at the maximum intensity level, thus permitting separation of missed points into relative and absolute defects, and in the Quantify Defects Strategy the threshold is measured in all missed points (Fig. 3). There is also a single intensity suprathreshold test.

3. Space-adaptive screening strategy. The space-adaptive screening test, called the Automatic Diagnostic Strategy, is an improved screening strategy with space adaptive properties. The first phase of this strategy consists of an 80 point threshold-related, supraliminal screening of the central 30° field. In

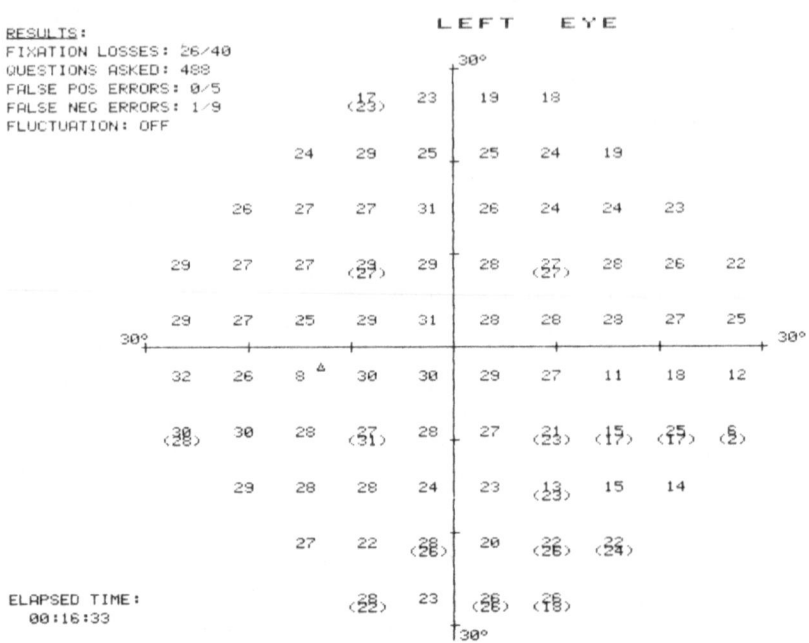

RESULTS:
FIXATION LOSSES: 26/40
QUESTIONS ASKED: 488
FALSE POS ERRORS: 0/5
FALSE NEG ERRORS: 1/9
FLUCTUATION: OFF

30°

17
(23)   23   19   18

24   29   25   25   24   19

26   27   27   31   26   24   24   23

29   27   27   (29/27)   29   28   (27/27)   28   26   22

30°   29   27   25   29   31   28   28   28   27   25   30°

32   26   8 △   30   30   29   27   11   18   12

(30/28)   30   28   (27/31)   28   27   (21/23)   (15/17)   (25/17)   (6/2)

29   28   28   24   23   (13/23)   15   14

27   22   (28/26)   20   (22/26)   (22/24)

ELAPSED TIME:
  00:16:33

(28/22)   23   (28/26)   (26/18)

30°

NO. = THRESHOLD IN DB
(NO.) = THRESHOLD IN DB (2ND/3RD TIME)

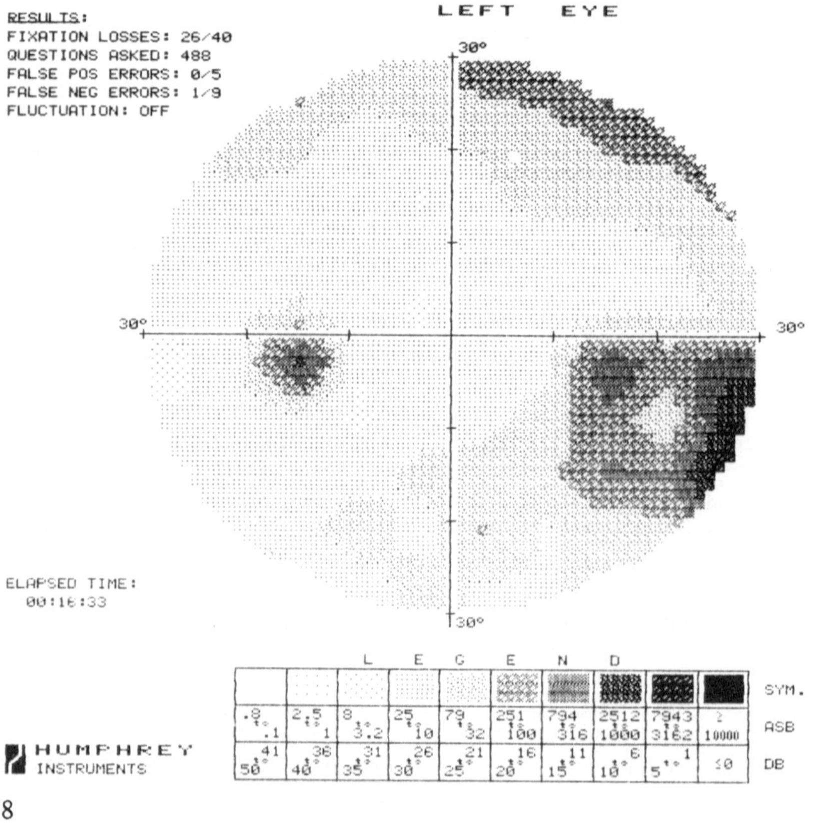

L E F T   E Y E

RESULTS:
FIXATION LOSSES: 26/40
QUESTIONS ASKED: 488
FALSE POS ERRORS: 0/5
FALSE NEG ERRORS: 1/9
FLUCTUATION: OFF

30°

30°   30°

ELAPSED TIME:
  00:16:33

30°

L E G E N D

										SYM.
.8 .1	2.5 1	8 3.2	25 10	79 32	251 100	794 316	2512 1000	7943 3162	2 10000	ASB
41 50°	36 40°	31 35°	26 30°	21 25°	16 20°	11 15°	6 10°	1 5°	10	DB

HUMPHREY
INSTRUMENTS

58

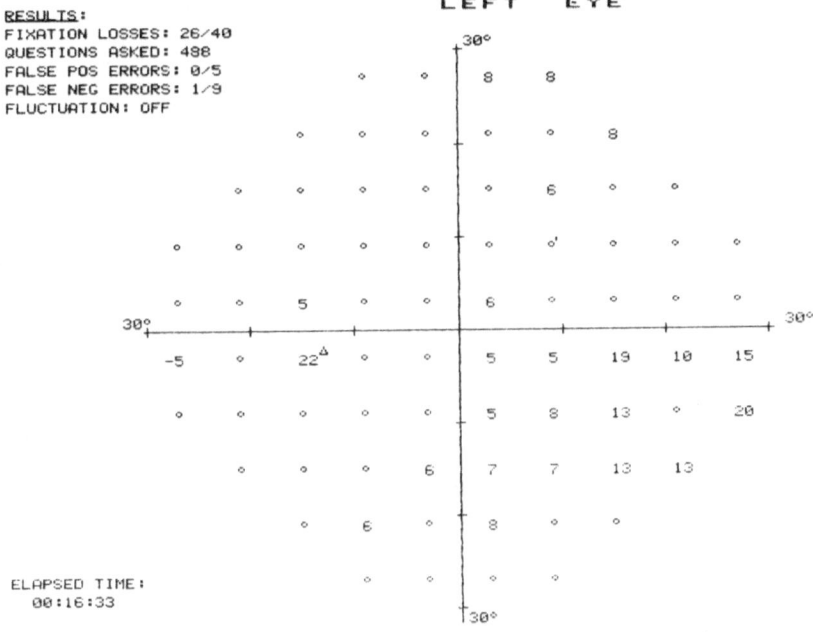

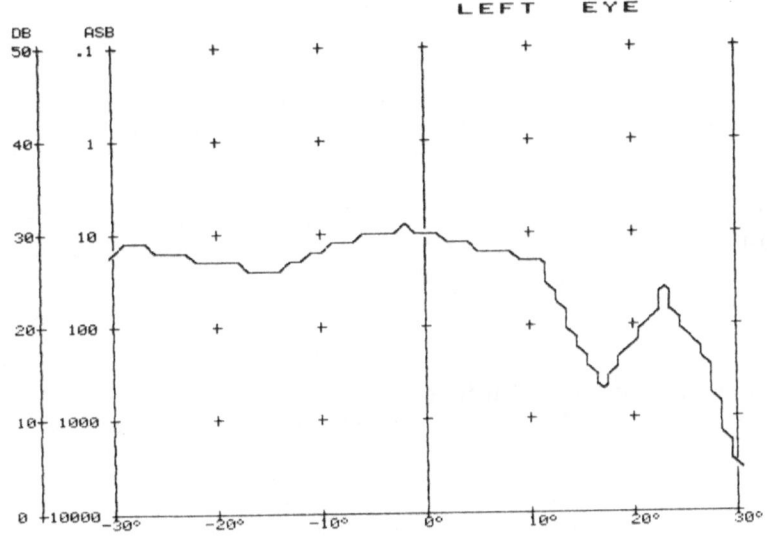

PROFILE OF MERIDIAN 160

RESULTS:
FIXATION LOSSES: 26/40
QUESTIONS ASKED: 488
FALSE POS ERRORS: 0/5
FALSE NEG ERRORS: 1/9

Fig. 2. Output formats for threshold tests. The result from a 30−2 test of glaucomatous eye displayed in four different ways: (a) Numeric representation of the thresholds in all measured points (in tenths of log units). (b) Greyscale representation. (c) Defect depth representation (in tenths of log units). (d) Interpolated profile through 160−340° meridan.

59

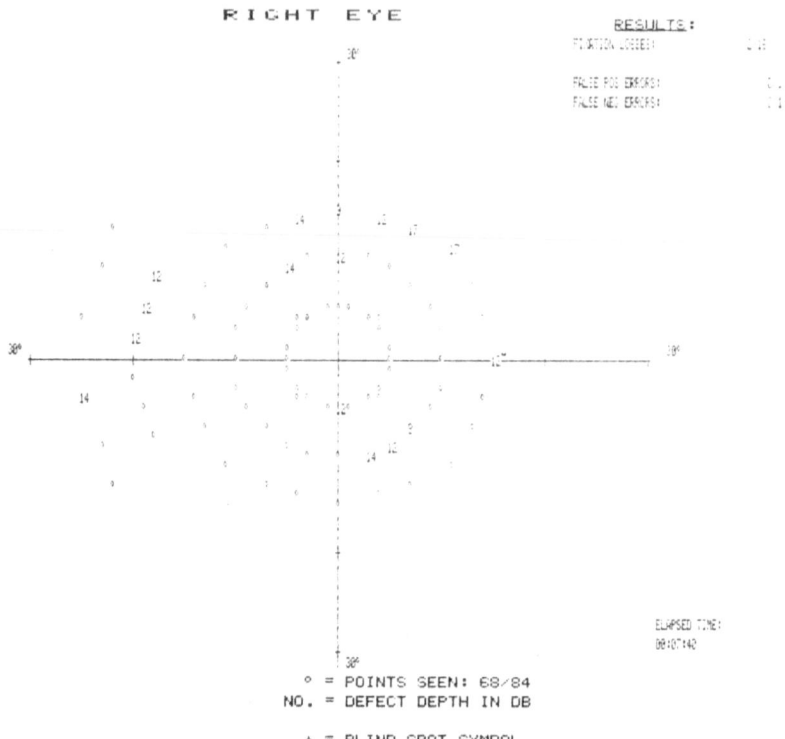

Fig. 3. Printout of Armaly Central Field screening test performed in the Quantify Defects mode. Normal points are indicated by circles. In pathological points the depth of the defect is indicated in tenths of log units.

phase II the depth of any detected defects is measured as in the Quantify Defects strategy. Additional points are then added around the pathological points. These are tested supraliminally (Fig. 4).

Point patterns

There are eight different patterns for threshold testing (Table 2) and nine screening patterns (Table 3). In addition there are several different possibilities

Table 2. Threshold programs

	Point density	No. of points
Central 30−1	6°	71
Central 30−2	6°	76
Peripheral 30/60−1	12°	63
Peripheral 30/60−2	12°	68
Temporal crescent	8, 5°	37
Neurological 20	N/A	16 tested 2× each
Neurological 50	N/A	22 tested 2× each
Macula	2°	16 tested 3× each
Custom	N/A	

Table 3. Screening programs

	Defect type	No. of points
Armaly Central	Glaucoma	84
Armaly Full Field	Glaucoma	98
RKPW Point Glaucoma Screen	Glaucoma	15–20
Central 40 Point	General	40
Central 80 Point	General	80
Central 166 Point	General	166
Full Field 81 Point	General	81
Full Field 120 Point	General	120
Full Field 246 Point	General	246
Custom	N/A	

to create custom programs. Thus meridional and circular profiles, high density grids and point clusters as well as single points may be tested both in threshold-measuring mode and supraliminally. The point density of the grids and profiles may be selected as well as the location in the visual field.

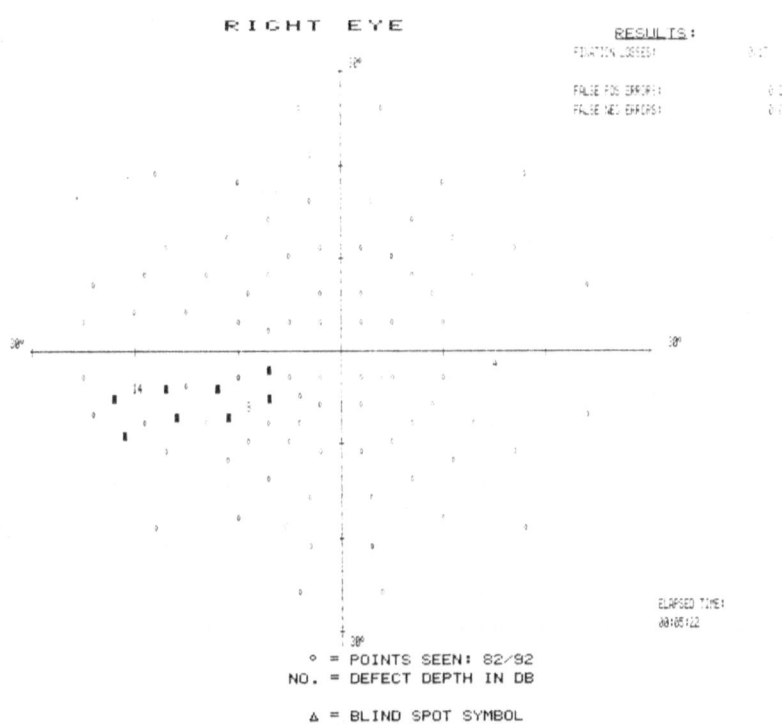

Fig. 4. An example of a space-adaptive screening test. In missed point in the 80-point pattern of phase I the defect depth is shown. The perimeter has automatically added extra points around the missed points; these extra points are indicated by squares if not seen, by circles if seen. The extra points confirm and help delineate the defect.

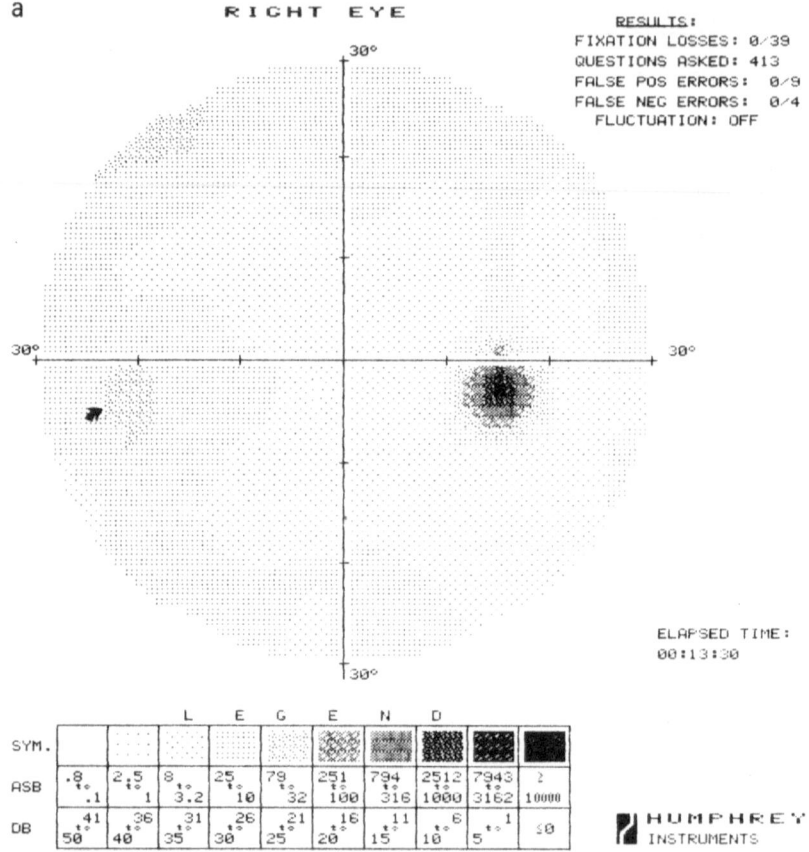

Fig. 5

MODES OF PRINTOUT

Most of the threshold tests may be displayed in four different ways, illustrated in Fig. 2. In the standard Suprathreshold Strategy and the One Level screening points are printed out as seen or missed. The Three Zone Strategy will separate between absolute and relative defects and The Quantify Defects Strategy will print out the defect depth in tenths of log units (Fig. 3). An example of a printout from the Automatic Diagnositc Strategy is shown in Fig. 4.

CLINICAL RESULTS

The HFA has been used at the University Department of Ophthalmology in Malmö for nine months. Results obtained mainly with the central threshold and the Armaly screening programs have shown good correspondance with

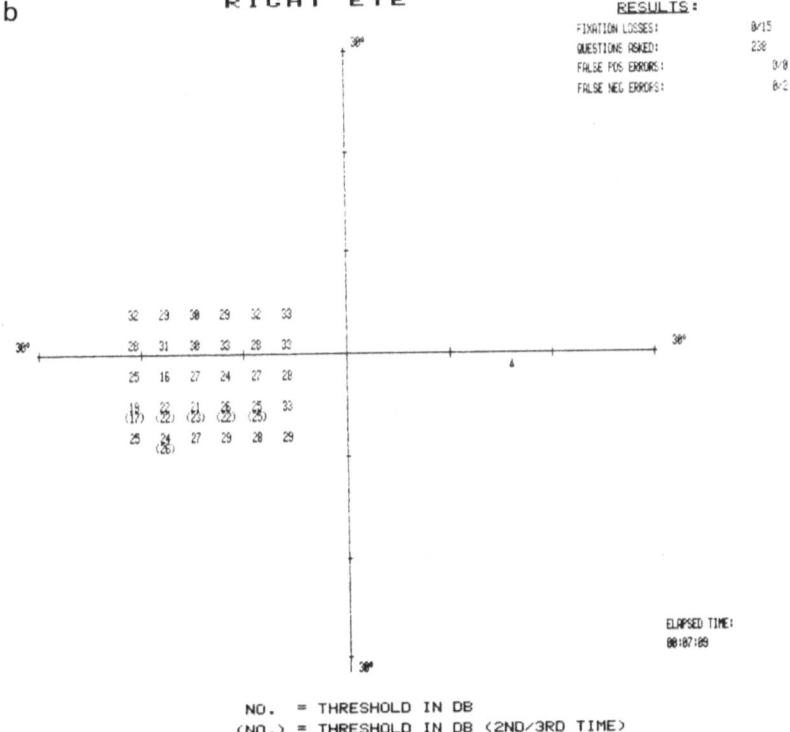

b

RIGHT EYE

RESULTS:
FIXATION LOSSES: 8/15
QUESTIONS ASKED: 238
FALSE POS ERRORS: 0/8
FALSE NEG ERRORS: 8/2

ELAPSED TIME:
00:07:09

NO. = THRESHOLD IN DB
<NO.> = THRESHOLD IN DB <2ND/3RD TIME>

Fig. 5. The central 30−2 threshold test (a) only arouses suspicion of a subtle inferior paracentral scotoma (arrow − same eye as in Fig. 4). A high density grid (b) in the questionable area confirms a shallow defect.

results from the Competer computerized perimeter and with Goldmann fields. The flexibility of the instrument in various clinical situations is more than adequate.

The threshold results have shown good reproducibility and the second threshold determination performed in points out of line with adjacent points have often contributed positively to the results. The threshold-related screening strategies seem to separate well between pathological and normal fields and the quantifying mode is often helpful in the interpretation of results. The space-adaptive program helps delineate identified defects and is particularly useful in cases with small defects (Fig. 4). The different custom programs, particularly the high density grids (Fig. 5) and the profiles are often very helpful in detailed analyses of small defects or questionable areas.

The light-pen/CRT system where programs and test parameters are selected and patient data entered is easy to use because of the hierarchical system of 'screens' of the instrument. Therefore very little time is needed for a technician to learn to operate the instrument. The multitude of strategies and point patterns, on the other hand, may require either familiarity with perimetric principles in general or rather long practical experience with the device before the ophthalmologist learns to use the facilities of the instrument in an optimal way.

The main shortcomings of the instrument are that the printer is rather slow and that the thresholding strategies might be quite time-consuming in pathological cases. The threshold tests will become faster in the near future because of some changes in the control of the projection system. The statistical package still only permits algebraical operations: averaging, merging and comparisons using subtraction fields. It is, however, expected to grow, permitting statistical analyses of changes in consecutive fields.

Author's address:
Dept. of Ophthalmology
Malmö General Hospital
S-21401 Malmö
Sweden

PERIMETRY IN CONGENITAL AND INFANTILE GLAUCOMA

M. ROLANDO, P. CAPRIS, E. GANDOLFO, C. BURTOLO,
G.A. CALABRIA and M. ZINGIRIAN

(Genoa, Italy)

ABSTRACT

By means of repeated kinetic (Goldmann) and static (Peritest and Perikon) perimetry, 53 eyes of congenital or infantile glaucoma patients have been followed. The visual field damage did not have the classic sequential progression of glaucoma in adults, but in 20% of cases the first sign was isopters contraction or fasciular defects in unusual positions. In 40% of eyes, sometimes as the first sign of damage, we have found a depression in the overall light sensibility. In 5.7% of cases when IOP has been controlled, regression of visual field defects has been shown. When both eyes were involved and the rise in IOP was symmetrical, visual field defects were not different from the characteristic adult open angle glaucoma defects. In asymmetric forms and in unilateral glaucoma, in the most affected eye, we noted together with the reported glaucoma defects, perimetric damages related to amblyopia.

INTRODUCTION

The clinical and anatomopathological features of congenital and infantile glaucomas are different from adult primary open angle glaucoma, but, like in any other class of glaucoma, perimetric follow-up is fundamental to assess the visual damage and to detect the progression of the disease or the efficacy of the therapy.

The perimetric findings of congenital and infantile glaucoma have some characteristic aspects which are different from adult open angle glaucoma both in the morphology and in the evolution of the defects (2–8).

MATERIAL AND METHODS

Thirty-one subjects (53 eyes) between 5 and 32 years of age, with diagnosis of infantile or congenital glaucoma assessed before 10 years of age, have been studied. In nine subjects (29%) the affection was monocular.

Perimetry has been performed in all the subjects, every eight months on average, at the Glaucoma Clinic of the Department of Ophthalmology of

E.L. Greve, W. Leydhecker & C. Raitta (eds.), Second European Glaucoma Symposium, Helsinki 1984.
© *1985, Dr. W. Junk Publishers, Dordrecht. ISBN 978-94-010-8934-0*

Genoa University. The eyes showing a higher risk of visual field worsening because of the difficulty in controlling intraocular pressure (IOP) or because of the presence of optic disc modifications, have been examined at closer intervals (every second or third month). The follow-up of the patients varied from 1 to 13 years (average: 6 years).

Twelve subjects (38.7%) have been observed for less than 10 years. The age of the first perimetric control varied from 5 to 28 years of age (average 16 years).

Perimetry has been performed by kinetic photopic method using an automatic computerized Goldmann perimeter: Perikon (Optikon) or by a static computerized multiple stimuli perimeter: Peritest (Rodenstock) when it became available (4).

RESULTS

The perimetric findings of the last control of the 53 eyes studied are reported in table 1. They show, together with the classic defects of adult open angle

Table 1. Infantile and congenital glaucoma

Perimetric defects	%
A Isopters contraction	64.1
B Nasal step	30.2
C Temporal bundle defect	18.9
D Arcuate scotoma	47.1
E Central scotoma	5.7
F Paracentral scotoma	22.6

glaucoma, some infrequent features characteristic of juvenile glaucoma, such as temporal or central scotomas.

In 34 eyes (64%) we have observed an overall depression of light sensibility. Such a depression, clearly detectable by static perimetry, appears as a lowering and flattening of the static profile if compared to normals. Often it does not come together to other, more defined, visual field defects, and, in kinetic perimetry appears as a concentric contraction of isopters.

In 16 eyes (30.1%) we did not notice any evolution of visual field defects, while in 27 eyes (50.9%) the defects followed the well-known sequence of adult open angle glaucoma (paracentral isolated scotomas, nasal step, bundle defects in nasal quadrants, etc.).

A more irregular and not sequential evolution of visual field defects was found in 6 eyes (11.3%), with overall depression of light sensibility and without the appearance of defects inside the 30° degrees of eccentricity or of any other 'classic' glaucoma defect.

In two eyes (3.8%) a central scotoma appeared and in three eyes (5.6%) superior temporal defects became detectable.

The evolution of visual field defects could not be correlated to the grade of IOP control. As a matter of fact we have observed a very good preservation of visual field in presence of uncontrolled IOP.

But also in presence of borderline or controlled IOP as soon as a worsening took place, the progression of visual field defects was very fast.

In three eyes (5.7%) when the IOP went under control after surgery a recovery of the visual field was detected.

We have noticed different features of perimetric defects depending on whether the disease is mono- or bilateral or if the IOP values have been asymmetrical for a long time.

DISCUSSION

In monolateral or bilateral asymmetric forms, it is conceivable that, together with the perimetric deficits caused by glaucoma, the alterations caused by amblyopia are present.

Amblyopia in these eyes could be related to corneal decompensation, anisometropia or eterotropia which are often present with these forms of glaucoma.

Amblyopia well explains the elevation of central sensitivity threshold, that sometimes becomes true central scotoma (1–3).

The difference from the known sequence of appearance of perimetric defects of adult open angle glaucoma could be correlated to the lack of blood perfusion deficits of the optic nerve head which are typical of older age (5) and to the elasticity of the ocular tissues which better absorb the noxa of IOP (6, 7).

The possibility of a sudden and rapid loss of visual field also in absence of huge IOP elevations, increases the danger of infantile glaucoma and stresses the importance of frequent perimetric controls.

The incidence of visual field defects related to amblyopia emphasizes that the control of IOP is just the first step of the visual rehabilitation of these young patients.

REFERENCES

1. Castellazzo, R., Fava, G.P., Capris, P. and Fioretto, M. 'Relationship between different kinds of functional amplyopia and perimetry'. Int. Symp. Strabismus Deditum. Florence, 1982, pp. 199–212.
2. Drance, S.M. 'The early visual field defects in glaucoma'. Invest. Ophthalmol. 8: 84–91 (1969).
3. Fava, G.P., Capris, P., Bisio, R. and Fioretto, M. 'L'ambliopia da inibizione e da anopsia: studio perimetrico e campimetrico'. Boll. Oculist. 63, suppl. 11/12: 325–333 (1984).
4. Greve, E.L., Dannheim, F. and Bakker, D. 'The Peritest, a new automatic and semi-automatic perimeter'. Int. Ophthalmol. 5: 201–214 (1982).
5. Hayreh, S.S., Review, I.H.S. and Edwards, J. 'Vasogenic origin of visual field defects and optic nerve changes in glaucoma'. Br. J. Ophthalmol. 54: 461–472 (1870).
6. Kessing, S.V. and Gregersen, E. 'The distended disc in early stages of congenital glaucoma'. Acta Ophthalmol. 55: 431–435 (1977).

7. Robin, A.L. and Quigley, H.A. 'Transient reversible cupping in juvenile-onset glaucoma'. Am. J. Ophthalmol. 88: 580–584 (1979).
8. Robin, A.L., Quigley, H.A., Pollack, I.P., Maumene, A.E. and Maumenee, I.H. 'An analysis of visual acuity, visual fields, and disk-cupping in childhood glaucoma'. Am. J. Ophthalmol. 88: 847–858 (1979).

Authors' address:
University Eye Clinic
Viale Benedetto XV, no. 5
16132 Genoa
Italy

COMPUTERIZED PERIMETRIC PROGRAM FOR DETECTION OF EARLY GLAUCOMATOUS DEFECTS

E. GANDOLFO, M. ZINGIRIAN and P. CAPRIS

(Genoa, Italy)

ABSTRACT

Among the static-kinetic programs, the Armaly-Drance strategy is universally accepted as a valid perimetric test for detecting early glaucomatous visual field defects. In our opinion, this program can be improved, thanks to recent progress in automated perimetry. The features of the Armaly-Drance program that can be modified are the following:
- Distribution of the tested points in the paracentral area: a more even arrangement of these points is desirable.
- Characteristics of the stimulus: individual threshold related stimuli can make the exam more accurate.
- Kinetic trajectories in the nasal v.f.: a greater number of kinetic stimuli can increase the probability of nasal step detection.
- Stimuli presentation sequence: a random stimuli presentation in recommended.

The Automatic Goldmann Perimeter (Perikon) permits a precise and rapid execution of the Armaly-Drance modified strategy. The results of clinical use of our computerized program 'Genoa Glaucoma Screening' are evaluated and compared with those of traditional procedures.

INTRODUCTION

Among the static-kinetic programs, the Armaly-Drance (A.D.) glaucoma screening technique is universally accepted as a valid perimetric strategy for detecting early glaucomatous visual field (v.f.) defects (1, 2, 3, 6).

In our opinion, the A.D. strategy can be improved, thanks to recent progress in automatic perimetry (8). The parameters of the A.D. program that can be modified are the following:

Distribution of the tested points in the paracentral area. The points on the 5° parallel, in fact, are closer than those on the 10° and 15° parallels. A more even arrangement of these points is desirable.

Characteristics of the stimulus. The stimulus adopted is the same in all points tested with static perimetry and often it is too supraliminal, especially for the 5° parallel explorations. A variation of stimulus luminance related

69

E.L. Greve, W. Leydhecker & C. Raitta (eds.), Second European Glaucoma Symposium, Helsinki 1984.
© *1985, Dr. W. Junk Publishers, Dordrecht. ISBN 978-94-010-8934-0*

to the individual threshold and to the eccentricity can make the exam more selective (3, 4).

Kinetic trajectories in the nasal visual field. A greater number of kinetic stimuli can increase the probability of detecting a nasal step (7).

Sequence of stimuli presentation. In the A.D. strategy, the static stimuli are presented in a sequential manner (clockwise arrangement). Also, kinetic trajectories for exploration of the blind spot and isopters follow an easily foreseeable sequence. A random presentation of static and kinetic stimuli is commonly recommended (4).

Obviously, only computerized perimetry allows us to perform all these modifications without increasing the time needed for the test. Automatic perimetry, on the other hand, has many advantages: the fixation control, the registration of results, the evaluation and classification of responses are automatically carried out (Figs. 1 & 2).

METHOD AND MATERIAL

The Automatic Goldmann Perimeter (8) (Perikon, Optikon Spa, Rome) has been the ideal apparatus to try and perfect our modified A.D. glaucoma screening strategy (Genoa Glaucoma Screening). The following characteristics have been adopted for our program:

Threshold determination. The individual threshold is tested in two points of the temporal v.f. at the eccentricity of 20° (emimeridians 285° and 75° in the R.E., emimeridians 105° and 255° in the L.E.). Every determination is repeated twice and the second best value is considered as the real 'basal threshold' of the individual. This stimulus is used for the points on the 5° parallel. For the 10° parallel points the luminance is increased on 0.2 L.U., an for the 15° parallel points on 0.4 L.U. The blind spot is examined with the same stimulus adopted for the 15° parallel. For the kinetic peripheral explorations the target adopted is 0.5 and 1 L.U. above basal threshold.

Static stimuli arrangement. The number of tested points on the 5° and 10° parallels has been reduced to 12 and 16, respectively in order to make the stimuli more evenly distributed in the paracentral v.f..

Kinetic trajectories characteristics. The kinetic exploration in the nasal v.f. has been increased up to 20 (1°, 3°, 5°, 10 and 30° above and below horizontal meridian). The temporal trajectories remained 2 (15° above and below the horizontal meridian). The velocity of target movement has been fixed at 5° per sec for peripheral determinations and at 2° per sec for blind spot (5).

Randomization of stimuli presentation. Both kinetic and static tests are randomized in order to eliminate the patient's tendency to lose fixation and to anticipate the response.

General course of the exam. The first phase of the test consists of a brief training program. Afterwards the program continues with individual threshold determination followed by blind spot mapping and random presentation of static stimuli in the paracentral area. Kinetic presentations in v.f. periphery conclude the test. The program automatically stops when it is necessary to

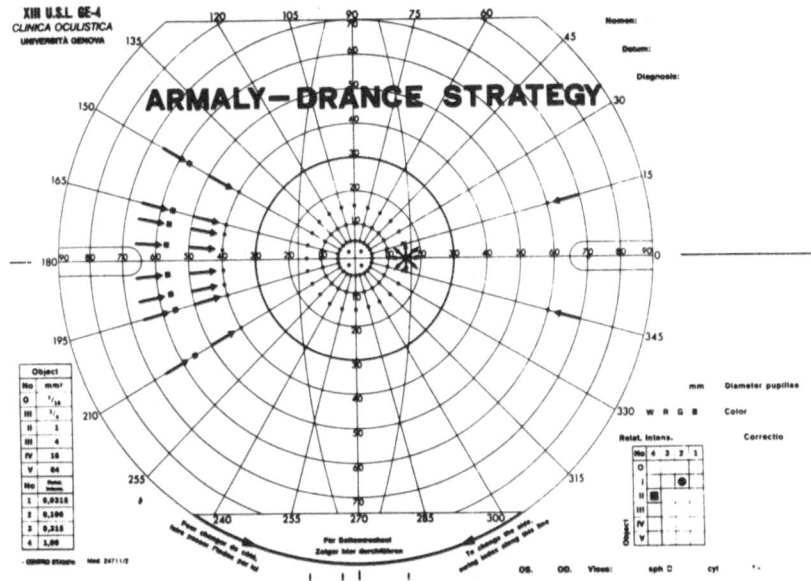

Fig. 1. Armaly-Drance 'Classic' strategy.

insert or remove correction lenses. At the end of the program, the computer evaluates the responses according to the following criteria:

Blind spot: It is considered normal if its margins do not exceed pre-determined limits (i.e.: R.E. = meridians $20°$ and $325°$, parallels $9°$ and $21°$; L.E. = meridians $170°$ and $215°$, parallels $9°$ and $21°$).

Paracentral defects: The loss of 1, 2 or 3 isolated points is not considered as defect. If more than 3 isolated points or 2 close points are lost, v.f. damage is suspected. If there are 3 or more missed close points or if 2 or more couples of 2 close points are lost, a certain paracentral defect is considered.

Nasal step: The presence of a nasal step is considered certain if the difference between the average eccentricities above and below the horizontal nasal meridian is more than $5°$. A nasal step is suspected when this difference is between $3°$ and $5°$.

Average isopteric eccentricity: A temporal isopter constriction to $40°$ or less is considered as a pathological sign. The nasal isopters are viewed as abnormal if their eccentricities are less than $25°$ and $35°$. The exam is con-sidered normal when all the following conditions are respected:
— The blind spot does not exceed the pre-fixed limits.
— There are no paracentral scotomata.
— Nasal and temporal isopters are wider than the minimum limits.
  The response is considered doubtful when:
— There is an enlargement of the blind spot, or
— there is a doubtful paracentral scotoma, or
— there is a doubtful nasal step, or
— there is isopteric contraction.

71

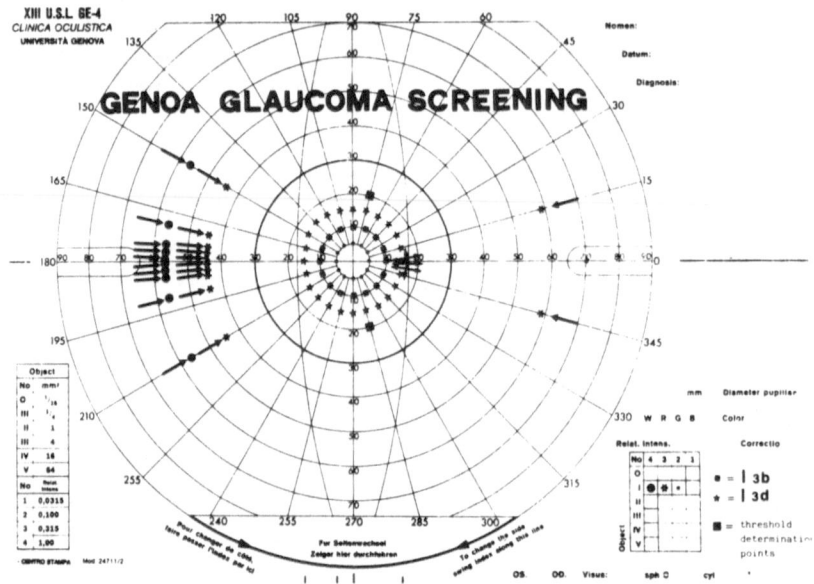

Fig. 2. 'Genoa Glaucoma Screening' strategy.

The response is pathological when:
— There is a definite paracentral scotoma, or
— there is a certain nasal step, or
— there is the presence of 2 or more doubtful signs.
Both results and diagnostic evaluation are printed out on a normal v.f. diagram by the plotter of the Perikon.

Our glaucoma screening program has been tested in 84 hypertensive eyes without glaucomatous defect during kinetic Goldmann perimetry. All the eyes also underwent a classic A.D. program and an accurate static-kinetic analysis of the whole v.f.

RESULTS

Among the 84 tested eyes the A.D. strategy has discovered 25 anomalies. Among these pathological eyes, an accurate v.f. analysis performed at later date showed 24 defects (1 false positive response). Among the 59 eyes classified as normal by A.D. test, the more complex controls showed 3 v.f. defects (3 false negative responses).

The Genoa Glaucoma Screening showed 31 pathological responses. Among these 31 eyes classified as glaucomatous or suspected by our program, 26 had their abnormality confirmed (5 false positive responses). Among the 53 eyes considered normal, only 1 showed glaucomatous alterations (1 false negative response).

72

COMMENT

In conclusion, our computerized glaucoma perimetric screening program has shown many advantages and few disadvantages compared with more traditional strategies.

The advantages are:

— the test is automatically performed by the computerized perimeter; therefore the exam conditions are more constant and standardized;
— the individual threshold determination allows us to carry out a slightly supraliminal test, that increases the probability of detecting a paracentral defect;
— the increased number of kinetic trajectories improves nasal step detection;
— the standardized criteria of result evaluation permit an immediate and automatic classification of defects.

The disadvantages are:

— there is a higher percentage of false positive responses;
— the cooperation required by the patient is slightly higher in comparison with A.D. strategy;
— it is necessary to buy a Perikon unit.

REFERENCES

1. Armaly, M.F. Ocular pressure and visual fields — A ten year follow-up study. Arch. Ophthalmol. 81: 25–40 (1969).
2. Armaly, M.F. Visual field defects in early open angle glaucoma. Trans. Am. Ophthalmol. Soc. 69: 147–159 (1971).
3. Bedwell, C.H. Visual fields. A basis for efficient investigation. London, Buterworth, 1982, pp. 14–15.
4. Fankhauser, F. Problems related to the design of automatic perimeters Doc. Ophthalmol. 47: 89–138 (1979).
5. Gandolfo, E. Contributo allo studio della soglia retinica differenziale in rapporto a stimoli cinetici. Boll. Oculist. 55: 385–396 (1976).
6. Rick, W.J., Drance, S.M. and Morgan, R.W. Modification of the Armaly visual field screening technique for glaucoma. Can. J. Ophthalmol. 6: 283–292 (1971).
7. Zingirian, M., Calabria, G. and Gandolfo, E. The nasal step: an early glaucomatous defect? Doc. Ophthalmol. Proc. 19: 273–278 (1979).
8. Zingirian, M., Gandolfo, E. and Orciuolo, M. Automation of the Goldmann perimeter. Doc. Ophthalmol. Proc. 35: 381–385 (1983).

Authors' address:
University Eye Clinic
Viale Benedetto XV, no. 5
16132 Genoa
Italy

EARLY GLAUCOMATOUS FIELD DEFECTS IN COMPUTERIZED PERIMETRY (OCTOPUS 201) AND TANGENT SCREEN (BJERRUM KAMPIMETRY)

JOHN THYGESEN and S.V. KESSING

(Copenhagen, Denmark)

ABSTRACT

A total of 120 visual fields of 90 chronic glaucoma patients exhibiting early glaucomatous field defects up to stage II according to Aulhorn were investigated to determine the frequency distribution of absolute and relative defects at the 72 test points of program 32 ($0°-30°$ eccentricity) of the computerized Octopus perimeter. The detection rate of Tangent screen in absolute and relative defects found in Octopus computer perimeter was investigated.

A. The following results in computerized Octopus perimetry were obtained:
1. The frequency distribution of absolute defects was highest in the lower nasal test points. Next was paracentral and peripheral absolute defects in the upper part of the visual field. The relative defects were also predominantly in the nasal testpoints, secondary they were found in the upper mid-periphery and not paracentral as the absolute defects.
2. The distribution of visual field defects (absolute and relative demonstrated a combination of paracentral and mid-peripheral defects (from $12°-30°$ eccentricity) in 52%, and exclusively mid-peripheral defects ($12°-30°$) in 40%. Exclusively paracentral defects were found in only 2% and exclusively enlarged blind spot in 6%, whereas enlarged blind spot in combination with paracentral or mid-peripheral defects was found in 34% of the field defects. Mid-peripheral nasal scotomas were found in only 6%. In contrast to the distribution of defects in eyes with combined absolute and relative defects the distribution of defects in eyes with exclusively relative defects were predominantly exclusively mid-peripheral (68%). Paracentral defects combined with mid-peripheral defects were found in only 16% and exclusively relative paracentral defects in 2%.
3. The frequency distribution of early glaucomatous absolute defects correspond to Aulhorn's reports based on manual perimetry, whereas the frequency distribution of relative defects is predominantly in the mid-periphery as nasal scotomas and superior arcuate scotomas and not paracentral as indicated by Aulhorn. These findings are in accordance with the reports of E. Gramer and colleagues.
B. The following results of Tangent screen were obtained:
1. The detection rate of absolute defects found in Octopus computer perimetry

75

E.L. Greve, W. Leydhecker & C. Raitta (eds.), Second European Glaucoma Symposium, Helsinki 1984.
© *1985, Dr. W. Junk Publishers, Dordrecht. ISBN 978-94-010-8934-0*

was in Tangent screen only 51%. Among these defects 65% were arcuate, 17.5% linear and 17.5% single point defects. Among the 49% absolute defects found by Octopus perimetry but not detected by Tangent screen 52% of the eyes had suspected optic disc in ophthalmoscopy. The Tangent screen detection rate of relative defects was only 16%.

REFERENCES

1. Aulhorn, E. Sensoric Functional Damage. Glaucoma. Conceptions of a Disease. Ed. Heilmann, K. and Richardson, K.T. Georg Thieme Publ., Stuttgart, pp. 157–168 (1978).
2. Gramer, E., Gerlach, R., Krieglstein, G.K. and Leydhecker, W. Zur Topographie früher glaukomatöser Gesichtsfeldausfälle bei der Computerperimetrie. Klin. Mbl. Augenheilk. 180: 515–523 (1982).

Authors' address:
University Glaucoma Clinic
Dept. of Ophthalmology
Rigshospitalet
DK-2100 Copenhagen Ø
Denmark

RABBIT IOP AND VITREOUS, LENS AND AQUEOUS WEIGHTS AFTER VARIOUS DIURETICS AND WATER LOADING TEST. THE INFLUENCE OF OPTIC NERVE TRANSECTION

A.D. PETOUNIS, J. LASKARATOS and J. FRONIMOPOULOS
(Athens, Greece)

ABSTRACT

The effect of osmotic and non-osmotic diuretics (mannitol, urea, glycerol, furosemide and acetazolamide) and water loading test on IOP and the weight of vitreous, lens and aqueous of frozen rabbits' eyeballs was studied. It was shown that all the administered diuretics resulted in reduction (or elevation) of either intraocular pressure or weight of vitreous, lens and aqueous humor, but in different percentages and time course. This relation (IOP/weight) was found to be analogous but not completely linear. The same procedures repeated after unilateral retrobulbar optic nerve transection and sham operation on the fellow eye.

Intraocular pressure of the eyes with transected optic nerve was significantly decreased on the 2nd postoperative day, probably due to no observable early vascular disorders of the eye. On the 7th and 30th postoperative day, no side differences in IOP were observed.

The administration of the above-mentioned drugs significantly changed the intraocular pressure of both eyes, without any side differences, from 2nd to 30th postoperative day.

The weights of vitreous, lens and aqueous responded proportionally to IOP alterations, but equally to both eyes. Our results do not support the hypothesis that osmotic agents act on a central neural regulation mechanism rather than producing a direct dehydrating effect on the ocular bulb.

INTRODUCTION

It is well known that intraocular pressure is influenced by osmotic stimuli. Some investigators suggested that osmotic agents act on a central neural regulation mechanism, rather than producing a direct dehydrating effect on the ocular globe. Water-drinking test in patients with unilateral optic nerve lesion produced a less pronounced increase of IOP on the damaged side than on the healthy one. This observation of Riise and Simonsen (10) was tested with a lot of experimental work in animals in order to confirm the theory of a central control of IOP.

Several results of older experiments (3, 13, 15) reported the existence of

77

E.L. Greve, W. Leydhecker & C. Raitta (eds.), Second European Glaucoma Symposium, Helsinki 1984.
© *1985, Dr. W. Junk Publishers, Dordrecht. ISBN 978-94-010-8934-0*

areas in the hypothalamus influencing the I.O.P. via efferent fibers in the optic nerve (12). Previous studies, reporting intraocular pressure response to various osmotic agents in experimental animals, are rather conflicting. In order to further investigate this matter we studied the changes of intraocular pressure in either normal eyes or those with transected optic nerve, in relation to changes of vitreous, aqueous and lens weight, following administration of osmotic and non osmotic diuretics.

METHODS

Male albino rabbits 2.5−3 kg were used. Intraocular pressure measurements were performed by a hand-held Perkins applanation tonometer, calibrated for the living rabbit eye (closed stopckock method), after a sufficient adaptation period of the animals. Retrobulbar optic nerve transection was carried out in one eye and a sham operation on the fellow eye, under Na-pentobarbital anaesthesia. Surgical technique prescribed by Krupin et al. (5) was followed. The optic nerve was isolated through a conjuctival incision in the superior temporal area and rotation of the globe by retraction of the lateral and superior rectus muscles. Care was taken to avoid damaging the central retinal artery which enters the optic nerve close to the globe.

The direct pupillary reaction to light, as well as the optic nerve head as observed by ophthalmoscopy proved the complete optic nerve transection (on the 30th postoperative day). Vitreous body, lens and aqueous weights were determined by the use of a freezing technique. This method, prescribed by Robbins and Galin (11) for vitreous body weight measurements, was 'extented' to lens and aqueous humor weights. The technique involves rapid enucleation of the eye, freezing it for 24 hours in dry ice at − 74°C, isolating the frozen vitreous, lens and aqueous by careful cross dissections of the globe and then weighing them to milligram accuracy. We considered that the reliability of our method for aqueous humor weight determination was not very high, due to its very short defrosting time. The effect of optic nerve transection on IOP was tested in three groups of 25 rabbits each, for the 2nd, 7th and 30th postoperative day respectively.

Groups of six rabbits each were used for the determinations of IOP and vitreous, lens and aqueous weights following the administration of various substances. Enucleation of the eyes for the weight measurements was performed at the time of maximum effect of each of the administered substances or intraocular pressure, as it has been determined in earlier pilot experiments.

SUBSTANCES ADMINISTERED

1. Mannitol: Solution 20%, given i.v., 4 g/kg, in 10−15 min.
2. Urea: Solution 30%, given i.v., 1.5 g/kg in 10 min.
3. Acetazolamide: Commercial vial, given i.v. in a bolus dose of 50 mg/kg.
4. Glycerol: Aqueous solution 50%, 6 g/kg via oral gastric tube, in 5 min.
5. Furosemide: Commercial i.v. solution, in a bolus dose of 40 mg/kg, in 2 min.

6. Water: For water loading test, via oral/gastric tube, in a dose of 100 mg/kg in 5 min.
Statistical evaluation was performed on all data using the t-test, paired/or unpaired, according to protocol.

RESULTS

1. Figure 1 shows the vitreous, aqueous and lens weights in control animals of various ages. It becomes clear that these weights, especially the vitreous one, are related to the age of the animals. This observation seems to be important, emphasizing the need of using animals of very similar age for the reliability of the results, and in order to avoid standard deviations.

   Table 1 lists the percentages of IOP changes in relation to alterations of vitreous, aqueous and lens weights following administration of osmotic and non-osmotic diuretics. It is evident that all the administered substances reduced either intraocular pressure (water loading test increased it, as it was expected) or vitreous, aqueous and lens weights, but in various percentages and time after administration, mainly due to different routes of administration. Also, the proportion of IOP reduction (or elevation) to globe, and especially to vitreous, dehydration, becomes clear.

2. No significant differences in intraocular pressure were noted between the eyes with transected optic nerve and their controls (sham operated) on the 7th and 30th postoperative day. On the 2nd postoperative day, the intraocular pressure of the eyes with transected optic nerve was found to be significantly lower ($P < 0.01$) than those of the fellow ones (Fig. 2 and 2a). Furthermore, the IOP responses to all administered substances were similar between the eyes with intact and transected optic nerves, on either the 2nd or 7th and 30th postoperative days (Fig. 3, 3a and 3b).

   Finally, the weights of vitreous, aqueous and lens were changed similarly, following the administration of the substances, in either eyes with transected optic nerves or the controlateral sham operated ones (Fig. 4), independent of the postoperative day tested.

DISCUSSION

Laboratory and clinical studies have confirmed that osmotic agents reduce intraocular pressure by dehydrating the globe. According to our data, water loss from the vitreous was the major factor in lowering IOP following administration of acetazolamide (and much less of furosemide) as well as the water loading, alter intraocular pressure, mainly by changing the aqueous humor volume, decreasing or increasing it respectively. Generally, the role of lens dehydration seems to be rather secondary, but greatly evaluated during intraocular surgery (cataract extraction, glaucoma), following administration of osmotic agents (e.g. mannitol).

However, lens dehydration following acetazolamide or even furosemide administration, creates the problem of possible 'cataractogenic effect' of

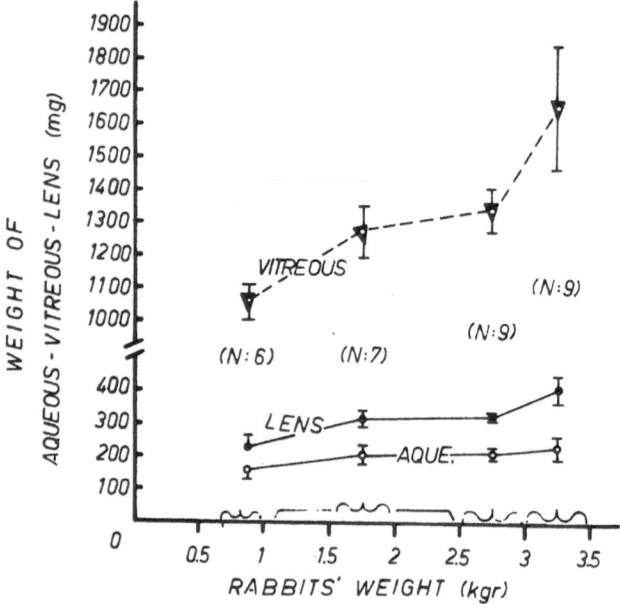

Fig. 1. Vitreous, aqueous and lens weights in control animals of various ages.

Table 1. Intraocular pressure changes in relation to vitreous aqueous and lens weight alterations, following administration of various diuretics (n : 6)

Substance	% I.O.P. change	Time ΔpMx	Differences in weights (mg)			
			Vitreous	Aqueous	Lens	Total
Mannitol	− 64	30	− 92.5*	− 19.5*	− 16.9*	128.9
Urea	− 53	30	− 82.0*	− 23.1*	− 7.7	112.8
Glycerol	− 59	50	− 88.8*	− 12.5	− 12.9*	114.2
Furosemide	− 17	30	− 28.5	− 20.6	− 5.6	56.4
Acetazolamide	− 39	15	− 16.7	− 39.6*	− 3.6	59.8
Water (loading test)	+ 28	30	+ 11.0	+ 31.0**	+ 3.0	45.0

* P < 0.01,   ** P < 0.05

these substances, following their chronic administration. Carbonic anhydrate distribution and activity in the lens is well known (2). Chronic administration of acetazolamide, conceivably inhibits it, dehydrating the lens. Since there is no control eye in systemic administration its possible effects on the lens is not known.

Finally, it can be concluded that the determination of weight of aqueous, vitreous and lens is a simple and accurate method for testing the mechanism of hypotonic action of either osmotic or non-osmotic diuretics.

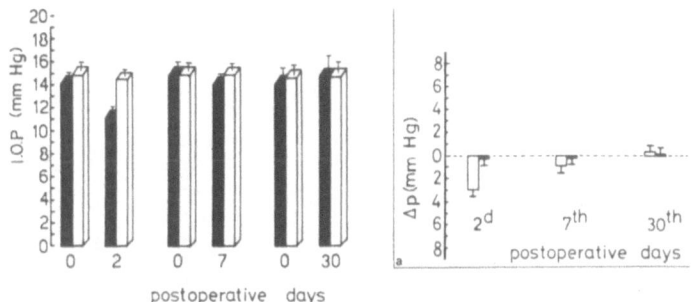

Fig. 2. Influence of unilateral optic nerve transection to intraocular pressure. Side differences were observed on the second postoperative day only. In Fig. 2a, the net effect on IOP is shown.

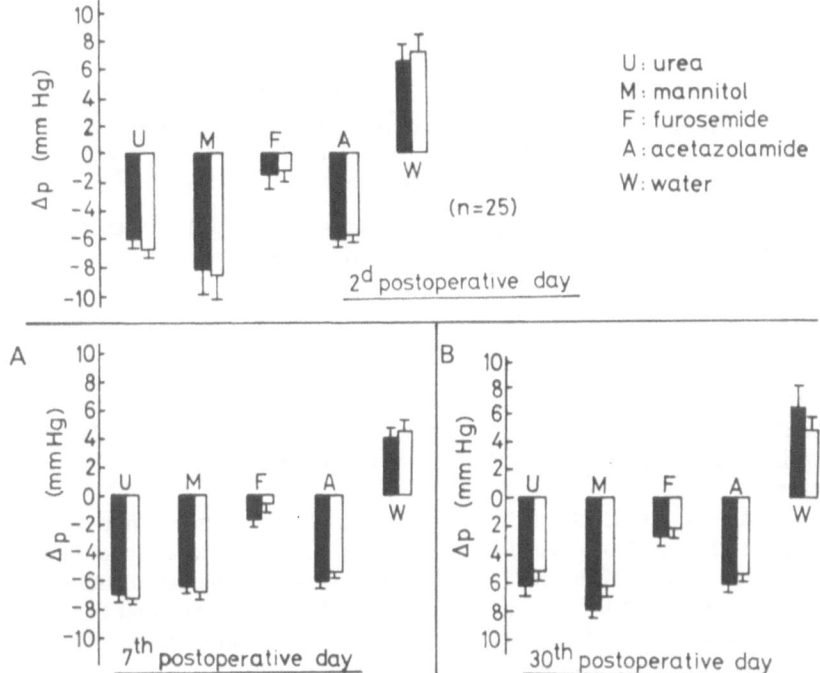

Fig. 3. Net effect of the substances administered on intraocular pressure, in eyes with either intact or transected optic nerve. No significant side differences between eyes were observed. (I = 1 SD). In Fig. 3a, 3b the effect on IOP is shown (n = 25.)

OPTIC NERVE TRANSECTION

According to our results, we found no side differences of steady-state intraocular pressure after unilateral optic nerve transection, on he 7th and 30th postoperative day. On the 2nd postoperative day a decrease of intraocular

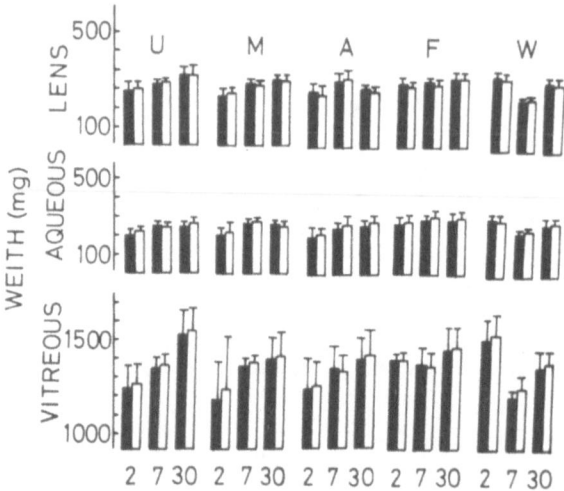

Fig. 4. Changes of vitreous, lens and aqueous weights following administration of various diuretics, in eyes with intact and transected optic nerves. No side differences were observed on any postoperative day (I = 1 SD).

pressure at the side of tensected optic nerve was observed. This was probably due to early (and non permanent) vascular disorders of the optic nerve vessels. This finding is not reported by other investigators, since the effect of the optic nerve transection on IOP was tested only on the 30th postoperative day.

Furthermore, in our group of experiments we were unable to demonstrate any differences in the responsiveness to osmotic agents between eyes with cut optic nerves and those with intact ones. Previous studies (4, 5) have demonstrated a decrease IOP response to osmotic agents in rabbit and monkey eyes with transected optic nerves, as compared to their controlateral sham operated eyes.

Thus, our results clearly do not support the idea that osmotic agents 'express' their IOP lowering effect through a central neural control, via efferent fibers carried by optic nerve (1, 9, 12). Our data support the recent studies by Serafano and Brubaker (14) and Lam et al. (6) who observed that the hypotensive effect of osmotic agents was not influenced by optic nerve transection.

However, the nonexistence of any side differences between eyes with transected and intact optic nerves, in weights of vitreous, aqueous and lens supports the theory that either osmotic or non osmotic diuretics lower IOP by extraction of intraocular water rather than by influencing a central neural mechanism.

REFERENCES

1. Becker, B., Krupin, T. and Podos, S.M. Phenobarbital and aqueous humor dynamics: effect in rabbits with intact and transected optic nerves. Am. J. Ophthalmol. 70: 686 (1970).

2. Canady, M. and Bonting, S. Carbonic anhydrase distribution in rabbit lens. Exper. Eye Res. 4: 283 (1965).
3. Gloster, J. and Greaves, D.P. Effect of diencephalic stimulation upon the intra-ocular pressure. Br. J. Ophthalmol. 41: 513 (1957).
4. Krupin, T., Podos, S.M. and Becker, B. Effect of optic nerve transection on osmotic alterations of intraocular pressure. Am. J. Ophthalmol. 70: 214 (1970).
5. Krupin, T., Podos, S.M., Lehman, R.A.W. and Becker, B. Effects of optic nerve transection on intraocular pressure in monkeys. Arch. Ophthalmol. 84: 668 (1970).
6. Lam, K.W., Shihab, Z., Fu, Y.A. and Lee, P.F. The effect of optic nerve transection upon the hypotensive action of ascorbate and mannitol. Ann. Ophthalmol. 12: 1102 (1980).
7. Podos, S.M., Krupin, T. and Becker, B. Optic nerve transection and intraocular pressure response to various drugs. Invest. Ophthalmol. 9: 492–495, 1970.
8. Podos, S.M., Krupin, T. and Becker, B. Effect of small-does hyperosmotic injection on intraocular pressure of small animals and man when optic nerves are transected and intact. Am. J. Ophthalmol. 71: 898 (1971a).
9. Podos, S.M., Krupin, T. and Becker, B. Mechanism of intraocular pressure response after optic nerve transection. Am. J. Ophthalmol. 72: 79 (1971b).
10. Riise, D., Simonsen, S.E. Intraocular pressure in unilateral optic nerve lesion. Acta Ophthalmol. 47: 750 (1969).
11. Robbins, R. and Galin, M. Effect of osmotic agents on the vitreous body. Arch. Ophthalmol. 82: 694 (1969).
12. Sacks, J.G. and Lindenberg, R. Efferent nerve fibers in the anterior visual pathways in bilateral congenital cystic eyeballs. Am. J. Ophthalmol. 68: 691, 1969.
13. Sallmann, L.V. and Lowenstein, O. Responses of intraocular pressure, blood pressure and cutaneous vessels to electric stimulation in the diencephalon. Am. J. Ophthalmol. 39: 11 (1955).
14. Serafano, D.M. and Brubaker, R.F. Intraocular pressure after optic nerve transection. Invest. Ophthalmol. Vis. Sci. 17: 68 (1978).
15. Waitzman, M.B. Hypothalamus and ocular pressure. Surv. Ophthalmol. 16: 1–23 (1971).

Authors' address:
Laboratory of Experimental Pharmacology
School of Medicine
Athens University
Athens, Greece

EFFECT OF ADRENERGIC AGONISTS AND $\beta_1\beta_2$ ANTAGONISTS ON INTRAOCULAR PRESSURE AND ADENYLATE CYCLASE IN RABBIT CILIARY PROCESSES

A. PALKAMA, H. UUSITALO, K. RAIJ and R. UUSITALO

(Helsinki, Finland)

ABSTRACT

The hypotensive effect of different adrenergic agonists and antagonists were screened both in normo- and hypertensive rabbit eyes. The drugs were applied topically and intraocular pressure (IOP) was monitored constantly with a manometric method. Subsequently the inhibitory effect of the antagonists on isoproterenol-stimulated adenylate cyclase activity in the ciliary processes was analyzed in vitro.

In normotensive eyes agonist isoproterenol (β) and antagonists labetalol ($\alpha\beta$), metoprolol (β_1) and acebutolol (β_1) decreased IOP significantly. In hypertensive eyes only isoproterenol and labetalol decrease IOP markedly. Timolol (β) did not decrease IOP although it inhibited adenylate cyclase activity as actively as labetalol. The other antagonists showed no inhibitory effect on in this respect.

The results indicated that α-activity (labetalol, $\alpha\beta$) seems to potentiate the β-activity (limolol, β) in decreasing IOP. Whether this α-effect is a presynaptic effect (adrenergic denervation destroys it) is not yet clear. Similarly the β_1-effect (metoprolol) decreased IOP without affecting adenylate cyclase activity. This might be due to presynaptic release of endogenous transmitter(s) which in turn stimulate postsynaptic adenylate cyclase and induce the decreased IOP. Besides this the possible role of blood vessels and CNS must also be kept in mind.

E.L. Greve, W. Leydhecker & C. Raitta (eds.), Second European Glaucoma Symposium, Helsinki 1984.
© 1985, Dr. W. Junk Publishers, Dordrecht. ISBN 978-94-010-8934-0

RELATIVE DISTRIBUTION OF EPINEPHRINE, PILOCARPINE AND TIMOLOL IN THE RABBIT EYE

L. SALMINEN and A. URTTI

(Turku and Kuopio, Finland)

ABSTRACT

After a single bilateral ocular application of epinephrine (EPI), pilocarpine (PLC) and timolol (TML), drug concentrations in the eye of pigmented rabbit were determined by radioactive technique. The corneal penetrability of PLC and TML was equal and greatly exceeded that of EPI. The aqueous EPI concentration at 3 h was half that of PLC and TML about one-sixth of the 0.5 h value. In the iris and ciliary body at 0.5 h, EPI and TML concentrations exceeded that of the aqueous. In the iris and ciliary body, the decline of EPI, PLC and TML concentrations was slower than in the aqueous. In the choroid and retina, the EP1 concentration at 0.5 h was equal and at 3 h higher than the aqueous value. EPI, PLC and TML concentrations in the lens were about one-twentieth of the aqueous value and exceeded those in the vitreous.

INTRODUCTION

The kinetics of topically applied ocular drugs in the anterior ocular structures, i.e. the conjunctival cul-de-sac, cornea and aqueous humor, have been subject to intensive and fruitful study during the last ten years (4, 6). Pharmacokinetic coefficients of the corneal permeability of the drugs and of drug absorption and elimination in the anterior chamber compartment describe the bioavailability of various topical drugs used in ophthalmic practice (4, 6). However, less is known of the distribution of topical ocular drugs outside the anterior chamber compartment. This drug distribution is generally irrelevant to the therapeutic effect but may have toxicological importance. In this study the ocular distribution of topically applied epinephrine (EPI), pilocarpine (PLC) and timolol (TML) was determined by radioactive technique.

Aqueous humor samples during intraocular operations offer a means of determining ocular drug penetration in humans (2, 7). The results of the present study are therefore presented as a ratio to the aqueous humor drug concentration at 0.5 h. Such information could contribute to the evaluation of the therapeutic and toxic effect of ocular drugs, if animal and human data were abundantly available.

85

E.L. Greve, W. Leydhecker & C. Raitta (eds.), Second European Glaucoma Symposium, Helsinki 1984.
© *1985, Dr. W. Junk Publishers, Dordrecht. ISBN 978-94-010-8934-0*

MATERIALS AND METHODS

Animals

The experimental animals consisted of 9, 8 and 4 adult mixed-breed pigmented rabbits for the study of EPI, PLC and TML, respectively. The rabbits were of both sexes. They were housed singly in cages under standard laboratory conditions.

Drugs

^{3}H-EPI with a specific activity of 68.0 Ci/mmol and ^{3}H-PLC with a specific activity of 10.0 Ci/mmol were obtained commercially (New England Nuclear, Boston, Mass.). ^{3}H-TML with a specific activity of 4.85 Ci/mmol was donated by Merck, Sharp and Dohme Research Lab., Rathway, N.J. The tracers were dissolved in 1% EPI ophthalmic solution containing 2% boric acid, 0.002% phenylmercury nitrate, 0.3% sodium pyrosulphite, and 0.001% oxychinoline sulphate, with a pH 7 adjusted by sodium hydroxide, in 2% PLC base solution which had been buffered to pH 6.4 with phosphates and in 0.5% TML ophthalmic solution (6.8 mg/ml of TML maleate) containing 0.1 mg/ml of benzalkonium chloride and with a pH of 6.8–7.0. The tracers did not significantly affect the drug content of the solutions.

Drug distribution studies

A 20 or 30 μl volume of the drug solution was instilled onto the upper corneo-scleral limbus of the cornea of both eyes of the rabbits. During instillation the upper lid was gently pulled away from the globe. The animals were sacrificed with i.v. injection of Nembutal at 0.5 and 3 h after the instillation. Aqueous humor samples were aspirated from the anterior chamber of the enucleated eyes and the eyes were promptly frozen in liquid nitrogen. The eyes were stored at $-20°C$ until dissection, which was carred out as described previously (8).

The radioactivity of the samples was determined by liquid scintillation counting (LSC). The tissue samples were digested with a solubilizer (Lumasolve®, Lumac B.V., Schaesberg, The Netherlands) in glass vials at 40–50°C; a scintillation liquid (Lipoluma®, Lumac) was then added and the samples were counted when the chemiluminescence had vanished. Another scintillation liquid (Lumagel®, Lumac) was added to the aqueous humor. All the samples were counted at 9°C in an LKB Wallac Rackbeta 125 liquid scintillation counter for 10 min or up to 10,000 counts.

The results for the aqueous humor at 0.5 h are expressed as means ± S.E.s of drug radioactivity equivalents (μg/g), denoted 'total drug concentration' in the text. The rest of the ocular results were divided by the 0.5 h aqueous humor total drug concentration and a relative distribution index of the drug in the eye was obtained.

RESULTS

The total drug concentrations in the aqueous humor at 0.5 h after topical application of ^{3}H-EPI, ^{3}H-PLC and ^{3}H-TML are presented in Table 1, and the relative drug distributions in the eye at 0.5 and 3 h in Table 2.

Table 1. Aqueous humor total drug concentration in pigmented rabbit eyes 0.5 h after ocular application of 30 μl of 1% ^{3}H-epinephrine, 30 μl of 2% ^{3}H-pilocarpine and 20 μl of 0.5% ^{3}H-timolol. Means (S.E.) of 14, 8 and 4 eyes are shown.

Drug	Dose applied (μg)	Total drug concentration (μg/g)
Epinephrine	250	0.12 ± 0.02
Pilocarpine	600	13.88 ± 2.03
Timolol	100	2.29 ± 0.17

Table 2. Relative distribution of radioactive material in pigmented rabbit eye at 0.5 h and 3 h after ocular application of ^{3}H-epinephrine, ^{3}H-pilocarpine and ^{3}H-timolol. Total drug concentration in the aqueous humor after each drug at 0.5 h (shown in Table 1) equals 1.

Tissue	Drug					
	Epinephrine		Pilocarpine		Timolol	
	0.5 h	3 h	0.5 h	3 h	0.5 h	3 h
Aqueous humor	1	0.50	1	0.15	1	0.16
Cornea	24.50	4.50	2.75	0.40	14.54	1.45
Iris	1.92	1.92	1.06	0.85	3.37	2.64
Ciliary body	2.50	2.00	0.78	0.63	1.66	1.22
Lens	0.075	0.083	0.016	0.009	0.012	0.028
Vitreous	0.025	0.050	0.006	0.005	0.003	0.017
Choroid and retina	1.00	4.83	0.15	0.15	0.49	0.15

DISCUSSION

The drug dose applied onto the ocular surface was greatest with PLC. Its penetrability into the aqueous humor equalled that of TML, which after a dose one-sixth the size produced a total drug aqueous humor concentration of the same relative range. Compared with PLC and TML, the aqueous humor penetration after topical EPI was minimal.

The corneal penetrability of TML, however, was better than that of PLC. This is in good agreement with the permeability constant of the epithelial barrier of the rabbit cornea calculated for various drugs (6). After ocular application TML formed a drug reservoir in the cornea. The permeability constant of the corneal epithelium is lowest for EPI (6). This was reflected in the low EPI total drug concentrations in the aqueous humor as well in the cornea, although EPI formed the highest proportionate corneal drug reservoir among the drugs studied. The EPI drug reservoir has recently been localized in the corneal stroma-endothelium (5). This depot was reflected in the high proportionate aqueous humor concentration at 3 h; while the PLC and TML aqueous concentrations at 3 h were about one-sixth of the 0.5 h value, that of EPI was only one-half. The decline of PLC and TML in the aqueous humor from 0.5 to 3 h agreed closely with the elimination rate constants of the drug from the anterior chamber compartment calculated from various isotope experiments (4, 6).

The accumulation of TML in the pigment-containing iris and ciliary body exceeded that of PLC, after which relative iris and ciliary body concentrations were also obtained, which were above aqueous humor values. This difference may reflect a greater melanin binding of TML compared with PLC, although in vitro PLC is accumulated in pigmented iris-ciliary body in great amounts (3). One explanation could be the relatively smaller amount of TML present in the aqueous humor. The binding of drugs to melanin, although different with various drugs, is also a concentration-dependent and saturable process (10). Of the low aqueous concentration of TML, a greater amount was bound to the iris and ciliary body than of the six-fold amount of PLC.

In the case of EPI, aqueous humor values were always exceeded in the iris and ciliary body, and there was no concentration decline during the elimination phase. In our earlier study on EPI distribution in albino and pigmented rabbit eye (11) we have suggested that these high concentrations of EPI in the iris and ciliary body do not reflect EPI pigment binding but rather EPI binding to adrenergic neurons. This specific binding of EPI was especially obvious in the choroid and retina, structures which have abundant adrenergic innervation. The accumulation of EPI in the choroid and retina has been reported earlier (1, 12) and has toxicological significance. It is also worth noting that all the topical drugs studied reached the choroid and retina and showed only a minor concentration decline during the 3 h observation period. Systematically absorbed EPI, PLC and TML obviously contributed greatly to the drug accumulation in the choroid and retina, since measurable topical drug concentrations have been observed in untreated eyes (9, 12).

The drug concentrations in the lens and vitreous were small. They increased, however, during the 3 h observation period, and at least with long time multiple dosing drug accumulations in these structures can be expected.

REFERENCES

1. Kramer, S.G. Epinephrine distribution after topical administration to phakic and aphakic eyes. Trans. Am. Ophthalmol. Soc. 78: 947 (1980).
2. Krohn, D.L. Flux of topical pilocarpine to the human aqueous. Tr. Am. Ophthalmol. Soc. 76: 502 (1978).
3. Lyons, J.S. and Krohn, D.L. Pilocarpine uptake by pigmented uveal tissue. Am. J. Ophthalmol. 75: 885 (1973).
4. Maurice, D.M. and Mishima, S. Ocular pharmacokinetics. In: Handbook of Experimental Pharmacology, Vol. 69, ed. M.L. Sears, Springer-Verlag, Berlin, Heidelberg, 1984.
5. Mindel, J.S., Smith, H., Jacobs, M., Kharlamb, A.B. and Friedman, A.H. Drug reservoirs in topical therapy. Invest. Ophthalmol. Vis. Sci. 25: 346 (1984).
6. Mishima, S. Clinical pharmacokinetics of the eye. Invest. Ophthalmol. Vis. Sci. 21: 504 (1981).

7. Phillips, C.I., Bartholomew, R.S., Kazi, G., Schmitt, C.J. and Vogel, R. Penetration of timolol eye drops into human aqueous humour. Br. J. Ophthalmol. 65: 593 (1981).
8. Salminen, L. Cloxacillin distribution in the rabbit eye after intravenous injection. Acta Ophthalmol. (Kbh.) 56: 11 (1978).
9. Salminen, L. and Urtti, A. Disposition of ophthalmic timolol in treated and untreated rabbit eyes. A multiple and single dose study. Exp. Eye Res. 38: 203 (1984).
10. Shimada, K., Baweja, R., Sokoloski, T. and Patil, P.N. Binding characteristics of drugs to synthetic levodopa melanin. J. Pharm. Sci. 65: 1057 (1976).
11. Urtti, A., Salminen, L. and Periviita, L. Ocular distribution of topically applied adrenaline in albino and pigmented rabbits. Acta. Ophthalmol. 62: 753 (1984).
12. Wei, C.P., Anderson, J.A. and Leopold, I. Ocular absorption and metabolism of topically applied epinephrine and a dipivalyl ester of epinephrine. Invest. Ophthalmol. Vis. Sc. 17: 315 (1978).

Authors' addresses:
Dr L. Salminen
Dept. of Ophthalmology
Turku University Central Hospital
SF-20520 Turku 52
Finland

Dr A. Urtti
Dept. of Pharmaceutical Technology
University of Kuopio
SF-70210 Kuopio 21
Finland

LOCATION OF β-ADRENERGIC RECEPTORS IN THE CORNEA AND CILIARY BODY OF THE RABBIT*

I. LEHTO., A. PALKAMA., K. RAIJ., H. UUSITALO and J. LEHTOSALO

(Helsinki, Finland)

ABSTRACT

Both β-adrenergic agonists and antagonists decrease intraocular pressure. This discrepancy has caused confusion, but one possible way to explain it is to assume that agonists are postsynaptically and antagonists presynaptically effective. To solve the regulatory mechanisms it is important to locate the β-adrenergic receptors at these two sites.

In preliminary experiments the effect of fixation on ligand binding was studied biochemically. Binding of 3-H-dihydroalprenolol (3-H-DHA) to isolated fresh or pre- and/or postfixed (1% paraformaldehyde, 0.75% glutaraldehyde for 15 min at 22°C) ciliary processes showed prefixation with 1% paraformaldehyde to decrease the specific binding least (19%). Autoradiographic technique was used to demonstrate the radio-ligand (3-H-DHA) binding to β-receptors in light microscopy. Paraformaldehyde fixed cryostate sections were incubated in presence of 4 nM of 3-H-DHA, pargyline, ascorbid acid and $CaCl_2$ in Tris-HCl for 60 min. Control specimens were preincubated with a hundredfold concentration of cold DHA and incubated with both cold and hot DHA. Both wet and dry mount autoradiographic techniques were used.

Silver grains showing specifically bound 3-H-DHA sites were found in the corneal epithelium and endothelium. In the ciliary processes the ligand was bound to non-pigmented epithelial cells. The mechanisms of action of β-receptors on the regulation of intraocular pressure will be discussed.

This study was supported by the Sigrid Jusélius Foundation, Helsinki, Finland.

*To be published in Experimental Eye Research.

E.L. Greve, W. Leydhecker & C. Raitta (eds.), Second European Glaucoma Symposium, Helsinki 1984.
© *1985, Dr. W. Junk Publishers, Dordrecht. ISBN 978-94-010-8934-0*

EFFECT OF OCULAR PIGMENTATION ON OCULAR DISPOSITION, METABOLISM AND BIOPHASIC AVAILABILITY OF PILOCARPINE

L. SALMINEN and A. URTTI

(Turku and Kuopio, Finland)

ABSTRACT

In albino and pigmented rabbit eyes, the ocular disposition, metabolism and biophasic availability of ocularly applied pilocarpine was studied by radioactive technique, TLC and by registration of pilocarpine-induced miosis. Pilocarpine disposition and biophasic availability, but not metabolism, were affected by ocular pigmentation. In the pigmented rabbit eye, pilocarpine was accumulated in the iris and ciliary body. In albino and pigmented rabbit eye, pilocarpine was efficiently and equally metabolized into pilocarpic acid. The biophasic availability of pilocarpine was greater in pigmented than in albino eyes after the application of large pilocarpine doses but not with small doses.

INTRODUCTION

Ocular response to topically applied pilocarpine is modified by the extent of ocular pigmentation. In brown-eyed subjects pilocarpine induced miosis was smaller (1) or of similar degree (11) and the time taken to reach peak effect was longer than in blue-eyed subjects (1, 11). In normal volunteers, the intraocular pressure of darkly pigmented eyes responded to a single dose of pilocarpine less than that of lightly pigmented eyes (8). In a multipledose study, darkly pigmented glaucomatous eyes showed a relative resistance to pilocarpine compared to lightly pigmented eyes (3).

It is unclear to what extent pilocarpine binding to ocular pigment (6, 7), differences in pilocarpine metabolism in the eye (5) and differences in the anatomical structure of darkly and lightly pigmented irides (2) contribute to the relative resistance of darkly pigmented eyes to pilocarpine effect. Our study was undertaken to determine the ocular pilocarpine concentration per mg of tissue in the site of action of pilocarpine, pilocarpine metabolism and pilocarpine induced response in albino and pigmented rabbit eyes. The results of this study are part of a project dealing with ophthalmic drug inserts (10, 12).

91

E.L. Greve, W. Leydhecker & C. Raitta (eds.), Second European Glaucoma Symposium, Helsinki 1984.
© *1985, Dr. W. Junk Publishers, Dordrecht. ISBN 978-94-010-8934-0*

MATERIAL AND METHODS

Animals. Fifteen adult New Zealand White albino rabbits and 14 adult mixed-breed pigmented rabbits were used.

Pilocarpine solutions. Four different aqueous pilocarpine hydrochloride solutions were used: 0.5% and 2.0% in Sorensen's phosphate buffer (pH 6.4), 4.0% commercial eye drops with 1.4% of poly(vinyl alcohol) (PVA) (pH 4.9), and 10.8% solution with 1.4% of PVA (pH 7.0). The commercial solution contained a preservative (0.004% of benzalkonium chloride).

^{3}H-pilocarpine alkaloid in alcohol with a specific activity of 10.0 Ci/mmol was obtained commercially (New England Nuclear, Boston, Mass.) and evaporated to dryness by vacuum distillation. The labelled material was dissolved in the 2% pilocarpine solution. The addition of ^{3}H-pilocarpine had no appreciable effect on the molarity of the drug solution. The radioactivity of the solution was 0.29 μCi/μl.

Drug distribution studies. During the experiment the rabbits were kept in wooden restraint boxes. A 30 μl volume of the labelled pilocarpine solution was instilled onto the upper corneoscleral limbus of both eyes. During instillation the upper lid was gently pulled away from the globe. The animals were sacrificed with i.v. injection of mebumal at 0.5 h or 3 h after ^{3}H-pilocarpine instillation. Aqueous humor samples were aspirated from the anterior chamber of the enucleated eyes and the eyes were promptly frozen in liquid nitrogen. Part of the aqueous humor was used for the TLC-analysis of pilocarpic acid. The eyes were stored at $-20°$C until dissection. The radioactivity of the samples was determined by LSC.

Metabolic studies. The relative volume of pilocarpine and pilocarpic acid in the aqueous humor samples was determined by TLC (5).

Studies of pilocarpine induced miosis. The rabbits were acclimatized to the wooden restraint boxes and dim lighting for two hours prior to the experiments. A 25 μl volume of the four pilocarpine solutions was pipetted onto the upper corneoscleral limbus of the eye. Only one eye of a rabbit was used in the test procedure. A minimum interval of one week was held between two tests with the same animal.

After application of the drug the eyes were photographed from a constant distance at fixed times. The negatives were enlarged with a microfilm reflector. The pupillary area was measured from the magnifications with a planimeter and the diameters of the pupils were calculated as though the pupils were circular.

Analysis of the time course of miosis. The biophasic pharmacokinetics of pilocarpine were analysed according to Yoshida and Mishima (14) and have been described in detail previously (12). The analysis is based on a response parameter (RP) which is related to the drug concentration surrounding the receptors (9, 13). The changes in pupillary diameter were converted to values of $RP = (D_0 - D)/(D - D_{min})$, where D_0 = the original pupillary diameter, D = the diameter at a given time and D_{min} = the minimum attainable diameter (maximal response). The values of RP were plotted against time. Actual data points were used to evaluate the magnitude of the peak response and its time delay. Relative biophasic availability (AUC) was measured as the area under the RP vs. time curve, using a trapezoidal rule with extrapolation to infinite time. The apparent elimination rate constant was determined by linear regression analysis from the ln(RP) vs. time representation.

Analysis of the results. In the pilocarpine distribution study the results are expressed as means ± S.E. of pilocarpine radioactivity equivalents (μg/g of tissue wet weight), denoted 'total pilocarpine concentration' in the text. The statistical significance of the differences between pigmented and albino rabbits was tested with Mann-Whitney's U-test. A P-value of less than 0.05 was considered to be significant.

RESULTS

The total pilocarpine concentration in the iris and ciliary body and the pharmacokinetic parameters of the miotic response after the application of pilocarpine eye drops are shown in Tables 1 and 2.

Table 1. Radioactive material distribution in albino and pigmented rabbit iris and ciliary body 0.5 h and 3 h after application of 30 μl of 2% aqueous ^{3}H-pilocarpine. Values show the means ± S.E. of nine albino and eight pigmented eyes

Tissue	Equivalent of pilocarpine (μg/g of tissue)			
	0.5 h		3 h	
	Albino	Pigmented	Albino	Pigmented
Iris	5.36 ± 1.88	14.64 ± 2.37**	1.79 ± 0.47	11.85 ± 2.92***
Ciliary body	3.48 ± 1.00	10.86 ± 2.15**	0.85 ± 0.14	8.77 ± 3.13***

**P < 0.01 vs. albino eyes
***P < 0.001 vs. albino eyes.

Table 2. Pharmacokinetic parameters of miotic response induced by 25 μl of 0.5%, 2%, 4% and 10.8% aqueous solution of pilocarpine in the eyes of albino and pigmented rabbits

Percentage of pilocarpine solution	Peak effect		AUC (RP·h)	Apparent elimination rate constant (h^{-1})	n
	Time delay (min)	Magnitude (RP)[a]			
0.5 (A)[b]	21.0 ± 1.9	0.94 ± 0.09	1.37 ± 0.09	0.69 ± 0.08	5
(P)[c]	64.0 ± 6.8**	0.51 ± 0.09**	1.62 ± 0.39	0.31 ± 0.08**	5
2.0 (A)	21.2 ± 2.0	1.12 ± 0.19	1.18 ± 0.18	0.58 ± 0.06	5
(P)	48.0 ± 7.8**	0.67 ± 0.08*	2.18 ± 0.55	0.42 ± 0.07	5
4.0 (A)	20.4 ± 2.8	1.51 ± 0.17	1.60 ± 0.15	0.79 ± 0.09	5
(P)	45.0 ± 0.0**	1.85 ± 0.26	5.22 ± 0.57**	0.43 ± 0.04**	6
10.8 (A)	20.0 ± 2.7	1.44 ± 0.08	2.45 ± 0.17	0.81 ± 0.05	5
(P)	21.7 ± 2.1	1.73 ± 0.18	5.12 ± 0.33**	0.38 ± 0.02**	6

[a]RP = response parameter = (original pupillary diameter − pupillary diameter)/(pupillary diameter − 2.16 mm)
[b]A = albino rabbits, [c]P = pigmented rabbits
*P < 0.05,   **P < 0.01 pigmented vs. albino eyes (Mann-Whitney's U-test)

The metabolism of pilocarpine was considerable in both albino and pigmented rabbits. At 0.5 h the percentage of total drug due to pilocarpic acid in the aqueous humor of albino rabbits was $30.2 \pm 6.8\%$ and that in pigmented ones $24.2 \pm 3.0\%$. At 3 h the corresponding values were $70.4 \pm 11.8\%$ and $64.0 \pm 6.9\%$. Significant differences between the two rabbit races in the relative amounts of pilocarpic acid were not observed in this study.

DISCUSSION

In our experiments, pilocarpine-induced miotic response was of smaller magnitude and the time taken to reach the peak effect after the application of 0.5% and 2.0% pilocarpine solutions was longer in the pigmented than in the albino eyes. After the application of 4% pilocarpine solution the peak RP magnitude was equal but again came later, and it was only after the application of a 10.8% solution that the two peak effect parameters were equal in both rabbit strains. These findings are identical to those observed in the human eye (1, 11). In brown-eyed subjects pilocarpine induced miosis was lesser and came later after the application of 0.5%, 1% and 4% aqueous pilocarpine (1), and while the miosis was equal in brown- and blue-eyed subjects after the application of 2% oily pilocarpine the time taken to reach the peak effect was longer in the former group (11). In the human eye the transcorneal penetration of pilocarpine is lesser than in the rabbit eye (4). Obviously only after the use of an oily pilocarpine solution was pilocarpine concentration in the biophase of the human eye sufficient to reach the drug concentration which was obtained in the rabbit eye with a 4% aqueous solution.

Contrary to observations after the application of low dose pilocarpine to pigmented rabbit eyes (5), we observed no differences in pilocarpine metabolism between the two rabbit strains.

The accumulation of pilocarpine in the biophase of pigmented eyes at the end of the drug absorption phase (0.5 h) and during the elimination phase (3 h) greatly exceeded that in the albino eyes. These total drug concentrations in the iris and ciliary body are in good agreement with the apparent elimination rate constants (Table 2), which have been calculated from the kinetics of pupil response. The 50% lower elimination rate constant and the up to 10-fold pilocarpine concentration in the iris-ciliary body in the pigmented compared to albino eye are due to the drug reservoir of ocular pigment tissue. After low pilocarpine doses the depot was able to neglect the competition between pilocarpine receptors and pigment tissue by producing equal AUC values and after high pilocarpine doses AUC values which greatly exceeded those in the albino eye.

From our study, no direct conclusions can be drawn as to the relative resistance of darkly pigmented eyes to the pilocarpine-induced lowering of intraocular pressure. However, a similar pigment-binding mechanism obviously also competes with pressure-lowering receptors as in the case of miosis.

94

REFERENCES

1. Borgmann, H. and Wurster, W. Der Einfluss unterschiedlicher Konzentrationen und Vehikel auf die Pilocarpin-Miosis I. Unterschiedliche Konzentrationen. Klin. Mbl. Augenheilk. 163: 44 (1973).
2. Emiru, V.P. Response to mydriatics in the African. Br. J. Ophthal. 55: 538 (1971).
3. Harris, L.S. and Galin, M.A. Effects of ocular pigmentation on hypotensive response to pilocarpine. Am. J. Ophthalmol. 72: 923 (1971).
4. Krohn, D.L. Flux of topical pilocarpine to the human aqueous. Trans. Am. Ophthalmol. Soc. 76: 502 (1978).
5. Lee, V.H.L., Hui, H.W. and Robinson, J.R. Corneal metabolism of pilocarpine in pigmented rabbits. Invest. Ophthalmol. Vis. Sci. 19: 210 (1980).
6. Lee, V.H.L. and Robinson, J.R. Disposition of pilocarpine in the pigmented rabbit eye. Int. J. Pharm. 11: 155 (1982).
7. Lyons, J.S. and Krohn, D.L. Pilocarpine uptake by pigmented uveal tissue. Am. J. Ophthalmol. 75: 885 (1973).
8. Melikian, H.E., Lieberman, T.W. and Leopold, I.H. Ocular pigmentation and pressure and outflow responses to pilocarpine and epinephrine. Am. J. Ophthalmol. 72: 70 (1971).
9. Ohara, K. Effects of cholinergic agonists on isolated iris sphincter muscles: a pharmacodynamic study. Jpn. J. Ophthalmol. 21: 516 (1977).
10. Salminen, L., Urtti, A. and Periviita, L. Effect of ocular pigmentation on pilocarpine pharmacology in the rabbit eye. I. Drug distribution and metabolism. Int. J. Pharm. 18: 17 (1984).
11. Smith, S.A., Smith, S.E. and Lazare, R. An increased effect of pilocarpine on the pupil by application of the drug in oil. Br. J. Ophthalmol. 62: 314 (1978).
12. Urtti, A., Salminen, L. Kujari, H and Jäntti, V. Effect of ocular pigmentation on pilocarpine pharmacology in the rabbit eye. II. Drug response. Int. J. Pharm. 19: 53 (1984).
13. Wagner, J.G. Kinetics of pharmacologic response. I Proposed relationship between response and drug concentration in the intact animal and man. J. Theor. Biol. 20: 173 (1968).
14. Yoshida, S. and Mishima, S. A pharmacokinetic analysis of the pupil response to topical pilocarpine and tropicamide. Jpn. J. Ophthalmol. 19: 121 (1975).

Authors' addresses:
Dr L. Salminen
Turku University Central Hospital
SF-20520 Turku 52
Finland

Dr A. Urtti
Dept. of Pharmaceutical Technology
University of Kuopio
SF-70210 Kuopio 21
Finland

THE COMPARATIVE OCULAR RESPONSES
OF PILOCARPINE OPHTHALMIC RODS
AND PILOCARPINE EYE DROPS

G.K. KRIEGLSTEIN, W. SCHREMS and R. DE NATALE

(Würzburg, F.R.G.)

ABSTRACT

Ophthalmic rods represent a solid dosage form for drugs to be used on the eye with distinct advantages over aqueous drug solutions. In a controlled clinical trial single doses of 500 μg or 200 μg of pilocarpine, either mounted on ophthalmic rods or in form of aqueous eyedrops were applied to a series of 20 ocular hypertensive or glaucomatous patients. Right eyes were treated with drops, left eyes with ophthalmic rods. The amount of drug in both preparations was randomized and blinded. IOPs and pupillary diameters were recorded before, and 30 min, 1 h, 2, 4, and 6 h after treatment. Both pilocarpine preparations mediated equivalent ocular responses, both on intraocular pressure and pupillary diameter.

INTRODUCTION

The aqueous preparation of drugs for topical application to the eye involves a series of problems: contamination, preservation, stability, pH adjustment, systemic absorption of the drug via drainage through tear canals, poor availability of drug at the intended site of action (1, 5). The ophthalmic rod delivery system is free of many of these problems and opens a new dimension of topical drug application to the human eye. The ophthalmic rod is a disposable, single-dose, sterile, solid drug preparation, which contains no preservatives. It is made of a small stick of acrylic plastic about 50 mm long, on which the drug is available as a thin layer at one end of the rod. The drug is applied to the rod by dipping it into the drug solution and drying it. The rod is packed air-tight and sterilized by radiation or ethylene oxide. By rolling the drug-covered end of the rod into the conjunctival sac the thin layer of drug is dissolved in the lacrimal fluid. It seemed logical to test these ophthalmic rods mounted with pilocarpine against pilocarpine eyedrops, an aqueous preparation of an antiglaucomatous drug widely used in ophthalmology (4).

The present study was designed to evaluate the I.O.P. and pupillary responses of an equivalent amount of pilocarpine dissolved in an aqueous preparation and in solid form on the ophthalmic rod.

97

E.L. Greve, W. Leydhecker & C. Raitta (eds.), Second European Glaucoma Symposium, Helsinki 1984.
© *1985, Dr. W. Junk Publishers, Dordrecht. ISBN 978-94-010-8934-0*

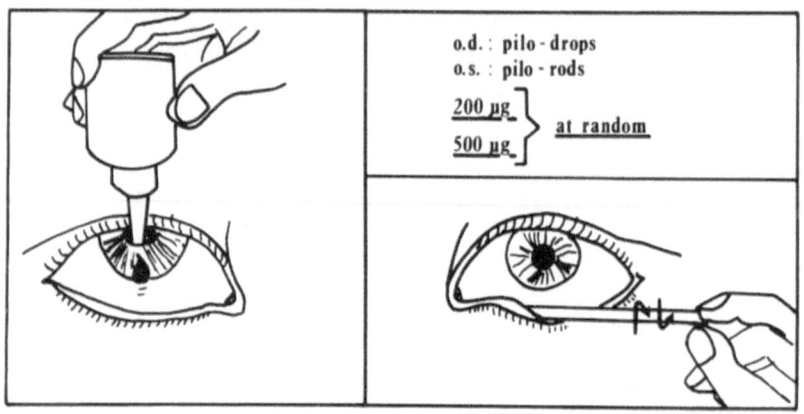

Fig. 1. Schematic study design: Pilocarpine eye drops containing either 200 μg or 500 μg active drug per drop were applied to the right eyes, pilocarpine mounted on ophthalmic rods (200 μg or 500 μg) was applied to the left eyes. The amount of active drug was randomized.

METHODS

Two groups of 10 patients each with bilateral ocular hypertension or primary open angle glaucoma were enrolled in the study. After enlightening the patient about the test procedure, a written consent form was obtained. The single dose trial was preceded by a wash-out period of previous antiglaucomatous drugs (miotics 24 h, epinephrine 1 week, topical betablockers 2 weeks). Four different drug preparations were used: pilocarpine eyedrops containing either 200 μg or 500 μg in one drop; pilocarpine ophthalmic rods mounted either with 200 μg or 500 μg of active drug. Throughout the study the pilocarpine drops were applied to the right eyes, the ophthalmic rods to the left eyes only. The type of preparation was uncontrolled to the patient and to the observer; however, the amount of drug present in the two preparations was controlled to both. A schematic drawing illustrates the study design in Fig. 1.

The single dose trial started for all patients at 8:00 a.m. Untreated IOP levels and pupillary diameters were identified at this time before drug application on both eyes. Intraocular pressure measurements were performed with the Goldmann applanation tonometer (duplicate readings, mean values considered for statistics), the pupillary diameters were measured at the observation tube of the Goldmann perimeter.

After drug application, the test parameters (I.O.P. and P.D.) were measured 30 min, 1 h, 2 h, 4 h, and 6 h after drug application. Bartlett test and analysis of variance were used to decide on the statistical relevance of the results.

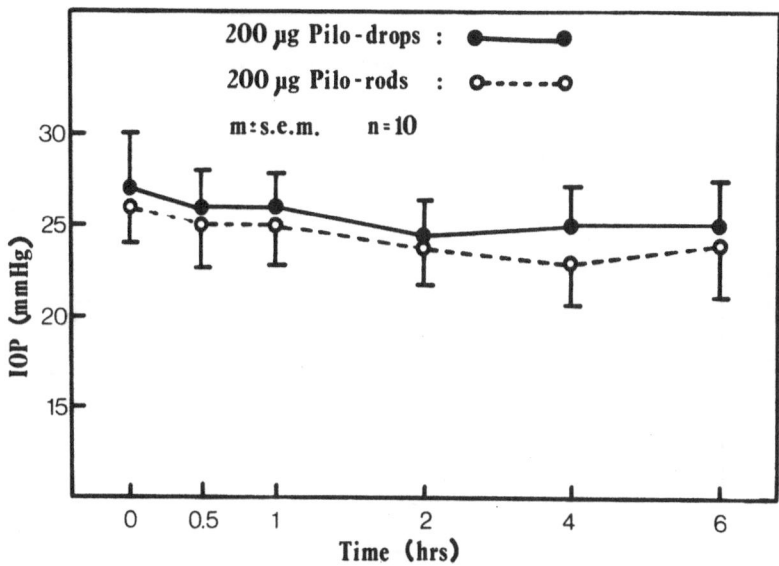

Fig. 2. The mean time course of IOP to 200 μg pilocarpine eyedrops and 200 μg pilocarpine rods in 10 glaucoma patients. The ordinate gives IOP, the abscissa time after treatment.

RESULTS

The mean I.O.P. responses of 200 μg pilocarpine in eyedrops and mounted on ophthalmic rods are compared in Fig. 2. There was only a slight pressure reduction with 200 μg of pilocarpine with either preparation (2.9 mmHg for the drops and 3.2 mmHg for the rods). There was no statistically significant difference between both preparations. The mean IOP responses to 500 μg pilocarpine in both preparations is given in Fig. 3. A highly significant IOP reduction could be noted for both preparations (5 mmHg for the drops and 6 mmHg for the rods). Again, there was no significant difference between the IOP responses of both preparations. By analysis of the IOP responses of the two dosages irrespective of the type of preparation it was shown that the dose dependence was not significant.

The miotic activity is given with the mean-time course of the pupillary diameter after drug application. 200 μg pilocarpine drops and 200 μg pilocarpine rods produced a significant miosis (Fig. 4). 500 μg of pilocarpine in both preparations induced a comparable miosis which was again statistically significant (Fig. 5). However, the mioses caused by the two dosages of either preparation were not significantly different.

Re-analyzation of active drug in the test solution and of residual drug on the rods after application confirmed the concentration of pilocarpine in the aqueous solution, and the fact that the major amount of the drug was dissolved from the rod into the aqueous environment of the conjunctival sac.

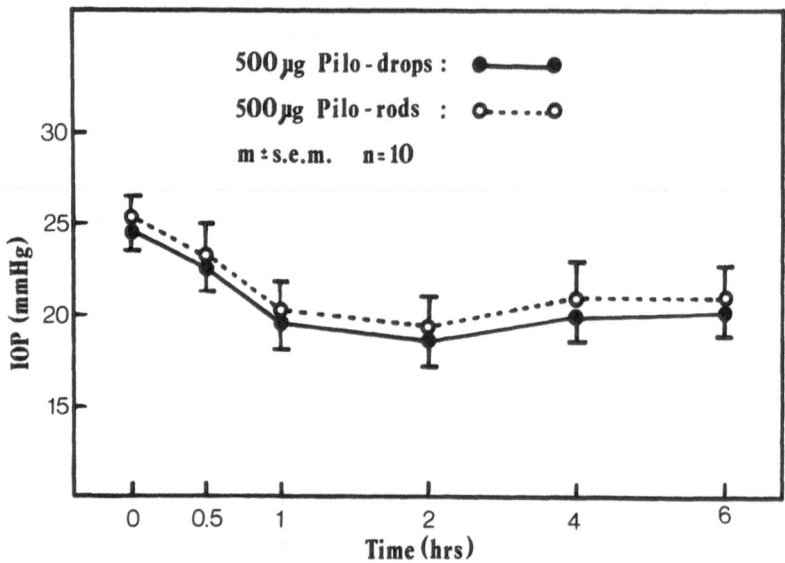

Fig. 3. The mean time course of I.O.P. to 500 μg pilocarpine eyedrops and 500 μg pilocarpine rods in 10 glaucoma patients. The ordinate gives IOP, the abscissa time after treatment.

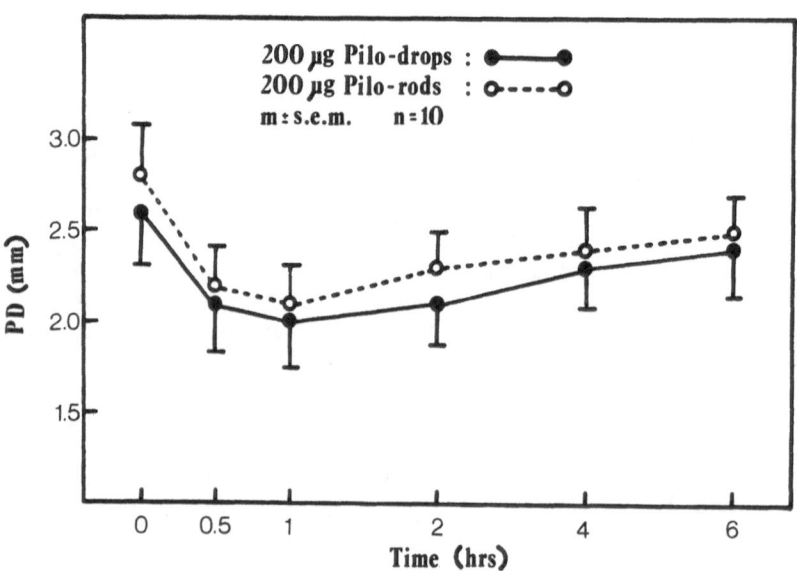

Fig. 4. The mean time course of pupillary diameter (PD) to 200 μg pilocarpine eye drops and 200 μg pilocarpine rods in 10 glaucoma patients. The ordinate gives the pupillary diameter, the abscissa time after treatment.

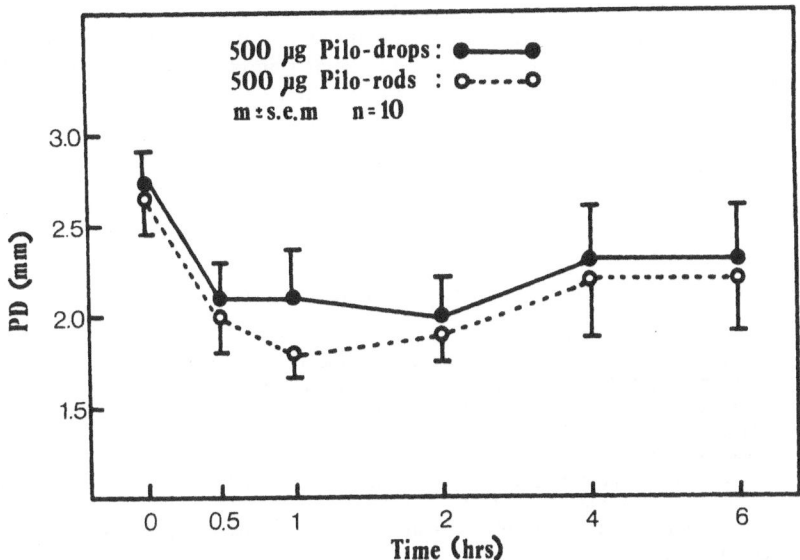

Fig. 5. The mean time course of pupillary diameter (PD) to 500 µg pilocarpine eyedrops and 500 µg pilocarpine rods in 10 glaucoma patients. The ordinate gives the pupillary diameter, the abscissa time after treatment.

DISCUSSION

Sensitization to preservatives in aqueous eye drug preparations is most common with antiglaucomatous drugs, since these agents usually have to be used throughout life (3). Amongst the antiglaucomatous compounds, the risk/benefit ratio is best established with pilocarpine (2). It was therefore an attractive approach to compare pilocarpine in the two preparations. It could be shown that pilocarpine gives equivalent ocular responses with respect to miosis and IOP reduction on the basis of a single dose trial for two dosages (200 µg and 500 µg pilocarpine either in one drop or on one ophthalmic rod).

However, the pressure-lowering effect with the low dose for both preparations was only marginal. There was no statistically significant dose-dependence for both preparations. It can be suggested that the group 1 of patients which was treated with the low dose was not miotic-sensitive enough to bring out a clear cut dose—response relationship. One can conclude that pilocarpine mounted on ophthalmic rods was at least as effective as an equivalent single dose in an aqueous solution for producing miosis and lowering IOP.

Considering the topical application of betablockers Nielsen (6) proved that 0.22 mg metoprolol on an ophthalmic rod produced a similar effect on intraocular pressure, blood pressure and heart rate as one eyedrop of 3% metoprolol. Alani (1) had encouraging results with diagnostic agents on ophthalmic rods as well. He used tropicamide as a mydriatic, oxybuprocaine hydrochloride and fluorescein sodium. Neither in the present study nor in the other studies quoted were there any ocular side effects to be attributed to the use of the ophthalmic rod. The advantages of this new disposable delivery device for ophthalmic drugs are obvious and should be considered for patients in whom sensitization to preservatives is known or in whom systemic absorption of the topically applied aqueous drug solution may be risky.

REFERENCES

1. Alani, D.S. The ophthalmic rod – description of a disposable ophthalmic drug delivery device. Acta Pharm. Suec. 15: 237 (1978).
2. Engelmayr, W. and Krieglstein, G.K. Pilokarpin. Ein Jahrhundert in der Glaukomtherapie. Dr. Reinhard-Kaden-Verlag/Heidelberg, 1980.
3. Krieglstein, G.K. Parasympathomimetika in der Therapie des chronischen Glaukoms. In: Die medikamentöse Behandlung des chronischen Glaukoms. Rundtischgespräch Univ. Augenklinik Münster, 1979.
4. Krieglstein, G.K. Die Therapie des chronischen Glaukoms. Dtsch Med. Wschr. 105: 398 (1980).
5. Krieglstein, G.K. Konservierungsstoffe in ophthalmologischen Arzneimitteln. Z prakt. Augenheilk. 2: 59 (1981).
6. Nielsen, N.V. A diurnal study of the ocular hypotensive effect of metoprolol mounted on ophthalmic rods compared to timolol eye drops in glaucoma patients. Acta Ophthalmol. 59: 495 (1981).

Authors' address:
Univ. Augenklinik
Josef-Schneider-Str. 11
D-8700 Würzburg
F.R.G.

THE INFLUENCE ON THE CAPILLARY BLOOD VOLUME OF THE OPTIC NERVE HEAD EXERTED BY BETA-BLOCKING AGENTS WITH AND WITHOUT INTRINSIC SYMPATOMIMETIC ACTIVITY

Y. ROBERT* and Ph. HENDRICKSON

(Basle, Switzerland)

ABSTRACT

Despite the good intraocular pressure-lowering effect of Timolol, glaucomatous damage of the visual field is known to progress. Lack of intrinsic sympato-mimetic activity is blamed as one of the causative factors, in the sense that perfusion pressure of the capillaries of the nerve head is impaired. Pindolol is a beta-blocking agent with a high intrinsic sympatomimetic activity and, as such, was used in this comparison study.

A randomized study on 14 healthy, elderly volunteers was carried out to investigate the effect of Pindolol (1%) and Timolol (0.5%) eye drops, as well as Pindolol tablets (Visken 5 mg) on the capillary blood volume of the optic nerve head. The volume of the capillaries was calculated as a function of the disappearance of their red colour when intraocular pressure was artifically elevated to the level of the perfusion pressure. The red colour was measured with a direct measuring device built into a Zeiss fundus camera.

INTRODUCTION

In the years intervening since beta-blockers became established in glaucoma therapy, suspicion has grown that, in spite of pressure-reducing effects, the progress of glaucoma is not retarded but continues instead, as seen in further deterioration of the visual field (2). A possible explanation (for the time being) for this phenomenon might be found in the fact that intraocular pressure reduction is accompanied by a decrease in perfusion on the optic nerve head. This hypothesis is supported by the fact that the beta-blocker most highly suspected in this regard, namely Timolol®, has the least 'intrinsic sympatomimetic activity' (4).

Quite naturally the question arises whether it is not possible to employ a substance which has the desired pressure-reducing properties without eliciting a deterioration of the perfusion at the papilla. It follows that such a substance should be one with maximum intrinsic sympatomimetic activity. It has been shown that application of Pindolol®, in contrast to Timolol, has no effect on cardiac output (7); therefore, perfusion pressure, as an indication of the perfusion at the papilla, must increase or, at least, not decrease.

*To whom requests for offprints should be addressed.

103

E.L. Greve, W. Leydhecker & C. Raitta (eds.), Second European Glaucoma Symposium, Helsinki 1984.
© 1985, Dr. W. Junk Publishers, Dordrecht. ISBN 978-94-010-8934-0

Perfusion cannot be directly measured clinically, but the content of the blood can be estimated by quantitative measurement of pallor of the nerve head evoked by artificial elevation of the intraocular pressure (5). The more filled the capillaries, the more marked will be pallor which is evoked during reduction of the perfusion pressure to zero. Additionally, the higher the perfusion pressure on the optic nerve head, the greater will be the influence of the autoregulative response of the small vessels by such artificial intraocular pressure elevation. Therefore, we have pondered whether we could differentiate between the influence on the perfusion pressure of two beta-blockers, one with and the other without intrinsic sympatomimetic activity, using pallor measurements during artificial intraocular pressure elevation. In other words, could we determine a difference in induced pallor of the papilla under artificially elevated intraocular pressure following application of these two types of beta-blockers?

MATERIALS AND METHODS

Fourteen healthy elderly persons of both genders (mean age = 60.5 ± 5.8 years) were included in this study. Following screening for glaucoma and vascular disease by means of ocular examination including visual acuity, tonometry, slit-lamp examination (with contact-glass observation of the chamber angle and posterior pole), the upper-arm blood pressure was determined, and the pupils were dilated to at least 6 mm diameter. Subsequently the brightness of the temporal rim of the papilla was measured by means of a photopapillometer (3). This device consists essentially of a light-sensitive resistor built into the image plane of a Zeiss fundus camera. After five control measurements were made in quick succession, the intraocular pressure was artificially elevated by means of a Müller ophthalmodynamometer, and the brightness measurements repeated. The intraocular pressure was raised in three steps: to 20 increments, to 40 increments, and to 70 increments on the ophthalmodynamometer scale.

Medication

A few days after the control examination, each subject returned to be measured again. Two hours before the actual measurements were repeated, one of the three medications was administered (Pindolol either as drops or tablets, or Timolol). At the beginning and end of that two hour period, intraocular- and blood pressures were taken. The order in which the medications were administered to any one subject was random. Pindolol and Timolol drops were given to all 14 subjects, whereas Pindolol tablets (Visken) were taken by only 11 of those 14 persons.

Perfusion pressure calculation

The perfusion pressures were calculated according to the formula of Weigelin (8):

Perfusion pressure = 0.73 (mean blood pressure) − IOP

At an ophthalmodynamometic increment reading of 70, the calculated perfusion pressure in every subject was zero.

Representation of relative brightness

Each brightness value (mean of five measurements) was related to its corresponding perfusion pressure. To express the pallor evoked, we calculated the 'area under the curve' for each series on each test person.

RESULTS

1. Pressures

Intraocular pressure. Table 1 depicts the pressure-reducing effects of the three medications. Topical Pindolol (1%) reduced the intraocular pressure by a mean value of 4.07 ± 3.22 mm Hg, whereas topical Tomolol (0.5%) caused a reduction of 5.64 ± 3.03 mm Hg. In the untreated contralateral eye of each case, the intraocular pressure was lowered 1.36 ± 2.34 mm Hg by both local medications. Pindolol tablets only slightly lowered the pressure (by an average of 1.91 ± 3.02 mm Hg in the right eyes and of 1.18 ± 4.49 mm Hg in the left eyes).

While the result in the treated eyes for both of the topical medications was significant ($p < 0.01$), that for the untreated, fellow eyes was only barely so ($p < 0.05$). For all 11 subjects receiving Pindolol tablets per os, the results for the right eyes were barely significant ($p < 0.05$) but those for the left eyes not at all so.

Perfusion pressure. Following administration of topical Pindolol, the perfusion pressure rose by a mean amount of 5.38 ± 3.08 mm Hg, and this increase following topical Timolol was 5.14 ± 5.87 mm Hg (Table 2). No improvement in the perfusion pressure was observed subsequent to administration of Pindolol tablets (mean change = 0.75 ± 7.9 mm Hg). This last value is not significant, but that for topical Timolol is significant on the 0.01 level, and that for topical Pindolol even more highly so ($p < 0.001$).

2. Brightness

Brightness with slight pressure increase. Pallor increasing subsequent to elevated intraocular pressure to values of 30 and 40 mm Hg is depicted in a 'box-and-whiskers' plot (Fig. 1). This synoptic overview representation shows at a glance that no change in brightness was seen in the papillas of healthy, elderly persons when the original intraocular pressure had been raised by about 20 mm Hg. The mean difference of median without medication was 0.787, with Timolol was 0.793, with Pindolol drops was 0.811, and for Pindolol per os 0.580 (relative brightness units (3)), as seen in Fig. 1. These values do not differ among themselves to a statistically significant extent.

Table 1. IOP-lowering effect of the three drugs

	Pindolol (1%)		Timolol (0.5%)		Pindolol-tablets (5 mg)	
	Treated eye	Fellow eye	Treated eye	Fellow eye	Right eye	Left eye
mm Hg ± SD	− 4.07 ± 3.22	− 1.36 ± 2.34	− 5.64 ± 3.03	− 1.36 ± 2.34	− 1.91 ± 3.02	− 1.18 ± 4.49
Statistical significance	++	+	++	+	(+)	−
Level	1%	5%	1%	5%	(5%)	−

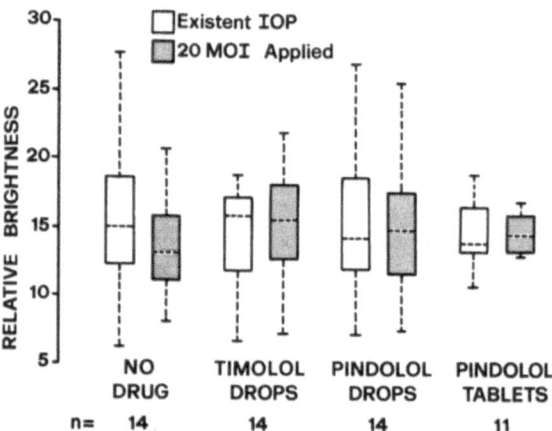

Fig. 1. Box-and-whiskers plot of relative brightness of the papillas of subjects under four medication conditions without and with applied ophthalmodynamometric pressure. (MOI = Müller Ophthalmodynamometric Increments)

Brightness with intraocular pressure raised to the level of the perfusion pressure. Since the pallor response (increase) with further raised intraocular pressure varies greatly, the area under to curve was calculated by the trapezoidal rule for each trial on each subject (Table 3). Comparison of these areas by means of a paired T-test yields a mean pallor increase of 6.23 ± 19.59% and 6.82 ± 24.68% for Timolol drops and Pindolol tablets, respectively, but 1.53 ± 21.68% for Pindolol drops.

With all three medications, the increase in pallor when compared to that of trials without medication was greater in half of the subjects and less in the other half.

DISCUSSION

As has already been shown in healthy subjects by Smith et al. (7) and Rowley et al. (5) and in glaucomatous patients by Andréasson and co-workers (1), Pindolol (1%) reduces the intraocular pressure by approximately the same

106

Table 2. Change of perfusion pressure after administration of three drugs

	Pindolol drops (1%)		Timolol drops (0.5%)		Pindolol tablets (5 mg)	
	Before	After	Before	After	Before	After
Mean perfusion pressure	53.07 ± 6.10	58.45 ± 7.78	55.11 ± 9.97	60.25 ± 11.72	56.59 ± 6.33	55.84 ± 7.37
Diff. of the mean	+ 5.38 ± 3.08		+ 5.14 ± 5.87		+ 0.75 ± 7.90	
T-value	6.5		3.28		0.31	
DF	13		13		10	
Significance	++		+		—	
Level	0.001		0.01			

Table 3. Area under the curve with different drugs

Person	Without drug	Pindolol drops (1%)	Difference (%)	Timolol drops (0.5%)	Difference (%)	Pindolol tablets (5 mg)	Difference (%)
1	890.70	784.05	− 12	1098.04	+ 23		
2	1231.46	1152.47	− 6	1230.71	− 0.06		
3	845.30	833.16	− 1	810.11	− 4		
4	694.06	553.64	− 20	739.64	+ 7	834.58	+ 20
5	916.04	834.27	− 9	829.34	− 9	889.50	− 3
6	1008.08	640.30	− 36	1199.31	+ 19	1114.60	+ 11
7	902.89	1106.93	+ 23	945.88	+ 5	878.15	− 3
8	662.67	665.36	+ 0.47	641.20	− 3	428.27	− 35
9	568.03	675.12	+ 19	572.06	− 10	591.99	+ 4
10	434.07	409.48	− 6	346.39	− 20	363.26	− 16
11	681.60	710.06	+ 4	839.06	+ 23	807.23	+ 18
12	903.92	851.34	− 6	770.58	− 15	807.31	− 11
13	463.58	540.60	+ 17	542.04	+ 17	642.38	+ 39
14	616.28	949.93	+ 54	950.53	+ 54	927.54	+ 51
Mean ± SD	772.76 ± 222.39	764.77 ± 210.59		818.21 ± 257.28		753.16 ± 224.40	
Diff. ± SD		− 8.00 ± 164.81	1.53 ± 21.68	45.44 ± 134.36	6.23 ± 19.59	39.42 ± 151.60	6.82 ± 24.68
T-value		− 0.18		+ 1.26		+ 0.86	
DF		13		13		10	

amount as does Timolol (0.5%). A pressure-reducing effect on the untreated contralateral eyes of our own volunteers could be measured as well. In spite of the fact that a single drop of Pindolol causes an almost unmeasurably low plasma-level, our trials with Pindolol tablets (which showed the same tendency toward pressure reduction as the drops in the untreated fellow eyes) nevertheless support the hypothesis suggested by Zimmerman and Kaufman (9), according to which this effect may be explained by systematic resorption.

Here it must be emphasized that the trials with Pindolol tablets, while demonstrating a tendency toward pressure reduction, did not do so to a statistically significant extent.

The actual difference between the two preparations (according to the different intrinsic sympatomimetic activities present) is expressed as different increases in perfusion pressure. Although a purely mathematical measure, this increase can be used as a reference against which the relationship between the intraocular pressure and the arterial blood pressure may be judged. The clearly greater increase in the perfusion pressure in the fundus following topical Pindolol administration could not be brought into direct correlation with measurements of the red colour of the papilla. This means that the theoretically better status of perfusion in the fundus following the administration of Pindolol than that following Timolol cannot be proven by means of an indirect method for estimating blood content. This holds true for pallor induced by slight artificial pressure elevation which simulates glaucomatous conditions as well as for pallor induced by means of greater artificial pressure increases which serve as an indication of the original blood volume.

CONCLUSIONS

The difference between the maximum brightness of induced pallor and the original brightness, that is, the blood content of the capillaries of the optic nerve (expressed as the area under the curve) was not significantly different in four experimental conditions, regardless of whether the perfusion pressure was improved or worsened by the medications.

Under the assumption that the measured pallor of the papilla's rim represents its blood content it means no less than perfusion can be held constant over extremely varying pressure levels in healthy subjects. However, it also means that the influence of the intrinsic sympatomimetic activity cannot be established directly on the optic nerve. Perhaps after examinations over a longer period of time can we gain an indication whether the intrinsic sympatomimetic activity is effective on the eye or not. For example, if the effect is accumulative, a longer period could reveal that the short-term regulation is no longer capable of compensating.

ACKNOWLEDGEMENTS

Pindolol eye drops and Visken tablets 5 mg were supplied by SANDOZ Produkte CH, Basle.

The authors thank Dr H. Prestele, Sandoz Ltd., Basle for his help with the statistical analysis.

REFERENCES

1. Andréasson, S. and Møller-Jensen, K. Effect of Pindolol on IOP in glaucoma: pilot study and a randomised comparison with Timolol. Br. J. Ophthalmol. 67: 228 (1983).

2. Demmler, N. and Müller-Bardorff, G. Zunahme von Gesichtsfelddefekten unter Timolol-Langzeitbehandlung bei Patienten in der augenärztlichen Praxis. Klin. Mbl. Augenheilk. 183: 53 (1983).
3. Hendrickson, Ph and Robert, Y. Direkte Messung der Papillenhelligkeit. Klin. Mbl. Augenheilk. (in press).
4. Man in 't velt, A.I. and Schalekamp, M.A.D.H. How ISA modulates the haemodynamic responses to beta-adrenoceptor antagonists. Br. J. clin. Pharmac. 13: 245S (1982).
5. Robert, Y., Niesel, P. and Ehrengruber, H. Measurement of the optic nerve head I: The pallor of the papilla in artificial ocular hypertension. Graefe's Arch. clin. exp. Ophthalmol. 219: 176 (1982).
6. Rowley, S., Staunton, J.E., Tosch, A., Steward-Jones, J.H., Edgar, D.F. and Turner, P. A noninvasive tonometer in the measurement of the effects of Pindolol and Timolol on IOP in normal subjects. Br. J. Ophthalmol. 65: 536 (1981).
7. Smith, S.E., Smith, A.S., Reynolds, F. and Whitmarsh, V.B. Ocular and cardiovascular effects of local and systemic Pindolol. Br. J. Ophthalmol. 63: 63 (1979).
8. Weigelin, E. and Lobstein, A. Ophthalmodynamometrie. S. Karger, Basel (1962).
9. Zimmermann, T.J. and Kaufman, H.E. Timolol – A beta-adrenergic blocking agent for the treatment of glaucoma. Arch. Ophthalmol. 96: 601 (1977).

Authors' address:
Univ.-Augenklinik
Mittlere Strasse 91
CH-4056 Basle
Switzerland

(−)-PROPRANOLOL IN THE ISOLATED RABBIT IRIS

H.A. FLEIG* and G.K. KRIEGLSTEIN

(Würzburg, F.R.G.)

ABSTRACT

There was no significant cocaine-sensitive or reserpine-sensitive accumulation of (−)-propranolol in the isolated rabbit iris. Veratridine did not increase the efflux of (−)-propranolol from the rabbit iris. The experiments are not in favour of a neuronal and/or vesicular accumulation of (−)-propranolol. Hence, our experiments are not in favour of an adrenergic neurone-blocking action of (−)-propranolol in the isolated rabbit iris.

Wash-out experiments with the isolated pigmented or non-pigmented (albino) iris, loaded with labelled (−)-propranolol, indicate that there exist binding sites of high affinity in or at pigment cells. These results can explain the long duration of action of beta-adrenoceptor-blockers in lowering the intraocular pressure in man.

INTRODUCTION

In the treatment of glaucoma, beta-adrenoceptor-blockers decrease the production of aqueous humor formation. Saelens et al. (8), Mysecharane and Raper, and Kaiho et al. (6) discussed the principles for the action of beta-adrenoceptor-blockers: beta-adrenoceptor-blockade, local anaesthetic effects, or adrenergic neurone blockade. It was of interest to know whether there is a neuronal uptake of propranolol into the adrenergic nerve endings and/or storage of propranolol in the vesicles. These experiments were performed to check the adrenergic neurone-blocking properties of beta-adrenoceptor-blockers.

The fact that beta-adrenoceptor-blockers take a long time to act in lowering intraocular pressure was used as an argument against the beta-adrenoceptor-mediated mechanism of action of these drugs (10). As shown by Patil, atropine, a highly lipophilic substance, is bound to a great extent in or at pigment cells of the rabbit iris. Although there is only a very slow dissociation from these binding sites, effective atropine concentrations are maintained in the aqueous humor for several days. Hence, in the second part of the study we investigated

*To whom requests for offprints should be addressed.

111

E.L. Greve, W. Leydhecker & C. Raitta (eds.), Second European Glaucoma Symposium, Helsinki 1984.
© *1985, Dr. W. Junk Publishers, Dordrecht. ISBN 978-94-010-8934-0*

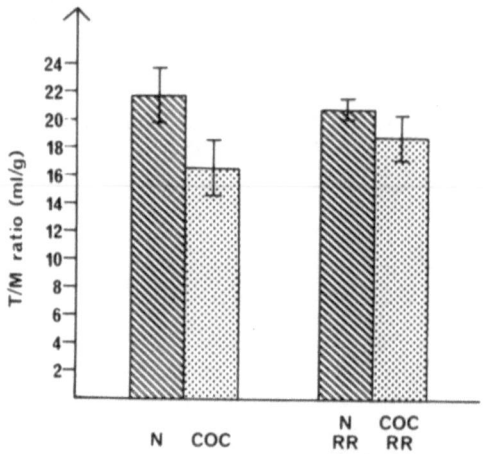

Fig. 1. The influence of cocaine, an inhibitor of neuronal uptake, on the accumulation of 0.1 μmol.l^{-1} ^{3}H-propranolol after 60 min incubation in the isolated albino rabbit iris. Height of columns: T/M ratio. Shown are means ($\pm$ s.e. as vertical bars; n = 5 each). Pairs of columns represent paired experiments with irides of the same animal. Symbols: N = controls, COC = in the presence of 30 μmol/l cocaine, RR = after pretreatment of the animals with reserpine.

the distribution of propranolol in the isolated rabbit iris. The comparison of the pigmented iris with the non-pigmented (albino) iris should reveal the binding of ($-$)-propranolol in or at pigment cells.

RESULTS

Incubation experiments and the action of reserpine and veratridine

The accumulation of ^{3}H-(−)-propranolol. Isolated albino irides were incubated with 0.1 μmol/l ^{3}H-propranolol for 60 min in the absence or presence of 30 μmol/l cocaine. Experiments were carried out with irides obtained from untreated and from reserpine-pretreated rabbits. Cocaine, a competitive inhibitor of the neuronal uptake mechanism, had no significant influence on the accumulation of propranolol in the tissue. As shown in Fig. 1, pretreatment with reserpine, an inhibitor of the accumulation of catecholamines in the storage vesicles, had no significant influence on the accumulation of propranolol in the tissue. After 60 min of incubation, very high T/M ratios (T/M ratios were calculated following equation − (concentration of the drug in the tissue in pmol/g)/(concentration of the drug in the medium in pmol/ml)) were observed for ^{3}H-(−)-propranolol, apparently not because of any distribution into adrenergic nerve endings. These remarkably high T/M ratios will be discussed below.

The effect of veratridine. After 60 min incubation of the tissue with 0.1 μmol/l ^{3}H-(−)-propranolol tissues were washed for 60 min with propranolol-free solution. After this period, the spontaneous efflux of ^{3}H-(−)-propranolol

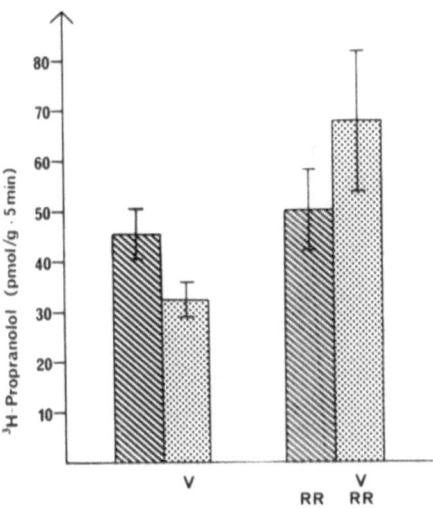

Fig. 2. The influence of veratridine on the spontaneous efflux of ³H-propranolol from isolated albino rabbit iris after 120 min incubation with 0.1 μmol.l⁻¹ ³H-propranolol and after 60 min wash-out with propranolol-free solution. One set of experiments was done with reserpine (RR) pretreated animals. Hatched columns show the spontaneous release of ³H-propranolol just before addition of veratridine (V). Dotted columns show the efflux of ³H-propranolol in the presence of 100 μmol.l⁻¹ veratridine. Ordinate: rate of efflux of ³H-propranolol (in pmol/g · 5 min).

from one half of the iris was measured for 5 min (hatched columns in Fig. 2). The pretreatment of the animals with reserpine had no influence on this spontaneous efflux (Fig. 2). The other half of the iris was exposed to 100 μmol/l veratridine for 5 min. It is known that veratridine opens the fast sodium channels. This leads by a rpaid influx of sodium to a depolarization of the adrenergic nerve endings, which causes an exocytotic release of the content of the storage vesicles. As shown in Fig. 2, the presence of veratridine failed to increase the efflux of ³H-(−)-propranolol (dotted columns).

Wash-out experiments with propranolol

Pigmented and albino isolated rabbit irides were incubated with 0.1 μmol/l ³H-(−)-propranolol for 120 min in the presence of 30 μmol/l cocaine to inhibit the neuronal uptake mechanism. After loading, the tissues were washed out with propranolol-free and cocaine-containing solution for 300 min. Wash-out curves are shown in Fig. 3. This figure shows the multiphasic efflux curves of ³H-(−)-propranolol from albino (open circles) and from pigmented irides (closed circles).

The results of the compartment analysis (following the method of Henseling et al. (5)) are shown in Table 1. Propranolol was distributed into at least four different compartments. Compartment I, characterized by a very short half-time, probably represents propranolol distributed into the extracellular space and adhering to the surface of the preparation. Compartment II probably represents an intracellular compartment; it is characterized

113

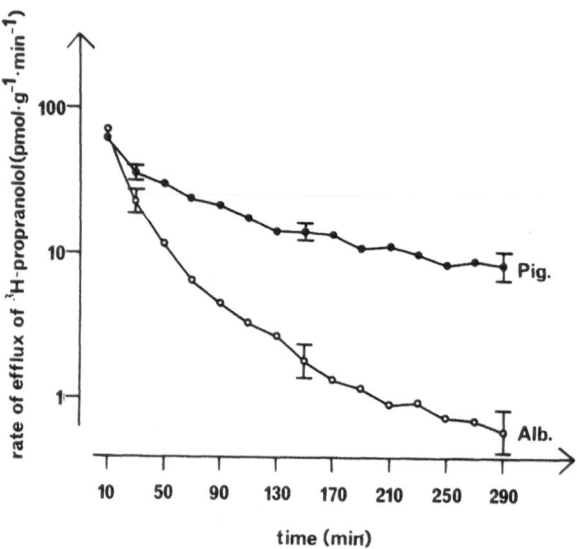

Fig. 3. Efflux of ^{3}H-propranolol from the isolated albino (Alb.) or pigmented (Pig.) rabbit iris during wash-out with propranolol-free solution. The tissues were exposed 120 min to 0.1 μmol. l^{-1} ^{3}H-propranolol before starting wash-out. Cocaine was always present. Ordinate: rate of efflux of ^{3}H-propranolol (in pmol. g^{-1}. min^{-1}, log scale); abscissa: time of wash-out (in min). Shown are geometric means of n = 4 ($\pm$ s.e. as vertical bars).

by a half-time of about 20–30 min. Compartment III is small in the albino iris, though it has a relatively long half-time for efflux from the tissue. Moreover, there exists no bound fraction in the albino iris. However, in the pigmented iris there exists a very large compartment III with a half-time of about 200 min and additionally a bound fraction of roughly 1000 pmol/g.

Table 1. Compartment analysis of the efflux of ^{3}H-propranolol from albino and pigmented irides (shown in Fig. 3) initially exposed to 0.1 μmol. l^{-1} ^{3}H-propranolol for 120 min; cocaine was present throughout the experiments. Shown are compartment size (in pmol. g^{-1}; arithmetic means $\pm$ S.E.) and half times of efflux (in min; geometric means with 95% confidence limits).

| | Albino iris | | Pigmented iris | |
	size (pmol/g)	half time (min)	size (pmol/g)	half time (min)
Total accumulation	2779.9 ± 252.0		8195.7 ± 549.2	
Compartment I	952.4 ± 393.1	7.7 (6.8; 8.7)	352.8 ± 169.8	
Compartment II	1288.0 ± 119.4	22.4 (20.1; 25.0)	1566.2 ± 780.5	31.8 (17.7; 57.1)
Compartment III	624.0 ± 168.3	129.1 (101.0; 164.8)	6318.6 ± 373.8	198.7 (139.1; 283.7)
Bound fraction	no bound fraction		953.0 ± 55.3	

114

But though the rate constant is low, there is a high rate of efflux from this compartment because of the very large size of compartment III. Furthermore, there is a compartment, the bound fraction, which does not contribute to the efflux from the tissue during the 300 min of wash-out. A look at compartment III and bound fraction in the albino and pigmented iris reveals a very pronounced difference between the two tissues. But already, the total accumulation amount shows that the pigmented iris accumulates much more propranolol than the albino iris.

DISCUSSION

(−)-propranolol and the adrenergic nerve ending

Saelens et al. (8) found that in addition to its adrenergic neurone-blocking properties, propranolol enhanced the spotaneous release of ^{3}H-neurotransmitter from the guinea-pig Vas deferens by a mechanism consistent with the direct interaction between propranolol and the synaptic storage vesicles.

Therefore, it was interesting to investigate the neuronal uptake and the neuronal storage of propranolol in the iris. The results shown in Fig. 1 indicate that there was no measurable cocaine-sensitive, i.e. carrier-mediated neuronal uptake of (−)-propranolol into the adrenergic nerve ending. Pretreatment of the animals with reserpine did not influence the accumulation of propranolol in the tissue. This is not in favour of any uptake of propranolol into the storage vesicles. But the neuronal uptake of an adrenergic neuron-blocking drug and its accumulation in the storage vesicles are conditions for this mechanism of action. Hence, our results are not in favour of a guanethidine-like adrenergic neurone-blocking action of propranolol. There exist, however, basic difficulties in the exact quantitative determination of a carrier-mediated transport of highly lipophilic substances. Thoenen et al. (11) were unable to demonstrate a carrier-mediated transport of (±)-amphetamine into adrenergic nerve endings of the isolated perfused heart of the rat. This means that, in an organ where adrenergic nerve endings represent only a very small fraction of the total tissue weight, it is impossible to see a carrier-mediated uptake of highly lipophilic substances. Looking at the high T/M ratios of (−)-propranolol in the tissue, a small degree of carrier-mediated uptake of propranolol into the adrenergic nerve endings might be masked by a rapid influx due to the lipophilicity of the beta-blocker.

According to Bönisch et al. (2), $100 \mu mol/l$ veratridine cause a very pronounced exocytotic release of noradrenaline from adrenergic nerve endings. As Fig. 2 shows, veratridine had no influence on the spontaneous efflux of propranolol from pre-loaded rabbit irides. Once more, these results are not in favour of a guanethidine-like uptake and accumulation of propranolol.

Wash-out experiments and the pigment cells of the rabbit iris

As shown in Table 1, the total accumultion of the beta-blocker in the pigmented iris is much higher than that in the albino iris. The compartment with the long half-time (III) and the bound fraction in the pigmented isolated rabbit iris exceed the corresponding compartments in the albino iris by a factor of 10. Though the rate constant for the efflux of propranolol is very low for this compartment, there is a measurable and long-lasting efflux because of the very large size of compartment III. Also, the bound fraction will finally participate in the efflux of propranolol from the tissue after 300 min of wash-out.

It is surprising that pigment cells generate T/M ratios up to 82. Furthermore, these T/M ratios refer to the entire tissue and the total tissue weight. If we take into account that roughly one tenth of the total weight of the pigmented rabbit iris represents the pigment cells (7), the T/M ratios are even much higher without any hint of a transport system.

The present results resemble the data presented by Patil. He found that atropine reaches a T/M ratio of 16 in the pigmented rabbit iris, and that the half-time for the efflux is roughly 200 min.

Both atropine and propranolol are highly lipophilic substances. As Hellenbrecht et al. (1979) showed, propranolol is one of the most lipophilic beta-adrenoceptor-blockers. It seems that lipophilicity of these basic compounds is important for their accumulation in pigment cells.

The long-lasting efflux of propranolol from compartment III and, at a later time, from the bound fraction might maintain a concentration of propranolol in the extracellular space of the iris and in the aqueous humor, which is able to block beta-adrenoceptors for many hours. Hence, in contrast to the conclusions of Sears (10), it is distinctly possible that beta-adrenoceptor-blockers lower intraocular pressure by an effect on beta-adrenoceptors.

ACKNOWLEDGEMENTS

The authors are grateful for the generous help of the Deutsche Forschungsgemeinschaft. They are also grateful for the donation of propranolol by ICI-Pharma, Heidelberg. The authors thank Frau Martina Fischer for her excellent technical assistance in the study.

REFERENCES

1. Bönisch, H. Evidence for a cocaine-sensitive and sodium-dependent uptake of amphetamine. Naunyn-Schmiedeberg's Arch. Pharmacol. 316: 214 (1981).
2. Bönisch, H., Graefe, K.H. and Keller, B. Tetrodotoxin-sensitive and -resistant effects of veratridine on the noradrenergic neurone of the rat vas deferens. Naunyn-Schmiedeberg's Arch. Pharmacol. 324: 264–270 (1983).
3. Daniell, H.B., Walle, T., Gaffney, T.E. and Webb, J.G. Stimulation-induced release of propranolol and norepinephrine from adrenergic neurons[1,2]. J. Pharmacol. Exp. Ther. 208: 354–359 (1979).
4. Hellenbrecht, D., Lemmer, G., Wiethold, G. and Grobecker, H. Measurement of hydrophobicity, surface activity, lokal anaesthesia, and myocardial conduction velocity as quantitative parameters of the non-specific membrane affinity of nine ß-adrenergic blocking agents. Naunyn-Schmiedeberg's Arch. Pharmacol. 277: 211–226 (1973).

5. Henseling, M., Eckert, E. and Trendelenburg, U. The distribution of ^{3}H-(+) noradrenaline in rabbit aortic strips after inhibition of the noradrenaline-metabolizing enzymes. Naunyn-Schmiedeberg's Arch. Pharmacol. 292: 205–217 (1976).
6. Kaiho, M., Kubo, T. and Misu, Y. Comparative studies of (–)-, (±), (+)-propranolol, atenolol, guanethidine, bretylium and tetracaine on adrenergic transmission. Br. J. Pharmacol. 74: 365–370 (1981).
7. Patil, P.N. and Trendelenburg, U. The extraneuronal uptake and metabolism of ^{3}H-isoprenaline in the rabbit iris. Naunyn-Schmiedeberg's Arch. Pharmacol. 318: 158–165 (1982).
8. Saelens, D.A., Daniell, H.B. and Webb, J.G. Studies on the interactions of propranolol with adrenergic neurons[1,2]. J. Pharmacol. Exp. Ther. 202: 635–645 (1977).
9. Salazar, M., Shimada, K. and Patil, P.N. Iris pigmentation and atropine mydriasis. J. Pharm. Exp. Ther. 197: 79–88 (1976).
10. Sears, M.L. Receptor control of aqueous humor formation. In: New Directions in Ophthalmic Research, Sears, M.L. (ed). New Haven and London, Yale University Press, p. 131 (1981).
11. Thoenen, H., Hürlimann, A. and Haefely, W. Mechanism of amphetamine accumulation in the isolated perfused heart of the rat. J. Pharm. Pharmacol. 20: 1–11 (1968).

Authors' address:
University Eye Hospital
Josef. Schneider-Str. 11
D-8700 Würzburg
F.R.G.

COMPARISON OF DIFFERENT β-BLOCKERS IN OPEN ANGLE GLAUCOMAS

J.R. STRYZ and H.-J. MERTÉ

(Munich, F.R.G.)

ABSTRACT

We compare the pressure lowering effect and side effects of Propranolol, Timolol, Bupranolol, Metipranolol, 1-Bunolol, Befunolol and Pindolol in the form of eye drops in the treatment of glaucoma. There is no difference with regard to the long-term pressure lowering effect. With regard to the one-drop-curve and to side effects, there are some slight differences.

For more than 100 years myopic drugs were the treatment of choice for glaucoma. Although many other substances were tested, e.g. Epinephrine, Clonidine or Guanethidine, none was able to compete with the miotics for first position. The detection of the IOP-lowering effect of Propranolol, however, challenged the leading position of Pilocarpine. The following report of our experience with various β-blockers shows the difference we found between the tested drugs.

About 10 years ago we started clinical investigations with Propranolol. Two special effects of the β-blockers, in addition to the absence of drug-related miosis and myopia, are the influence on IOP either in non-glaucomatous eyes or of systemic application.

The first of these drugs which we gave topically to patients with open angle glaucomas was Propranolol. The effect of the one-drop-curve on IOP was relatively slow and not as strong as it was after repeated applications for a longer period.

The blood pressure and pulse rate show a significant decrease within one year. An influence on tear production was not clinically evident; the effect on corneal sensitivity is well known. Often a satisfactory control of IOP was only obtainable with frequent applications.

One drop of Timolol showed a fast pressure-lowering effect with a maximum after 4 hours and a duration of 12 to 24 or more hours. The long-term reduction was about 30%. Neither higher concentrations than 0.5% nor more applications than twice a day could increase this effect. The heart rate demonstrated an average decrease of 12%, the systolic blood-pressure of 3.8% and the diastolic of 2.8%.

A comparison of Propranolol, Timolol and Bupranolol, which we tested

119

E.L. Greve, W. Leydhecker & C. Raitta (eds.), Second European Glaucoma Symposium, Helsinki 1984.
© *1985, Dr. W. Junk Publishers, Dordrecht. ISBN 978-94-010-8934-0*

only in a small orientating study, showed a slightly stronger effect of Timolol on IOP and a clearly smaller effect with regard to the undesired corneal anaesthesia. For other studies with new β-blockers we mainly used Timolol, which in the meantime appeared on the market as a reference.

Metipranolol, a non selective β-blocker without intrinsic sympathomimetic activity like Timolol, showed no difference compared to Timolol in the one-drop-curve. Multicenter cross-over studies with Metipranolol and Timolol demonstrated no statistically significant difference between IOP, blood pressure, pulse rate and corneal sensitivity.

The subjective experience of the patients showed small differences. More patients of the Metipranolol-groups reported a slight and short burning sensation after the application of the drug. But in no case was that a reason to discontinue treatment.

In another double-masked study with 45 patients randomized into three parallel groups we compared 0.5% l-Bunolol and 1.0% l-Bunolol with Timolol 0.5%. L-Bunolol eye drops — like Timolol — have only the left-turning part of the racemat. They have no receptor-selectivity and no intrinsic sympathomimetic activity. In all three groups the documented parameters such as one-drop-curve, long-term pressure-lowering effect, blood pressure, pulse rate, corneal sensitivity, tear-production, visual acuity, visual fields, biomicroscopy, ophthalmoscopy, diameters of pupils and compliance were not significantly different. Application twice a day was sufficient to achieve the best pressure-lowering effect.

Pharmacologically the next two drugs are different from those reported above. Befunolol and Pindolol have an intrinsic sympathomimetic activity.

Befunolol showed an IOP-lowering effect in the one-drop-curve, which seemed to be dose-related. The 0.25% concentration did not work as strong as the 0.5% concentration. The duration was over 12 hours. In contrast with the other drugs tested we did not find any statistically significant influence on pulse and blood pressure systolic or diastolic over a one-year period.

Referring to the other parameters there is no difference between Befunolol and the other reported drugs after 3 months and after 1 year. Comparing the 3-month results with the results after 1 year we see there is no diminuation of the effect of Befunolol on IOP in this period.

Pindolol 1.0% solution in comparison with Timolol 0.5% initially showed a smaller effect on IOP in the one-drop-curve and during the first days of treatment. After 8 weeks it reached the level of Timolol. The influence on blood pressure and pulse was not significantly different from Timolol. All other parameters showed no difference except some more allergic reactions to Pindolol. Dorow and Bleckmann (2) reported that Pindolol 1.0% eye drops did not influence the ventilation resistance, the 1-sec-capacity, the peak-expiratory flow, the thoracic volume and the inspiratory vital capacity in contrast to Timolol 0.5% eye drops. They explained the difference by the intrinsic sympathomimetic activity of Pindolol. We do not yet have experience with these parameters.

Let me try to compare the data on these different β-blocking drugs (Tables 1 and 2). The task is not easy, as the studies are different in design and in number of patients.

120

Table 1. Comparison of the effect on IOP

	Propranolol 0.5%	Timolol 0.5%	Metipranolol 0.6%	L-Bunolol 0.5%	L-Bunolol 1.0%	Befunolol 0.25%	Befunolol 0.5%	Pindolol 1.0%
One-drop-curve ΔIOP [−%] Time [H]	20 4	39 4	39 3	38.5 3	38.5 3	32 2	39 3	27.5 3
ΔIOP [−%] After 8 days	X	24.5	≙ Timolol	≙ T.	— ≙ T.	22.1	18	23
ΔIOP [−%] After 3 months	X	22	≙ Timolol	≙ T.	≙ T.	17.5	17.5	≙ Timolol
ΔIOP [−%] After 6 months	X	23	X	≙ T.	≙ T.	X	X	≙ Timolol
ΔIOP [−%] After 1 year	34.6	22	X	≙ T.	≙ T.	21	X	≙ Timolol

Table 2. Comparison of the effects on pulse, blood pressure and corneal sensitivity

	Propranolol 0.5%	Timolol 0.5%	Metipranolol 0.6%	L-Bunolol 0.5%	L-Bunolol 1.0%	Befunolol 0.25%	Befunolol 0.5%	Pindolol 1%
Δ Pulse [−%]								
After 3 months	8.5	7.0	≅ Timolol	≅ T.	≅ T.	N.S.	N.S.	≅ Timolol
After 1 year		11.5	≅ Timolol	≅ T.	≅ T.	N.S.	N.S.	≅ Timolol
Δ RR systolic [−%]								
After 3 months	N.S.	10.5	≅ Timolol	≅ T.	≅ T.	N.S.	N.S.	≅ Timolol
After 1 year		N.S.		≅ T.	≅ T.	N.S.	N.S.	≅ Timolol
Δ RR diastolic [−%]								
After 3 months	N.S.	6.7	≅ Timolol	≅ T	≅ T.	N.S.	N.S.	≅ Timolol
After 1 year		N.S.	≅ Timolol	≅ T.	≅ T.	N.S.	N.S.	≅ Timolol
Corneal Anaesthesia	+	(−)	(−)	(−)	(−)	(−)	(−)	(−)

N.S. = not statistically different from baseline
$P < 0.05$

122

If we compare the one-drop-curves we see that for Timolol, Metipranolol, l-Bunolol and Befunolol the reducation of the IOP is of the same magnitude: about 39%. Propranolol shows a minor effect of 20% and Pindolol of 27.5%.

After 8 days the effects of Timolol, Metipranolol and l-Bunolol are not statistically different. Befunolol and Pindolol are a little less efficient. After a treatment period of 1 year all substances have the same level of IOP reduction. Only Propranolol lies higher. This could be explained by the fact that none of the patients of the propanol study had been treated with a β-blocker before.

The influence on pulse and blood pressure of the tested solutions is only different for the Befunolol-group. In our studies Befunolol had no statistically significant effect on these parameters. The other drugs show a small but statistically significant depression of heart rate and blood pressure within the first 3 months.

With our method of touching the center of the cornea with a wisp of cotton, a corneal anaesthesia we only found for Propranolol. But we know that with more accurate examination techniques, such as the aesthesiometer of Draeger, an effect on the corneal sensitivity exists for the other drugs too.

In conclusion, in the documented parameters the tested solutions differ only slightly. In the future we also have to look at other parameters such as pulmonaly function to find advantages of a new β-blocker for glaucomas.

REFERENCES

1. Bleckmann, H. and Dorow, P. Die Wirkung von Timolol- und Pindolol-Augentropfen auf den intraokularen Druck und den Atemwegswiderstand. In: Krieglstein, G.K., W. Leydhecker (eds.), Medikamentöse Glaukomtherapie. Bergmann, München (1982).
2. Dorow, P. and Bleckmann, H. Die Wirkung von Timolol- und Pindolol-Augentropfen auf die großen und kleinen Atemwege bei Patienten mit chronisch obstruktiver Bronchitis. In: Krieglstein, G.K., W. Leydhecker (eds.), Medikamentöse Glaukomtherapie. Bergmann, München (1982).
3. Merté, H.-J. and Merkle, W. Propranolol-Augentropfen in der Glaukom-Dauertherapie. Klin. Mbl. Augenheilk. 177: 437−442 (1980).
4. Merté, H.-J. and Merkle, W. Timolol-Augentropfen in der Glaukombehandlung, Ergebnisse einer Langzeitstudie. Klin. Mbl. Augenheilk. 177: 562−571 (1980).
5. Merté, H.-J. (ed.). Metipranolol − Parmakologie der β-Blocker und ophthalmologische Anwendung von Metipranolol. Springer, en-New York (1983).
6. Merté, H.-J. and Stryz, J.R. Erste Erfahrungen mit dem Beta-Blocker Befunolol bei Glaukomen mit weitem Kammerwinkel in Europa. Klin. Mbl. Augenheilk. 184: 55−58 (1984).
7. Merté, H.-J., Stryz, J.R. and Mertz, M. Pindolol-Augentropfen − Halbjahresergebnisse einer Glaukomtherapie. Klin. Mbl. Augenheilk. 184: 227−232.
8. Merté, H.-J. and Stryz, J.R. Weitere Erfahrungen mit dem Beta-Blocker Befunolol bei Glaukomen mit weitem Kammerwinkel über einen Zeitraum von einem Jahr. Klin. Mbl. Augenheilk. 184: 316−317 (1984).

Authors' address:
Augenklinik und-poliklinik rechts der Isar
der Technischen Universitat
Ismaninger Strasse 22
D-800 München 80
F.R.G.

THE EFFECT OF *d*-TIMOLOL ON INTRAOCULAR PRESSURE IN PATIENTS WITH OCULAR HYPERTENSION*

EDWIN U. KEATES and RICHARD STONE

(Philadelphia, Pennsylvania)

ABSTRACT

The stereoisomer form of timolol used in the treatment of glaucoma is *l*-timolol. Although *d*-timolol is a less potent beta-adrenergic receptor blocker than *l*-timolol, several laboratory studies have found that *d*-timolol has ocular hypotensive effects. Thus, *d*-timolol may be a useful therapeutic agent for glaucoma that has fewer systemic side effects than *l*-timolol.

We conducted a randomized, double-masked, single-drop study of the effects of *d*-timolol and placebo on intraocular pressure in 34 patients with ocular hypertension. *d*-Timolol significantly lowered intraocular pressure for the six-hour duration of the study. No patients receiving the drug reported subjective side effects. There was no change in visual acuity, pupil size, or results of external ocular or slit-lamp examinations during the study. No changes in pulse rate or blood pressure were attributable to the drug.

*Paper published in full in Am. J. Ophthalmol. 98: 73–78 (1984).

E.L. Greve, W. Leydhecker & C. Raitta (eds.), Second European Glaucoma Symposium, Helsinki 1984.
© 1985, Dr. W. Junk Publishers, Dordrecht. ISBN 978-94-010-8934-0

THE EFFECTS OF TIMOLOL USE IN GLAUCOMA PATIENTS UNDER THE AGE OF 17 YEARS*

H. DUNBAR HOSKINS, Jr., JOHN HETHERINGTON, Jr.,
SCOTT D. MAGEE, RAISA NAYKHIN and CARL MIGLIAZZO

(San Francisco, California, U.S.A.)

ABSTRACT

Sixty-seven patients (100 eyes) with childhood glaucoma were treated with timolol maleate. Thirty-one eyes required additional surgery and 24 of these reinstituted timolol therapy postoperatively. In 13 eyes timolol therapy was discontinued because of successful surgery, noncompliance, complications, or lack of apparent effect. Forty eyes treated with timolol did not require additional surgery or medications. Seventy-eight percent of this group had a pressure drop; 45% had a pressure drop greater than 10 mm Hg. Timolol maleate appears to be beneficial and warranted in the treatment of pediatric glaucoma. Screening of patients for potential contraindications and making the parents aware of potential side effects are important.

INTRODUCTION

The use of timolol in the treatment of glaucoma in adults has been the subject of multiple and detailed studies which have shown that timolol is an effective and safe medication (5, 7, 9, 10). Few publications, however, are available on the use of timolol in pediatric glaucoma patients (1, 2, 3, 4, 6, 8, 11).

Olson (6) and Williams (8) each describe one instance of severe side effects in children treated with timolol. Zimmerman (11) and McMahon (4) observed complications in five children after the use of timolol, and Boger (1, 2) reports one such patient. With the exception of Zimmerman (11), these studies have short follow-up periods of 6 weeks to 14 months. Zimmerman reports four cases with follow-up periods longer than 40 months.

This study re-evaluates McMahon's (4) original population some 4 years later and includes additional cases to further understand complications and efficacy of timolol treatment in children.

*Supported by NIH Research Grant #EY01559 and by The Foundation for Glaucoma Research, San Francisco.

E.L. Greve, W. Leydhecker & C. Raitta (eds.), Second European Glaucoma Symposium, Helsinki 1984.
© 1985, Dr. W. Junk Publishers, Dordrecht. ISBN 978-94-010-8934-0

MATERIALS AND METHODS

Sixty-seven patients (100 eyes) started topical timolol therapy before the age of seventeen (Table 1). These patients include the original 38 cases reported by McMahon. Sixty-four eyes had glaucoma surgery which had failed prior to institution of timolol therapy. From patient records we noted

Table 1. Agen when timolol was started

Age	Number of eyes
NB–1 yr.	26
1–4 yrs.	16
5–8 yrs.	17
9–12 yrs.	11
13–17 yrs.	30
Total	100

Mean age $= 7.5 \pm 6.4$ years

birthdate, ocular diagnosis, glaucoma medications, and dosage of the initial timolol treatment. We also obtained the most recent IOP before stopping timolol, final or most recent timolol dosage, last number of glaucoma medications, and reason for stopping timolol.

Side effects and complications were classified as were all post treatment surgeries. In the event that timolol was not discontinued, we recorded the last available information in the chart. Table 2 summarizes the follow-up periods for these patients which ranged from 5 days to $5\frac{1}{2}$ years with a mean follow-up period of $2\frac{1}{2}$ years.

Table 2. Length of time on timolol

Length of time on timolol	Number of eyes
Less than 6 months	14
6 months– 1 yr.	13
1–2 yrs.	13
2–3 yrs.	19
3–4 yrs.	16
4–5 yrs.	14
5+ yrs.	13
Total	100

RESULTS

Of the 67 patients, seven experienced an adverse reaction to timolol (Table 3). Only two of these patients stopped the medication because of side effects. One 10-year-old boy reported a severe asthma attack following the start of timolol therapy. The other, a 17-year-old boy, had marked reduction in pulse rate. The remaining five patients suffered mild transitory reactions from

126

Table 3. Summary of complications

Type of complication	Number of children
None	60
Central nervous	4
Cardiovascular	1
Respiratory	2
Ocular	0
Total	67

timolol therapy. These included two cases of dizziness, one case each of asthma, drowsiness and hyperactivity.

Of the 100 eyes initially starting timolol therapy, 31 required additional surgery. Of those, 24 reinstituted timolol post-operatively, indicating the severity of these glaucomas.

Thirteen of the original 100 eyes had timolol discontinued because of successful surgery (7), non-compliance (2), complications (2), or lack of apparent effect (2).

Eighty-seven eyes continued timolol at the end of the study. Of these, 40 eyes had not undergone surgery and were on the same or fewer medications than prior to initiating timolol (Fig. 1). Of these, 78% had lowered IOP; 45% percent had a decrease in IOP in excess of 10 mm Hg. The average pre-timolol IOP of these 40 eyes was 30.1 ± 9.5 mm Hg with final IOP of 22.7 ± 8.5 mm Hg ($p < .001$).

DISCUSSION

Discontinuation of timolol because of side effects or complications occurred in only two of our patients. It is interesting that these two patients were those previously reported by McMahon et al. (4). We have not seen serious complications of timolol therapy since that report. We believe that this is due to the exclusion of patients with history of cardiac arrhythmias or bronchospasm as candidates for timolol therapy.

Compliance with timolol therapy has been good. Only one of the children failed to comply with timolol usage as far as we are aware. This is indicative of the generally well-tolerated nature of the drug.

It is difficult to assess efficacy in the pediatric age group. Intraocular pressure measurements are often hard to obtain and, in the very young children, must often be measured under general anesthesia. In addition, many childhood glaucomas are particularly severe, requiring multiple medications and surgeries.

To isolate the effects of timolol therapy, we identified a subset of children (40 eyes) who did not have further surgery nor did they increase medications following the start of timolol therapy (Fig. 1). Seventy-eight percent of these eyes showed evidence of reduction of intraocular pressure while 45% showed a reduction of pressure in excess of 10 mm Hg. This is a good pressure response in these difficult cases of glaucoma.

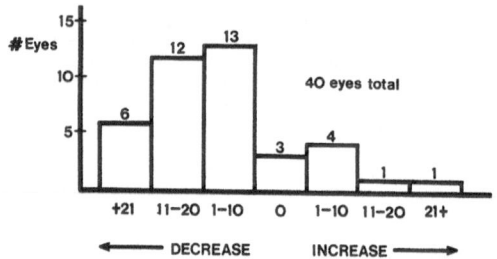

Fig. 1. Intraocular pressure response of eyes receiving timolol therapy not requiring surgery using the same or less medications.

Although we cannot state with statistical certainty that .25% timolol is as effective as .5% timolol, the majority of patients who ultimately achieved stability with timolol did so with the .25% solution. More importantly, all of the patients with complications were using the .5% solution. For these reasons, our current recommendations are to initiate therapy with the .25% solution and increase to the .5% only if the effect is not adequate. Utilization of a single drop and obstruction of the nasolacrimal passage may help reduce systemic absorption as recomended by Zimmerman (11).

Timolol maleate appears to be a safe and effective drug for the treatment of childhood glaucoma. The usual precautions of excluding patients with contraindications and using the minimal effective dosage are particularly important in the use of this drug in childhood. It is also impòrtant to notify the parents of potential side effects so they can immediately discontinue the drug should these occur.

The Food and Drug Administration has not ruled on the safety or efficacy of this drug in children, and it would seem wise to make parents aware of this. However, the sequellae of uncontrolled glaucoma are such that the advantages of this therapy, when it is effective, warrant its use.

REFERENCES

1. Boger, W.P. Timolol in childhood glaucoma. Surv. Ophthalmol. 28: 259 (1983).
2. Boger, W.P. and Walton, D.S. Timolol in uncontrolled childhood glaucomas. Ophthalmol. 88(3): 253 (1981).
3. Demailly, Ph. La place du maleate de timolol dans le traitment de l'hypertonie residuelle post-operatoire du glaucome congenital. J. Fr. Ophthalmol. 2(10): 543 (1979).
4. McMahon, C.D., Hetherington, J., Hoskins, H.D. and Shaffer, R.N. Timolol and pediatric glaucomas. Ophthalmol. 88(3): 249 (1981).
5. McMahon, C.D., Shaffer, R.N., Hoskins, H.D. and Hetherington, J. Adverse effects experienced by patients taking timolol. Am. J. Ophthalmol. 88: 736 (1979).
6. Olson, R.J., Bromberg, B.B. and Zimmerman, T.J. Apneic spells associated with timolol therapy in a neonate. Am. J. Ophthalmol. 88: 120 (1979).
7. VanBuskirk, E.M. Adverse reactions from timolol administration. Ophthalmol. 87: 447 (1980).
8. Williams, T. and Ginther, W.H. Hazards of ophthalmic timolol. N. Engl. J. Med. 306: 1485 (1982).
9. Wilson, R.P., Spaeth, G.L. and Poryzees, E. The place of timolol in the practice of ophthalmology. Ophthalmol. 87: 451 (1980).

10. Zimmerman, T.J., Baumann, J.D. and Hetherington, J. Side effects of timolol. Surv. Ophthalmol. 28: 243 (1983).
11. Zimmerman, T.J., Kooner, K.S. and Morgan, K.S. Safety and efficacy of timolol in pediatric glaucoma. Surv. Ophthalmol. 28: 262 (1983).

Authors' address:
Glaucoma Research
Clinical Eye Research Center
UC Medical Center
374 Parnassus Avenue
San Francisco, CA 94143
U.S.A.

LEVOBUNOLOL: MINIMUM CONCENTRATION REQUIRED TO CONTROL IOP IN SUBJECTS WITH PRIMARY OPEN-ANGLE GLAUCOMA OR OCULAR HYPERTENSION

E. DUZMAN, D. LONG, G. SPAETH and G.D. NOVACK

(Irvine, California, U.S.A.)

ABSTRACT

Levobunolol (LBUN) is a non-cardioselective β_1 and β_2 adrenoceptor antagonist. Topically applied LBUN has been reported to decrease IOP in subjects with primary open-angle glaucoma (POAG) for periods of up to 1 month.

We evaluated the efficacy of LBUN in 51 subjects with POAG or ocular hypertension. Subjects were washed out of antiglaucoma medications, and, in a double-masked fashion, assigned to receive LBUN (0.25, 0.5 and 1.0%) or timolol (TIM) (0.125, 0.25 and 0.5%). If the lowest concentration was inadequate to control IOP (i.e. did not decrease IOP ~ 20%), the concentration of drug was doubled, and, if required, doubled again.

Approximately 65% of subjects were controlled for 3 months at the lowest concentration of LBUN or TIM and an additional 8% at higher concentrations. Mean IOP decreases at each follow-up visit ranged from 5.4 to 8.5 mmHg, with no significant differences among treatment groups.

Untoward reactions observed with LBUN treatments were similar to those previously reported for TIM.

The results of this study suggest: a) LBUN was an effective agent for the treatment of elevated IOP, b) low concentrations of LBUN or TIM can effectively control IOP for 3 months, and c) subjects not controlled with a low concentration of a beta-adrenoceptor antagonist may not be controlled with much higher concentrations.

130

E.L. Greve, W. Leydhecker & C. Raitta (eds.), Second European Glaucoma Symposium, Helsinki 1984.
© *1985, Dr. W. Junk Publishers, Dordrecht. ISBN 978-94-010-8934-0*

LONG-TERM TREATMENT OF CHRONIC OPEN ANGLE GLAUCOMA WITH TOPICAL PINDOLOL 1%

M. GOETHALS, L. MISSOTTEN and K. WESTELINCK

(Leuven, Belgium)

ABSTRACT

This study gives the results of a six months double-blind randomised trial comparing the effect on intraocular pressure of Pindolol 1% (9 patients, 18 eyes) and Timolol 0.5% (10 patients, 20 eyes). The Pindolol patients were followed for more than six months in an open study. The intraocular pressure reduction during the first days was more pronounced with Timolol. After one month the effect of the two drugs was comparable.

The mean intraocular pressure reduction of Timolol was 10.1 mm. and of Pindolol 6.8 mm Hg.

INTRODUCTION

Beta-adrenergic blocking agents have been investigated for their ability to reduce intraocular pressure (9). One of them, Pindolol, is a non-selecting beta-blocking agent, blocking both $beta_1$ and $beta_2$ receptors. It has no local anaesthetic activity and is the only beta-blocking agent on the market with a intrinsic sympathomimetic activity (7).

Several studies has shown that Pindolol has the activity to reduce IOP for a short period (1, 2, 4, 8). The present study gives the results of six months of double-blind randomised trials comparing the intraocular pressure lowering effect of Pindolol 1%, (9 patients, 18 eyes) and Timolol 0.5% (10 patients, 20 eyes). The Pindolol patients were followed for six more months in an open study.

MATERIAL AND METHODS

Patients with open-angle glaucoma who were already being treated on topical antiglaucoma medication or were new patients were considered for the study. Patients with a history of cardiovascular disease or bronchospasm were omitted, as were patients with other ocular diseases or previous ocular surgical treatment. Nineteen patients (38 eyes) were included (12 female, 7 male; mean age: 64.4 years, S.D. 7.8). After a 10-day wash-out period for those

131

E.L. Greve, W. Leydhecker & C. Raitta (eds.), Second European Glaucoma Symposium, Helsinki 1984.
© *1985, Dr. W. Junk Publishers, Dordrecht. ISBN 978-94-010-8934-0*

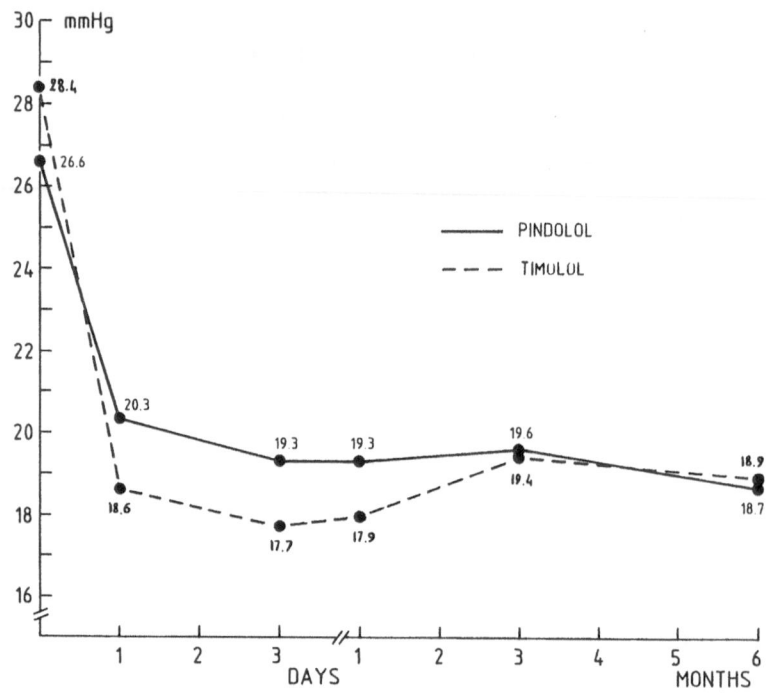

Fig. 1. Mean intraocular pressure before (day 0) and during treatment (day 1, day 3, month 3, and month 6) of 19 patients with glaucoma treated with Timolol 0.5% (dotted line) or Pindolol 1% (solid line).

patients on topical antiglaucoma treatment, a day-curve of intraocular pressures recorded at 09:00, 10:00, 13:00, and 17:00 was established for each patient. The IOP was measured at 09:00 within the next few days and treatment started either with Timolol solution 0.5% or Pindolol 1% solution applied twice daily in each eye in a double-blind procedure. On the same day, intraocular pressure was measured at 10:00, 13:00, and 17:00. All patients were reviewed at Day 3, Month 1, Month 3 and Month 6 and a day-curve established by readings at 09:00, 10:00, 13:00, and 17:00. Each time the pressure was measured twice with Goldmann applanation and the Haag-Streit slitlamp. The vital signs (sitting blood pressure and resting heart rate) were' recorded at the end of wash-out, on Day 3, Month 1, and Month 6. Visual acuity, tear production (Schirmer, cm/5 mm), the C/D ratio, corneal sensitivity, and the pupil diameter were recorded. The visual fields were measured on Day 0, Month 1, and Month 6 (Friedmann and Goldmann perimeter). The code was broken when the patient had completed six months of follow-up. Nine of the ten Pindolol patients participated in an additional 6 months of open study. All the parameters were measured at Month 9 and Month 12.

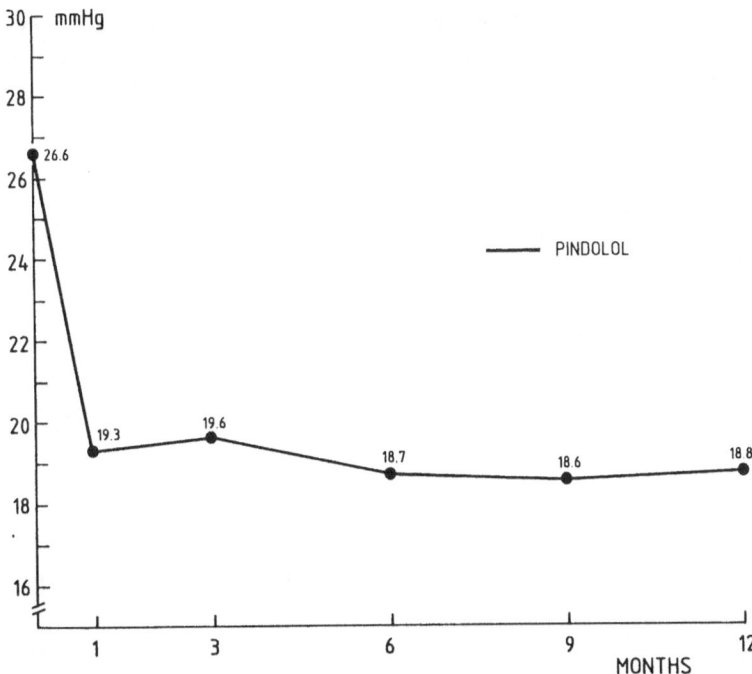

Fig. 2. Mean intraocular pressure of 9 patients with chronic open-angle glaucoma with Pindolol before and during treatment (months 1, 3, 6, 9 and 12).

RESULTS

Figure 1 gives the results of the double-blind study. All the patients showed a marked decrease of intraocular pressure on the fourth day of treatment, but less as the treatment continued. The pressure drop was slightly more pronounced in the Timolol group. All the control parameters remained the same. Figure 2 gives the results of the open study with topical Pindolol 1%. The intraocular pressure for all nine patients was under control with no additional treatment. The parameters at Month 9 and Month 12 were comparable. No local or general side effects were noted.

DISCUSSION

The purpose of the randomised double blind study and the open study was to investigate the effect of Pindolol, a beta-adrenergic blocking agent, on intraocular pressure in the treatment of chronic open angle glaucoma for a one-year period. The double blind study shows that both Pindolol and Timolol reduced intraocular pressure during the 6 month treatment period (5, 6).

No significant difference was found between Timolol 0.5% and Pindolol

1% administrated twice a day. The pressure drop the first days with Timolol 0.5% was more pronounced than with Pindolol, but after a month, the data were comparable. The mean pressure drop with Timolol was 10.1 mmHg and with Pindolol 6.8 mmHg. After six months, the mean pressure was 18.8 mmHg with both agents.

The open study with Pindolol revealed no tachyfhylaxis, and the mean pressure of the patient group remained at 18.8 mmHg.

Both preparations were well tolerated by all the patients, and no local or general side-effects were noted.

REFERENCES

1. Andreasson, S. and Jensen, K.M. Effect of Pindolol on intraocular pressure in glaucoma: pilot study and a randomised comparison with Timolol. Br. J. Ophthalmol. 67: 228–230 (1983).
2. Bonomi, L. and Steindler, P. Effect of Pindolol on intraocular pressure. Br. J. Ophthalmol. 59: 301–303 (1975).
3. Goethals, M. and Missotten, L. Long term trial of Timolol in different forms of glaucoma. Bull. Soc. belge Ophthalmol. 179: 95–101 (1977).
4. Heckenhahn, K., Levermann, H., Tauchert, A. and Wolf, A. Pindolol-Augentrophen, ein neuer beta-Rezeptorenblocker zur therapie der Weitwinkel glaukoms. Eine vergleichsstudie uber 4 Wochen Dauer. Med. Welt. 34: 676–678 (1983).
5. Rowley, S., Staunton, J.E., Tosch, A., Stewart-Jones, J.H., Edgar, D.F. and Turner, P. A non-invasive tonometer in the measurement of the effects of Pindolol and Timolol on intraocular pressure in normal subjects. Br. J. Ophthalmol. 65: 536–538 (1981).
6. Smith, R.J., Blamires, T., Nagasubramanian, S., Watkins, R. and Poinoosawmy, D. Addition of Pindolol to routine medical therapy: a clinical trial. Br. J. Ophthalmol. 66: 102–108 (1982).
7. Smith, S.E., Smith, S.A., Reynolds, F. and Whitmarsh, V.B. Ocular and cardiovascular effects of local and systemic Pindolol. Br. J. Ophthalmol. 63: 63–66 (1979).
8. Tyas, C., Stewart-Jones, J.H., Edgar, D.F. and Turner, P. The effect of 0.25% and 0.5% Pindolol on intraocular pressure in normal human volunteers. Curr. Med. Res. Opin. 7: 550–552 (1981).
9. Zimmerman, T.J. and Boger, W.P. The beta-adrenergic blocking agents and the treatment of glaucoma. Surv. Ophthalmol. 23: 347–362 (1979).

Authors' address:
Dept. of Ophthalmology
Universitair Ziekenhuis St Rafaël
Kapucijnenvoer 7
B-3000 Leuven
Belgium

MAXIMAL MEDICAL TREATED GLAUCOMA PATIENTS

M. SEFIĆ, A. PIŠTELJIĆ and R. ALAJBEGOVIĆ

(Banjaluha Sarajevo, Yugoslavia)

ABSTRACT

The study describes 64 eyes in 50 patients with primary open angle glaucoma. The intraocular pressure in these patients, despite the application of maximal tolerated medical therapy, remained above the allowed limits. In 61% of eyes we succeeded in avoiding operation by including timolol in the practised therapy, which brought down intraocular pressure to normal limits.

INTRODUCTION

Many reports have been published on the efficiency of timolol in the treatment of glaucoma. Likewise, it has already been reported that the addition of timolol to the maximal medical therapy has caused a further reduction of the intraocular pressure (1–7). The objective of this paper is to evaluate its additional hypotensive effect and how it may be used to avoid operative treatment in many patients with severe glaucoma.

MATERIAL AND METHOD

The study comprised 50 patients suffering from primary open angle glaucoma, with 64 eyes available for testing. The patients, before undergoing appropriate tests, were subjected to the most thorough examinations, such as visual acuity with and without correction, intraocular applanation pressure, size of the pupil, gonioscopy and tonography tests, detailed ophthalmoscopy of the fundus, perimetry and Schirmer's test, pulse, blood pressure and pulmonary tests.

The age of our patients ranged from 48 to 81 years, with an average of 69 years. The disease was known to exist from 7 months to 6 years (3.9 years average) and was treated with medical therapy, as shown in Table 1.

Despite this treatment the intraocular pressure in these patients remained above the allowed level, i.e., between 27 and 44 mm Hg. The mean intraocular pressure was 35.21 mm Hg. Each measurement of the intraocular pressure

135

E.L. Greve, W. Leydhecker & C. Raitta (eds.), Second European Glaucoma Symposium, Helsinki 1984.
© *1985, Dr. W. Junk Publishers, Dordrecht. ISBN 978-94-010-8934-0*

Table 1. Combinations of medication continued with addition of timolol

Medication	No. of eyes
Pilocarpine + noradrenaline	12
Pilocarpine + carbonic anhydrase inhibitors	13
Pilocarpine + noradrenaline + carbonic anhydrase inhibitors	37
Pilocarpine + carbachol + carbonic anhydrase inhibitors	2
Total	64

was made twice with a 15 minute time interval and afterwards the mean value was taken. The testing lasted for 12 months. These 'maximal' treated glaucoma patients were given timolol 0.25–0.50% solution twice a week.

RESULTS

Table 2. Results of timolol additive therapy

Ranges in IOP reduction	No. of eyes
1–5 mm Hg	19
6–10 mm Hg	27
11–15 mm Hg	15
16 mm Hg and above	3
Total	64

Table 2 shows the results produced by timolol application treatment. The mean intraocular pressure for 64 eyes was 35.21 ± 5.62 mm Hg in the pre-timolol period and 21.92 ± 7.94 mm Hg during timolol therapy.

In our study we failed to bring down intraocular pressure below 22 mm Hg in 25 eyes (39%) in spite of maximal medical treatment, which made us decide to operate on these eyes.

DISCUSSION

The results show that timolol has exercised a remarkable additional hypotensive effect in 61% of eyes that had an insufficient reaction to the existing maximal tolerated medical treatment. These patients, before undergoing timolol therapy, would have been operated. Neither sex nor age of patients had any influence whatsoever upon the concerned effect. Our results are in agreement with those of other authors such as Zimmerman (6, 7) for 50% of patients, Sonty (5) for 64.5%, Nagasubramanian (3) for 69% and Ashburn (1) for 76% and Kass (2) for 76%.

Side effects such as rhinitis catharrhalis and mild conjunctival hypaeremy, were negligible and there were no changes noticed in pulse and blood pressure.

Thanks to the combined maximal medication and timolol therapy nearly two-thirds of the patients could avoid an operation during the period of the study. Only 39% of the patients, where timolol therapy, in addition to the maximal medical one, failed to produce the desired effects, had to be treated surgically.

REFERENCES

1. Ashburn, F.S., Gillespie, J.E., Kass, M.A. and Becker, B. Timolol plus maximum tolerated antiglaucoma therapy. A one year followup study. Surv. Ophthalmol. 23: 389–394 (1979).
2. Kass, M.A. Medical therapy for glaucoma. Perspectives on current glaucoma therapy. Excerpta Med. 2: 15–24 (1980).
3. Nagasubramanian, S. The role of sympathetic beta-blocking agents in glaucoma therapy. Res. Clin. For. 2: 159–164 (1980).
4. Sefić, M. and Pišteljić, A. Djelovanje Metablena kod bolesnika refrakternih na dosadašnju terapiju. Simpozijum o beta-blokatorima u liječenju glaukoma. Proc. Series 1: 57–60 (1980).
5. Sonty, S. and Schwartz, B. The additive effect of Timolol on open angle glaucoma patients on maximal medical therapy. Surv. Ophthalmol. 23: 381–388 (1979).
6. Zimmerman, T. Basic pharmacology of some glaucoma drugs with emphasis on new developments. Glaucoma 21: 89–98 (1980).
7. Zimmerman, T.J., Gillespie, J.E., Kass, M.A., Yablonski, M.E. and Becker, B. Timolol plus maximum-tolerated antiglaucoma therapy. Arch. Ophthalmol. 97: 278–279 (1979).

Authors' addresses:
Prof. Dr M. Sefić
Prof. Dr A. Pišteljić
Eye Clinic, Medical School
Z. Korde 1
78,000 Banjaluka
Yugoslavia

Prof. Dr R. Alajbegović
Eye Clinic, Medical School
M. Pijade 12
71,000 Sarajevo
Yugoslavia

LEVOBUNOLOL: A NEW BETA-ADRENOCEPTOR ANTAGONIST FOR THE TREATMENT OF GLAUCOMA

G.D. NOVACK, E. DUZMAN, D.S. ROBINS and J.C. LUE

(Irvine, California, U.S.A.)

ABSTRACT

Levobunolol is a new non-cardioselective beta-adrenoceptor antagonist. Such agents are rapidly gaining acceptance in the treatment of elevated intraocular pressure (IOP). Levobunolol has been shown to have a long duration of action, and is well absorbed after both systemic and ocular administration, and has been reported effective for the treatment of systemic hypertension.

We compared the ocular hypotensive efficacy and systemic and ocular safety of levobunolol, 0.5% and 1.0%, b.i.d., with 0.5% timolol in two long-term double-masked studies in 463 subjects with glaucoma or ocular hypertension. Subjects received the test medication for up to 20 months.

Both concentrations of levobunolol reduced mean IOP 7–9 mmHg for up to 20 months, similar to timolol. Slight decreases in mean heart rate and blood pressure were observed. No unexpected adverse systemic or ocular reactions were reported.

The results of these studies suggest that levobunolol may be an effective therapy for the treatment of glaucoma.

E.L. Greve, W. Leydhecker & C. Raitta (eds.), Second European Glaucoma Symposium, Helsinki 1984.
© 1985, Dr. W. Junk Publishers, Dordrecht. ISBN 978-94-010-8934-0

EYE IRRITATION CAUSED BY TOPICAL BETA-BLOCKER THERAPY. A NEW METHODOLOGICAL SCREENING APPROACH

G.K. KRIEGLSTEIN and B. SCOVILLE

(Würzburg, F.R.G.)

ABSTRACT

A double blind single-dose trial screening for eye irritation caused by topical beta-blocker therapy is presented. In 36 healthy subjects eye irritation was measured, comparing carteolol, 1% and 2%, timolol, 0.5%, and balanced salt solution as a placebo reference. The evaluation was based on eye irritation scores by means of a self-evaluation analogue scale and a negative preference score. Eye irritation scores were obtained with a 10 point scale (three minutes after treatment) through observer evaluation as well. The results indicate that immediately after topical application, timolol 0.5% is more irritating than carteolol 2%, and carteolol 2% more irritating than carteolol 1%. Three minutes after treatment and 10 minutes after treatment eye irritation on self-evaluation analogue scales were not different between test solutions. It is concluded that the present screening approach is valid and informative for differentiation of topical beta-blockers in ophthalmology with respect to subjective symptoms related to the anesthetic properties of the drugs.

INTRODUCTION

Beta-blockers represent one of the cornerstones of modern antiglaucomatous drug treatment (7). These compounds do not lead to visual disturbances associated with miotics and are free from most of the adverse effects of epinephrine-like agents. They are believed to cause side effects rarely, provided high-risk patients with systemic contraindications are carefully excluded from therapy. However, there is one pharmacological property of beta-blockers which may induce irritation of the eye; the membrane-stabilizing activity or the local anesthetic character. This unfavourable effect for the human eye is peculiar to the broad spectrum of beta-blockers in a very different degree. Although many beta-blockers have been suggested to be free of a relevant local anaesthetic action on the eye, corneal hypoesthesia occurred in some of them, indicating that the threshold for the phenomenon on the eye is different from experimental models. Carteolol is one of the newer beta-blockers that is believed to have very little membrane-stabilizing activity (9). The present study was designed to test the anaesthesia-mediated side effects of carteolol

139

E.L. Greve, W. Leydhecker & C. Raitta (eds.), Second European Glaucoma Symposium, Helsinki 1984.
© *1985, Dr. W. Junk Publishers, Dordrecht. ISBN 978-94-010-8934-0*

Left eye \ Right eye	S	C 1%	C 2%	T
S		x	x	x
C 1%	x		x	x
C 2%	x	x		x
T	x	x	x	

S: BSS-Solution
C 1%: Carteolol 1%
C 2%: Carteolol 2%
T: Timolol 0.5%

Fig. 1. Treatment assignment and randomization of four different test solutions for identification of local anaesthetic side effects of different beta-blockers in comparison to the placebo solution BSS.

in comparison to timolol in terms of subjective symptoms on the basis of a self-evaluation analysis.

METHODS

The present study comprises 36 healthy volunteers for this single-dose trial. Four treatments were tested with respect to eye irritation in a double blind design: timolol 0.5%, carteolol 1% or 2%, and balanced salt solution (BSS/Alcon Pharma/Freiburg). One drop of the above preparations was applied to each eye of each subject. Balanced salt solution was used as placebo. Treatment assignment and blinding design are given in Fig. 1. After application of one drop of test solution to each eye, local irritation to the subject was measured with a self-evaluation analogue scale and a negative preference score. In the analogue scale the subject indicated with a cross his personal interpretation between no discomfort and severe irritation on a line of standard length. In the negative preference score, the subject had to decide between no difference or more discomfort either in the left or in the right eye. These self-evaluation forms were marked immediately after drug application, after 3 min and finally, after 10 min from administration. On the basis of a small number of questions 3 min after drug application, the observer provided a measure of standardization of responses across the subjects. Blood pressures and pulses were measured before treatment, 30, 60, and 120 min after treatment. Esthesiometry was performed using a Cochet-Bonnet instrument which measures corneal sensitivity in a semi-quantitative manner with a nylon filament. Westlake incomplete block design analysis was used to decide on the statistical significance of the results.

RESULTS

All subjects who had entered the study completed it. Immediately after administration of the test solutions a statistically significant effect could be noted. There was more irritation in the timolol-treated eyes than with carteolol

Table 1. Group mean scores of eye irritation after topical application of different test solutions. Mean values and standard errors of the means are presented.

Drug	Eye irritation scores (time after treatment)		
	Immediate	3 min	10 min
BSS	8.8 ± 3.5	2.8 ± 1.0	1.7 ± 0.8
Carteolol 1%	10.2 ± 3.0	8.0 ± 2.6	3.2 ± 0.9
Carteolol 2%	16.2 ± 5.2	8.7 ± 3.1	6.2 ± 2.6
Timolol 0.5%	30.1 ± 6.6	9.2 ± 3.1	5.7 ± 2.2

2%. Again, carteolol 2% was more irritating than carteolol 1%. There was no significant difference between carteolol 1% and saline solution immediately after treatment (Table 1). Three minutes and 10 min after treatment there were no significant differences among the three test solutions. Figure 2 shows the negative preference scores of eye discomfort after treatment, the subjects identifying the more painful eye by self-evaluation. The overall results of the eye irritation scores could be confirmed by this measure. Immediately after treatment, timolol 0.5% produced greater pain significantly more frequently. Again, 3 and 10 min after administration the differences were insignificant. Figure 3 illustrates the eye irritation scores after treatment on the basis of the observer's evaluation by means of a 10 point scale 3 min after treatment. There is a gradual increase in the irritation score from salt solution to carteolol 1%, to carteolol 2% and timolol 0.5%. The results concerning systemic blood pressure (systolic and diastolic) as well as pulse rates are summarized in Fig. 4. There were no statistically significant changes from baseline to post-treatment values 30 min, 60 min and 120 min after treatment.

DISCUSSION

Ocular side effects of topical beta-blocker therapy related to the membrane-stabilizing properties of these drugs are corneal anaesthesia (2, 3), punctate keratitis (1), and transitory manifestations of dry eyes syndromes (10). We found that corneal hypoesthesia associated with beta-blocker therapy (6) may limit the clinical usefulness of certain beta-blocking agents. Draeger et al. (4) used a new quantitative esthesiometer to investigate anaesthetic actions of beta-blockers and identified some subliminal anaesthesia with all the commercially available beta-blockers in ophthalmology. Even when there are no morphological changes of the corneal surface, subjective side effects like burning and foreign body sensation will signal some impact on corneal innervation. In this respect, Mertz (8) identified in a double blind crossover trial more burning sensation with metipranolol than with timolol. Pecori-Giraldi et al. (11) found a drop-out rate of 15% from propranolol long-term therapy because of the local anaesthetic properties of the drug. Carteolol eyedrops are supposed to have very little anaesthetic properties, and it was not surprising that Kitazawa et al. (5) observed essentially fewer topical side

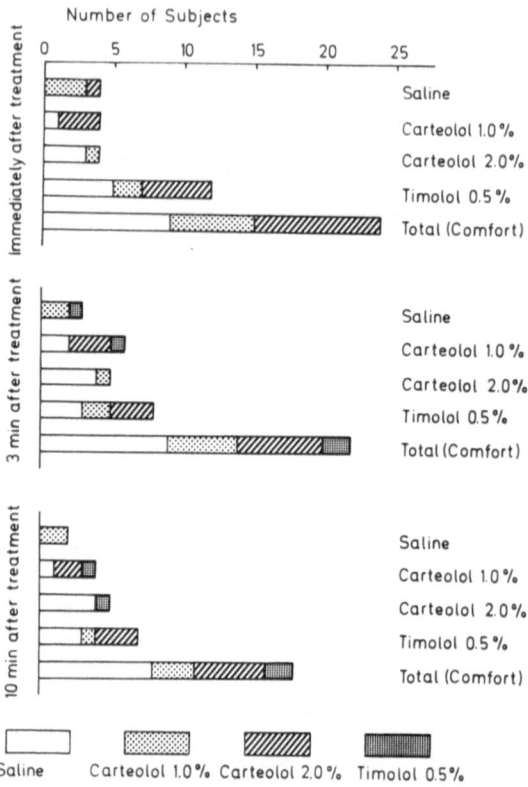

Fig. 2. The negative preference scores of eye discomfort after treatment is presented. The ordinate gives the time after treatment, the abscissa the number of subjects who identified the more painful eye by self-evaluation.

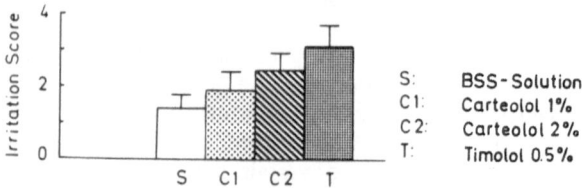

Fig. 3. The eye irritation scores after treatment by observer's evaluation using a 10 point scale three minutes after treatment. Again, the ordinate shows the irritation score, the abscissa the different test solutions.

effects with carteolol and befunolol in comparison to timolol. All these results indicate that the availability of a simple, valid screening test for the anaesthetic side effects of beta-blocker therapy is clinically very relevant. The clinical assay given in this study proved to fulfil the expectations of the therapist to expose his patients to as few problems as possible when prescribing beta-blockers for antiglaucomatous treatment. The beta-blocking

142

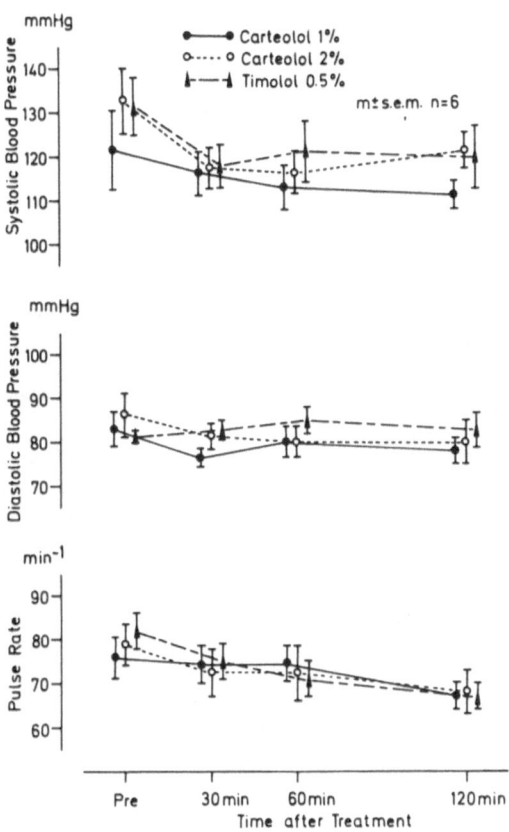

Fig. 4. The mean systolic and diastolic blood pressure and the pulse rate as found before and after treatment with carteolol 1% and 2% as well as after timolol 0.5%.

agent carteolol indeed turned out to have very little membrane-stabilizing activity on the human eye, but still a dose-dependence of local irritation could be identified, which points out the sensitivity of the test.

REFERENCES

1. Bischoff, P. Erfahrungen mit Timolol in der Glaukomtherapie. Klin. Mbl. Augenheilk. 173: 202 (1978).
2. Buskirk, van E.M. Corneal anaesthesia after timolol maleate therapy. Am. J. Ophthalmol. 88: 739 (1979).
3. Calissendorff, B. Corneal anaesthesia after topical treatment with timolol maleate. Acta Ophthalmol. 59: 347 (1981).
4. Draeger, J., Buhr-Unger, H. and Winter, R. Die Wirkung von Betarezeptoren-Blockern auf die Hornhautsensibilität. In: G.K. Krieglstein, W. Leydhecker (eds.) Medikamentöse Glaukomtherapie. J.F. Bergmann Verlag/München, 1982, pp. 195–199.
5. Kitazawa, Y., Horie, T. and Shirato, S. Ocular and systemic effects of new beta-blocking agents, Carteolol and Befunolol. In: G.K. Krieglstein, W. Leydhecker

(eds.) Medikamentöse Glaukomtherapie. J.F. Bergmann Verlag/München, 1982, pp. 183–187.

6. Krieglstein, G.K., Sold-Darseff, J. and Leydhecker, W. The intraocular pressure response of glaucomatous eyes to topically applied bupranolol. A pilot study. Albrecht V. Graefe's Arch. Klin. Exp. Ophthalmol. 202: 81 (1977).

7. Krieglstein, G.K. Betablocker-Therapie der Glaukome. In: G.K. Krieglstein, W. Leydhecker (eds.) Medikamentöse Glaukomtherapie. J.F. Bergmann Verlag/ München, 1982, pp. 29–40.

8. Mertz, M. Ergebnisse einer multizentrischen Doppelblindprüfung Metipranolol/ Timolol über 6 Wochen. In: H.-J. Merté (ed.) Metipranol. Pharmakologie der Betablocker und ophthalmologische Anwendung von Metipranolol. Springer Verlag/ Wien-New York, 1983, pp. 93–105.

9. Negishi, C., Kanai, A., Nakajima, A., Funahashi, M. and Kitazawa, Y. Ocular effects of the betablocking agent Carteolol on healthy volunteers and glaucoma patients. Jpn. J. Ophthalmol. 25: 464 (1981).

10. Nielsen, N.V. and Eriksen, J.S. Timolol induced transitory manifestations of dry eyes in long-term treatment. Acta Ophthalmol. 57: 418 (1979).

11. Pecori-Giraldi, J., Pellegrino, N. and Virno, M. Propranolol-Augentropfen in der Glaukombehandlung (fünfzehnjährige Erfahrungen) und Untersuchungen über den Wirkungsmechanismus. In: G.K. Krieglstein, W. Leydhecker (eds.) Medikamentöse Glaukomtherapie. J.F. Bergmann Verlag/München, 1982, pp. 173–178.

Authors' addresses:
Dr G.K. Krieglstein
Univ. Augenklinik
Josef-Schneider-Str. 11
D-8700 Würzburg
F.R.G.

Dr B. Scoville
Otsuka Research Office
Mainzer Landstraße 46
D-6000 Frankfurt/Main
F.R.G.

LASER TRABECULOPLASTY

PEKKA POHJANPELTO
(Lahti, Finland)

ABSTRACT

A review of the literature is presented. The technique, complications and results of the laser trabeculoplasty are discussed. Our own experiences with a follow-up from 24 months to 54 months are presented.

The first reports on laser treatment of open angle glaucoma appeared more than ten years ago (5, 8). Originally the attempt was to create holes through the trabecular meshwork leading into Schlemm's canal. Some rate of more or less long-standing success was achieved with multiple punctures covering about one quadrant of the chamber angle (6, 24, 28).

The present interest in laser treatment of open angle glaucoma arose mainly after Wise and Witter in 1979 reported on their promising experiences with multiple circumferential low-energy laser treatment without attempting to penetrate into the canal of Schlemm (35). The results were soon confirmed by others (4, 13, 20). The method has often been called laser trabeculoplasty (LTP).

The original technique of LTP is to place through a contact lens about one hundred burns all round the chamber angle into the pigmented trabecular band with a $50\,\mu$ beam diameter and 0.1 sec exposure time. The lowest power level required to produce a visible reaction in the chamber angle is used. The power setting is usually between 600 to 1800 mW.

Later some modifications were made. It seems that about 50 applications to 180° of the chamber angle decreases the pressure as effectively as the original technique with one hundred burns (22, 31). If the number of coagulations is only 25 and they are spaced to one quadrant, the effect decreases (21) but positive short-term results have also been reported (33).

The exact place of application does not influence the pressure reducing effect of LTP. Treatment of the anterior trabecular meshwork yields the same pressure lowering effect as coagulations directed at the posterior part of the trabecular meshwork (22).

The exact mechanism of pressure reduction is not known. There is histological evidence that no direct connection between the anterior chamber and

145

E.L. Greve, W. Leydhecker & C. Raitta (eds.), Second European Glaucoma Symposium, Helsinki 1984.
© *1985, Dr. W. Junk Publishers, Dordrecht. ISBN 978-94-010-8934-0*

Schlemm's canal is created with the energy levels used in LTP (18, 36). Experimental studies have shown that if such an opening is made by laser, scar formation closes the gap (23). Intraocular pressure (IOP) is not always reduced immediately after the intervention. On the contrary there may occur a transient hypertensive stage. The effect of treatment is often not seen until several weeks after LTP. In exceptional cases more than a month may elapse before the tension lowers (13).

The present view is that the coagulations produced in the chamber angle shrink immediately or on being cicatrised and thus stretch and open the surrounding, obstructed trabecular meshwork. This mechanism might also explain the success of the earlier multiple trabeculopunctures better than a creation of open channels. Be that as it may, many studies have shown that the tonographic facility of outflow improves after LTP (1, 13, 21, 26).

The reported rates of success in treating IOP in simple glaucoma with LTP are usually between 70 and 85%. The mean result of the materials presented in Table 1 is 82%. The criteria for success vary slightly among the different clinics and the results are usually based on a short-term follow-up.

Table 1. Success rates of laser trabeculoplasty. Primary open-angle glaucoma

No. of eyes	Success	%	Ref.
27	20	74	Gross & McCole 1981
35	34	97	Schwartz et al. 1981
58	49	84	Forbes & Bansal 1981
237	202	85	Thomas et al. 1982
31	29	94	Strasser & Witzmann 1982
74	59	80	Lieberman et al. 1983
76	58	76	Pohjanpelto 1983
66	52	79	Schwartz & Kopelman 1983
52	34	65	Tuulonen & Airaksinen 1983

LTP seems well adapted to the IOP lowering treatment of capsular glaucoma (Table 2). Usually the rate of success is between 75 and 90%. In some of the reports, late failures of treatment have been described, but mainly the results are based only on a short-term follow-up.

LTP treatment of secondary glaucomas has been somewhat less successful. The figures in Table 3 have been compiled from several small materials. The best results have been achieved in pigmentary glaucoma. According to available literature LTP seems to be unadapted to treatment of juvenile glaucoma. Cases of impairment after treatment have been reported (34).

Earlier, failed trabeculectomy has no unfavourable influence on the pressure reducing effect of LTP (11, 17, 21, 29). There is evidence that the outcome is not as good in aphacia as with phacic eyes (36). The old age of a patient appears to be a positive factor (21).

Little is known about the long-term results so far. In simple glaucoma the pressure reducing effect of LTP has been noted to be fully effective up to four years (36). Cases of recurring hypertension have also been described (11). This is true especially for eyes with the exfoliation syndrome (14, 15).

Table 2. Success rates of laser trabeculoplasty. Exfoliation syndrome +

No. of eyes	Success	%	Ref.
3	3	100	Schwartz et al. 1981
4	4	100	Forbes & Bansal 1982
16	12	75	Lee et al. 1982
5	5	100	Strasser & Witzmann 1982
34	33	97	Thomas et al. 1982
7	5	71	Lieberman et al. 1983
97	86	89	Pohjanpelto 1983
15	12	80	Rich & Podos 1983
4	4	100	Robin & Pollack 1983
9	8	89	Schwarz & Kopelman 1983
79	54	68	Tuulonen & Airaksinen 1983

Table 3. Laser trabeculoplasty. Success rates in secondary glaucomas

Category	No. of eyes	Success	%
Pigmentary glaucoma	75	50	67
Post-traumatic glaucoma	23	11	48
Glaucoma secondary to uveitis	27	8	30
Juvenile glaucoma	11	0	0

Figures have been collected from various small publications.

Several complications during and after LTP have been encountered.

White epithelial spots in the cornea are not rare during the procedure. They disappear within one or two days.

A small haemorrhage may occur from the application site during the intervention. The bleeding usually stops on its own and the laser procedure can be finished routinely. Some authors recommend immediate coagulation of the bleeding point with large spot size and lower power.

Transient post-laser pressure increase has been reported to appear in up to 75% of treated eyes (21). This phenomenon seems to be more common in capsular glaucoma than in simple glaucoma (13, 30). It may last from a few hours to several weeks. The reason for the post-treatment pressure increase is not known but a possible oedema of the trabecular meshwork after coagulations (13) or the influence of post-operative inflammation (19) have been postulated. Recently a histopathologic study disclosed abundant inflammatory changes and tissue debris within the trabecular meshwork of patients with elevation of IOP following LTP (3). The incidence of pressure increase can be reduced by directing the burns to the anterior part of the trabecular meshwork (21, 22, 27). Treatment of only half the angle with about 50 applications lowers the magnitude of the pressure increases and perhaps the frequency (7, 31). The transient hypertension does not essentially influence the final pressure reducing effect of LTP but individual cases of visual field deterioration have been observed (10, 26, 31).

Rare cases of persistently elevated tension after LTP have been reported.

It is possible that a small percentage of eyes are made worse by LTP (33).

Slight iritis is common after the intervention. Iritis lasting over one week is infrequent but occasional cases of prolonged uveitis leading to extensive anterior synechiae and increase of pressure have been reported (7, 33). Many surgeons use topical corticosteroid drops routinely about one week after treatment.

The reported incidence of periferal anterios synechiae ranges up to 47.5% (26). The synechiae are usually small and they have not been noted to adversely influence the pressure reducing effect of LTP.

In addition to these main complications, one more can be mentioned — cystoid macular oedema. Isolated cases have been encountered after LTP of aphacic eyes but direct connection with laser treatment has yet to be verified (7).

We have employed LTP in our clinic since May, 1979. I will present our experiences of the treatment of simple glaucoma and capsular glaucoma with follow-up periods from 24 to 54 months (mean 35 months). The method was mainly the same as Wise's but the number of burns was smaller, usually from 70 to 90 situated all round the chamber angle.

The present material consists of 94 eyes of 80 patients with simple glaucoma and 120 eyes of 108 patients with the exfoliation syndrome. The treatment was regarded as successful if the pressure level decreased at least 20% and, furthermore, if with adequate medical treatment, there were no pressure peaks over 22 mmHg.

Six months after LTP the mean pressure decrease in eyes with simple glaucoma which initially responded to treatment was about 35% (Table 4). The results obtained in various other clinics are astonishingly similar. The tension reduction in eyes with the exfoliation syndrome was about 40%.

For eyes with simple glaucoma the success rate was 72% six months after the treatment (Table 5). Medical therapy was discontinued in 20% of eyes. The results were almost unchanged at the end of the follow-up. In four eyes the pressure reincreased during the follow-up. One of these responded to repeated laser treatment, three others were classified as late failures.

In Table 6 the results are presented separately for eyes with pretreatment pressure level of 30 mmHg and over and for eyes with pressures below 30 mmHg. The pressure level of an individual eye was taken to consist of the mean value of three consecutive outpatient examinations preceding LTP during maximal tolerated medical therapy. The outcome seemed to be worse if the pretreatment pressure was high. The difference between the groups, however, remained statistically nonsignificant.

For eyes with the exfoliation syndrome the short-term results were good

Table 4. Mean tensions in eyes which initially responded to laser trabeculoplasty

Category	No. of eyes	Intraocular pressure (mmHg)	
		Before treatment	Six months after treatment
Primary open-angle glaucoma	68	25.1	16.4
Exfoliation syndrome +	114	26.8	16.0

Table 5. Results of laser trabeculoplasty. Primary open-angle glaucoma

Time after treatment	No. of eyes	Response	Failure
6 months	94	68 (72%)	26
At the end of follow-up (mean 35 months)	94	65 (69%)	29

Table 6. Pretreatment pressure level and the results of laser trabeculoplasty at the end of the follow-up. Primary open-angle glaucoma

Pressure level (mmHg)	No. of eyes	Response	Failure
< 30	80	58 (73%)	22
⩾ 30	14	8 (57%)	6

Table 7. Results of laser trabeculoplasty. Exfoliation syndrome +

Time after treatment	No. of eyes	Response	Failure
6 months	120	114 (95%)	6
At the end of follow-up (mean 35 months)	120	91 (76%)	29

Table 8. Pretreatment pressure level and the results of laser trabeculoplasty at the end of the follow-up. Exfoliation syndrome +

Pressure level (mmHg)	No. of eyes	Response	Failure
< 30	92	75 (82%)	17
⩾ 30	28	16 (57%)	12

(Table 7). Ninety-five percent responded to laser, and medical therapy was discontinued in 30% of eyes. The figures were different, however, at the end of the follow-up. The increased pressure recurred in 25 eyes. Eighteen of these were classified as late failures. Seven responded to repeated laser treatment or to reinstituted or increased medical therapy. There were in addition five eyes with one or two pressure spikes over 22 mmHg without a general rise of pressure level and according to the original criteria they were classified as failures. Still the rate of favourable response was 86% and 25% of eyes remained without medical treatment.

In Table 8 the results are presented separately according to pretreatment pressure level. Although the difference between the groups remained statistically nonsignificant, it is possible that a high pretreatment pressure level constitutes negative prediction for the final outcome. This is due to the late recurrences. These reached a total of 46% among the initial responders. In the low-pressure group, the corresponding figure was 16%. The short-term success rate was similar in the two tension groups.

Cases of recurring high pressure appeared at a steady rate during the first three years after therapy. In only one case, which was an eye with simple

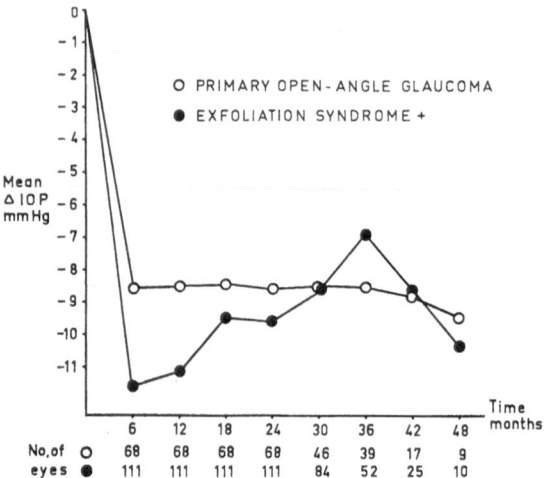

Fig. 1. Mean reductions of intraocular pressure after laser trabeculoplasty in eyes which initially responded to treatment.

glaucoma did pressure, elevation appear later, 39 months post-laser. It seems that relapses are rare after three years but no definite conclusions can be made because of the small number of eyes with such long follow-up. Only 19 eyes were observed 48 months or more.

The mean pressure decrease in eyes with simple glaucoma was constant during the follow-up (Fig. 1). For eyes with the exfoliation syndrome the mean result deteriorates gradually up to 36 months. After that the pressure decrease is better again. In most of the eyes the pressure level was quite stable over time. The rise of the curve is due to late recurrences. No new cases occurred after 36 months and the earlier relapses were partly dropped out because of an operation or pressure at a lower level with increased therapy.

No serious complications as a direct result of LTP were observed in this material. The minor complications were similar to those reported earlier. The incidence of peripheral anterior synechiae was 17%.

The pressure reducing effect of LTP seems to be rather good with few complications, but what happens to the main thing – visual fields? (Table 9). Small changes are also taken into account in these figures, and although there may be some fluctuation of the individual results, the tendency toward deterioration is quite evident. There were many eyes that showed a definite, progressive deterioration of visual fields in spite of a good pressure decrease after treatment.

Some reports describe isolated cases of field impairment due to the transient post-treatment pressure increase (10, 26, 31). In this material no evidence of connection between field loss and transient postlaser hypertension has emerged. There were 29 eyes with pressure increase of 5 mmHg or more on the day after treatment. In three of them the visual field was found to be impaired in the next examination after LTP, usually about one year

Table 9. Changes in visual fields after laser trabeculoplasty in eyes that responded to treatment

Category	No. of eyes	Unchanged	Worse	Better
Primary open-angle glaucoma	64	42	21 (33%)	1
Exfoliation syndrome +	102	60	41 (40%)	1

after treatment. This incidence does not exceed that found among the remaining patients. The pressure values were not taken hourly after the treatment, therefore some pressure peaks may have escaped notice.

LTP can be considered a safe and effective method of reducing intraocular pressure. It is well adapted to the treatment of increased 10 P in simple glaucoma and, in spite of some late failures to the reduction of 10 P in capsular glaucoma. It is also worth a try in some other forms of secondary glaucoma. The optimal mode of treatment is not known exactly but at present it seems that about 50 appiications to 180° of the anterior part of the trabecular meshwork is preferable. Long-term reports are needed before a definite estimation of the value of LTP in preventing or delaying the progress of glaucomatous damage can be made.

REFERENCES

1. Brubaker, R.F. and Liesegang, T.J. Effect of trabecular photo-coagulation on the aqueous humor dynamics of the human eye. Am. J. Ophthalmol. 96:139–147 (1983).
2. Forbes, M. and Bansal, R.K. Argon laser goniophotocoagulation of the trabecular meshwork in open angle glaucoma. Glaucoma 4:100–107 (1982).
3. Greenidge, K.C., Rodrigues, M.M., Spaeth, G.L., Traverso, C.E. and Weinreb, S. Acute intraocular pressure elevation after argon laser trabeculoplasty and iridectomy: A clinicopathologic study. Ophthalmic Surg. 15:105–110 (1984).
4. Gross, B.R. and McCole, C.E. Argon laser trabecular photocoagulation in the treatment of chronic open angle glaucoma: A preliminary report. Glaucoma 3:283–281 (1981).
5. Hager, H. Besondere mikrochirurgische Eingriffe. II. Erste Erfarungen mit dem Argon-Laser–Gerät 800. Klin. Monatsbl. Augenheilk. 162:437–450 (1973).
6. deHeer, L.J. Three years clinical application of laser trabeculopuncture (L.T.P.) in glaucomatous human eyes: Technique, indications and results. Proceedings of the 13 Hellen Ophthalmol. Congr. Glaucoma: 212–220 (1980).
7. Hoskins, H.D. Jr., Hetherington, J..Jr., Minckler, D.S., Liberman, M.F. and Shaffer, R.N. Complications of laser trabeculoplasty. Ophthalmology 90:796–799 (1983).
8. Krasnov, M.M. Laseropuncture of anterior chamber angle in glaucoma. Am. J. Ophthalmol. 75:674–678 (1973).
9. Lee, P.F., Shihab, Z.M. and Lin, Y.H. Laser trabeculoplasty in the management of open-angle glaucoma. Invest. Ophthalmol. (suppl) 22:128–132 (1982).
10. Levene, R. Major early complications of laser trabeculoplasty. Ophthalmic Surg. 14:947–953 (1983).
11. Lieberman, M.F., Hoskins, H.D. Jr. and Hetherington, J. Jr. Laser trabeculoplasty and the glaucomas. Ophthalmology 90:790–795 (1983).
12. Lunde, M.W. Argon laser trabeculoplasty in pigmentary dispersion syndrome with glaucoma. Am. J. Ophthalmol. 96:721–725 (1983).
13. Pohjanpelto, P. Argon laser treatment of the anterior chamber angle for increased intraocular pressure. Acta Ophthalmol. 59:211–220 (1981).

14. Pohjanpelto, P. Late results of laser trabeculoplasty for increased intraocular pressure. Acta Ophthalmol. 61:998–1008 (1983).
15. Rich R. and Podos, S. Laser trabeculoplasty in the exfoliation syndrome. Bull. NY Acad. Med. 59:339–344 (1983).
16. Rich, R. and Podos, S. Argon laser trabeculoplasty in secondary glaucomas. In: Frontiers in Ocular Surgery. W.B. Saunders Co, Philadelphia (in press).
17. Robin, A.L. and Pollack, I.P. Argon laser trabeculoplasty in secondary forms of open-angle glaucoma. Arch. Ophthalmol. 101:382–384 (1983).
18. Rodrigues, M.M., Spaeth, G.L. and Donohov, P. Electron microscopy of argon laser therapy in phacic open-angle glaucoma. Ophthalmology 89:198–210 (1982).
19. Ruderman, J.M., Zweig, K.O., Wilensky, J.T. and Weinreb, R.N. Effects of corticosteroid pretreatment on argon laser trabeculoplasty. Am. J. Ophthalmol. 96:84–89 (1983).
20. Schwartz, A.L., Whitten, M.E., Bleiman, B. and Martin, D. Argon laser trabecular surgery in uncontrolled phacic open-angle glaucoma. Ophthalmology 88: 203–212 (1981).
21. Schwartz, A.L. and Kopelman, J. Four-year experience with argon laser trabecular surgery in uncontrolled open-angle glaucoma. Ophthalmology 90:771–780 (1983).
22. Schwartz, L.W., Spaeth, G.L., Traverso, C. and Greenidge, K.C. Variation of techniques on the results of argon laser trabeculoplasty. Ophthalmology 90:781–784 (1983).
23. Spitznas, M. and Kreiger, A.E. Experimentelle Argonlaser-Trabekulopunktur an Rhesusaffen. Klin. Monatsbl. Augenheilk. 165:165–170 (1974).
24. Stiegler, G. Laser-Trabekulotomie und Laser-Iridektomie. Drei Jahre Erfahrung mit dem Glaukom-Research-Laser (Britt.). Klin. Monatsbl. Augenheilk. 175:333–340 (1979).
25. Strasser, G. and Witzmann, K. Laserbehandlung zur Straffung des Trabeculum corneosclerale bei Offenwinkelglaukom. (Trabekuloplastik). Klin. Monatsbl. Augenheilk. 181:411–413 (1982).
26. Thomas, J.V., Simmons, R.J. and Belcher, C.D. III. Argon laser trabeculoplasty in the pre-surgical glaucoma patient. Ophthalmology 89:187–197 (1982).
27. Thomas, J.V., Simmons, R.J. and Belcher, C.D. III. Complications of argon laser trabeculoplasty. Glaucoma 4:50–52 (1982).
28. Ticho, U. and Zaubermann, H. Argon laser application to the angle structures in the glaucomas. Arch. Ophthalmol. 94:61–64 (1976).
29. Tuulonen, A. and Airaksinen, P.J. Laser trabeculoplasty I in simple and capsular glaucoma. Acta Ophthalmol. 61:1009–1015 (1983).
30. Tuulonen, A. and Airaksinen, P.J. Laser trabeculoplasty II in secondary glaucoma and after failed trabeculectomy in primary open angle glaucoma. Acta Ophthalmol. 61:1016–1020 (1983).
31. Weinreb, R.N., Ruderman, J., Juster, R. and Zweig, K. Immediate intraocular pressure response to argon laser trabeculoplasty. Am. J. Ophthalmol. 95:279–286 (1983).
32. Weinreb, R.N., Ruderman, J., Juster, R. and Wilensky, J. Influence of the number of laser burns administered on the early results of argon laser trabeculoplasty. Am. J. Ophthalmol. 95:287–292 (1983).
33. Wilensky, J.T. and Weinreb, R.N. Low dose trabeculoplasty. Am. J. Ophthalmol. 95:423–426 (1983).
34. Wilensky, J.T. and Weinreb, R.N. Early and late failures of argon laser trabeculoplasty. Arch. Ophthalmol. 101:895–897 (1983).
35. Wise, J.B. and Witter, S.L. Argon laser therapy for open-angle glaucoma. A pilot study. Arch. Ophthalmol. 97:319–322 (1979).
36. Wise, J.B. Long-term control of adult open angle glaucoma by argon laser treatment. Ophthalmology 88:197–202 (1981).

Author's address:
Dr P. Pohjanpelto
Honkapirtinkatu 11
Lahti 95
Finland

152

COMPUTERIZED PERIMETRY BEFORE AND AFTER TRABECULOPLASTY. A STUDY OF THE SHORT-TERM EFFECT

CATHARINA HOLMIN and BIRGITTA BAUER
(Lund, Sweden)

Key words. Laser trabeculoplasty, computerized perimetry, glaucoma, short term study.

ABSTRACT

Argon laser trabeculoplasty was performed in 48 eyes with glaucomatous visual field defects. Applanation tonometry and computerized perimetry (Competer) were carried out shortly before and about one month after the treatment. A satisfying pressure control was generally achieved. There was no support of the hypothesis that an improvement of the visual field may follow a pressure reduction.

INTRODUCTION

All therapy in glaucoma is based on the idea that the intraocular pressure is too high and has to be lowered. The common opinion is that a substantial reduction of the pressure may prevent progression of visual field loss. It has even been claimed that an improvement of the visual field may follow a pressure reduction. In a study using manual perimetry Heilmann comes to the conclusion that an immediate reduction of defects may follow the administration of acetazolamid (1). However, in a controlled study based on computerized perimetry and with timolol as the pressure reducing agent no such favourable influence could be demonstrated (2).

The aim of the present study was to assess the possible influence on the visual field of an efficient and more long-standing pressure reduction. Since there is always a risk of non-compliance in medical therapy, laser trabeculoplasty which is a safe and efficient way of reducing the pressure was found to be the method of choice.

MATERIAL AND METHODS

In 48 eyes (48 patients) with glaucomatous visual field defects laser trabeculoplasty was performed. The indications for the treatment were as a rule a

153

E.L. Greve, W. Leydhecker & C. Raitta (eds.), Second European Glaucoma Symposium, Helsinki 1984.
© *1985, Dr. W. Junk Publishers, Dordrecht. ISBN 978-94-010-8934-0*

progression of the visual field loss or a high intraocular pressure ($\geqslant 30$ mm Hg) or both.

In most cases (40 eyes) pressure reducing therapy was already provided and, in order to keep the test conditions unchanged, this therapy was continued after trabeculoplasty.

Computerized perimetry and applanatory readings were performed before (mean 15 days) and in most cases about one month (mean 39 days) after trabeculoplasty. The interval between the two observations was in all cases < 3 months. A checkup of IOP was done one day as well as 2 weeks postoperatively.

With an argon laser about fifty evenly scattered burns (0.1 sec, 50 μm, 800–1000 mW) were placed in the trabecular meshwork within 180 degrees. In the first 16 eyes this procedure was repeated after one week. All eyes were treated with topical steroids during the first post-operative week.

The computerized perimeter (Competer) was used for the visual fields. All cases were well acquainted with this method previously. With the Competer the threshold values at 64 points inside 20 degrees are determined and given as numerical values. A high value corresponds to a high sensitivity and vice versa. Further a "performance" value (P) is calculated as the sum of all the 64 threshold values. With a few exceptions the IOP's represent the mean values of diurnal curves comprising three readings.

RESULTS

IOP

Preoperatively the mean IOP was 27 mm Hg (range 19–39). In all eyes but four the pressure exceeded 20 mm Hg. A significant lowering of the IOP (mean 8.96 mm Hg sem 0.68) was achieved after the trabeculoplasty. Even on the first postoperative day as well as at the two weeks control there was a minor but still significant pressure reduction (mean 7.72 sem 0.83 and mean 7.96 sem 0.80 respectively). The postoperative IOP and the extent of the pressure reduction for each eye are shown in Fig. 1.

The intervention was harmless as far as we could observe, with only a slight transitory irritation in a few cases.

Visual fields

The mean P-value was lower after the treatment than before but the difference was not significant (8.3 sem 6.47). With a mean interval between the two tests of 1.75 months this difference corresponds to a decay of 5.3 units/month.

The P-values varied from high values corresponding to small relative defects to very low values representing seriously damaged fields (Fig. 2). No correlation was found between the P-value and the P_{diff} ($P_{post} - P_{pre}$) ($r = 0.02$) which means that those with smaller defects were not better or worse off after the treatment than the more advanced cases. Further, no correlation was

154

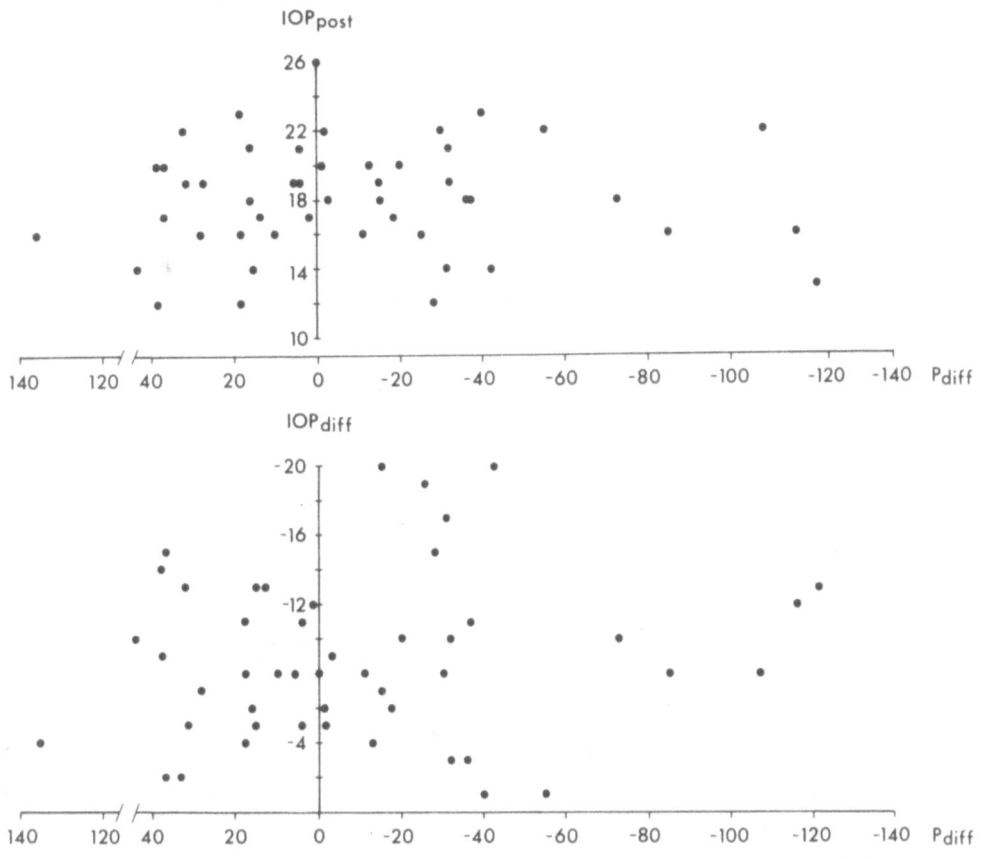

Fig. 1. Change of the performance values plotted against the postoperative IOP (above) and the pressure reduction (below) in mm Hg. A negative sign means that the P-value has been reduced postoperatively.

found between the change of the P-value (P_{diff}), neither to the extent of the pressure reduction nor to the postoperative IOP (Fig. 1).

DISCUSSION

In the present material of glaucomatous eyes the effect of laser trabeculo-plasty on the IOP was on the whole satisfactory.

Despite the pressure reduction no favourable influence on the visual field could be demonstrated. Actually we found a lower visual field performance after the treatment than before, but the difference was not significant.

Our material covered a range from small, relative to large, mainly absolute defects. The idea that a pressure reduction has a favourable effect especially in early cases, however, was not supported.

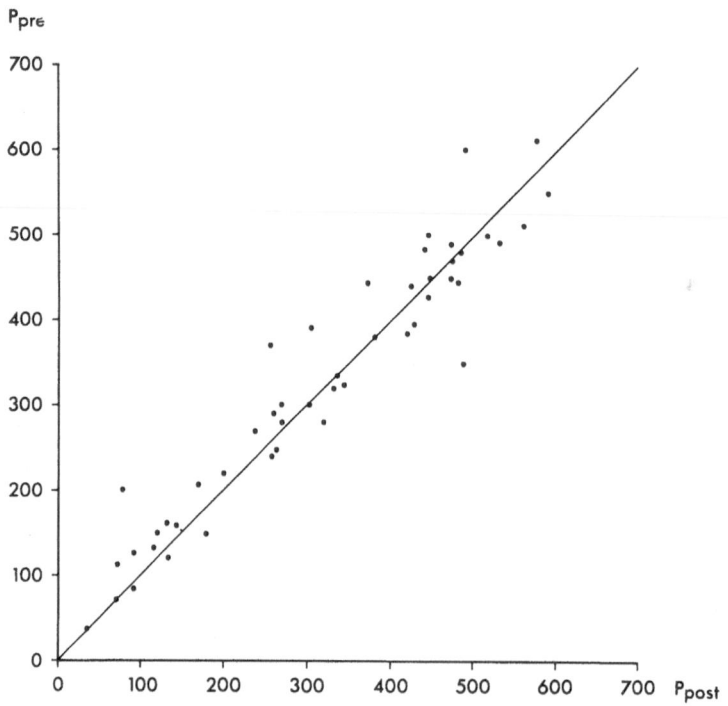

Fig. 2. Pre- and postoperative performance values. A low P value corresponds to a large defect and vice versa. Dots below the line represent fields with a higher performance after the treatment and vice versa.

A spontaneous variation in defects from time to time is in our experience more a rule than an exception in glaucoma, and if neglected this may lead an investigator astray. Certainly, in this group some cases appeared as "improvements" and others as "deteriorations". These changes showed no correlation neither to the extent of the pressure reduction nor to the pressure level and it is likely that this is merely an expression for a random variation.

To conclude: the view that there is an immediate or short-term improvement of the visual field after pressure reduction was no more supported by this study than it was by that using timolol for reducing the IOP.

REFERENCES

1. Heilmann, K. Augendruck, Blutdruck und Glaukomschaden. Buech. Augenarzt. 61, Enke, Stuttgart (1972).
2. Holmin, C. and Krakau, C.E.T. Short term effects of timolol in chronic glaucoma. Acta Ophthal. 60:337–346 (1982).

Authors' address:
Dept. of Experimental Ophthalmology
University Eye Clinic
S-221 85 Lund
Sweden

156

EFFECT OF ARGON LASER TRABECULOPLASTY IN OPEN ANGLE GLAUCOMA: OUR EXPERIENCE

CARLO E. TRAVERSO, GEORGE L. SPAETH, RICHARD J. STARITA,
RONALD L. FELLMAN, KEVIN C. GREENIDGE and EFFIE PORYZEES

(Philadelphia, Pennsylvania, U.S.A.)

ABSTRACT

Argon laser trabeculoplasty (ALT) was performed in 232 eyes of 180 patients affected by uncontrolled primary open angle glaucoma (POAG), exfoliation syndrome glaucoma (ESG) or pigment dispersion syndrome glaucoma (PDSG). Mean follow-up was 9 months (3, 22). Mean IOP change was -21.6% (± 19) from the initial value. The effect on IOP was larger in patients with ESG, PDSG, and in POAG cases with more pigmented trabecular meshwork. No relationship was found between IOP changes and age of patients. An Octopus computerized perimeter was used for pre- and post-treatment visual field tests. In 113 eyes Octopus exams met the requirements for quantitative analysis. In this group 17% of visual fields improved, 55% remained stable and 28% worsened. A good functional response was more frequent among the eyes with less advanced disease.

INTRODUCTION

Argon laser trabeculoplasty (ALT) is an effective method for lowering intraocular pressure (IOP) in primary open angle glaucoma (POAG) (1, 8, 10). Numerous investigators have reported long-lasting lowering of IOP; modifications of the original technique by Wise and Witter have been proposed in order to decrease complications (6). The purpose of this prospective study was to determine the effect of ALT on the progression of glaucomatous disease, evaluating some of the characteristics of the eye that might influence the pressure lowering effect of the procedure.

PATIENTS AND METHODS

All patients were selected from the private practice of one of the authors (G.L.S.), and entered the study after an informed consent was obtained. Indication for treatment was progressive visual field loss due to glaucoma, despite maximum tolerated medical treatment. Argon laser trabeculoplasty was performed using a Britt 152 Argon Laser in the "thermal" mode; the

157

E.L. Greve, W. Leydhecker & C. Raitta (eds.), Second European Glaucoma Symposium, Helsinki 1984.
© *1985, Dr. W. Junk Publishers, Dordrecht. ISBN 978-94-010-8934-0*

Wise technique was adopted, but with placement of the burns on the anterior portion of the trabecular meshwork. Laser settings were as follows: $50\,\mu$ diameter, 0.1 sec exposure time and 0.7–1.3 watt power. Power adjustments were made in order to keep the trabecular reaction to a blanching or to the smallest visible vapor bubble. 360 degrees of the angle were treated with 50 to 100 burns. All patients were examined 2 hours, 1 day, 1 week after laser treatment, and at an average of 3 month intervals thereafter. All were maintained on the same antiglaucoma medications, with the addition of fluorometholone topically q.i.d. for 1 week after ALT. Pre- and post-treatment visits included gonioscopy, applanation tonometry, disc drawings and/or stereophotography. When visual acuity was adequate visual fields were obtained with an Octopus computerized perimeter, using programs 31 and 32. In order to quantify visual field changes 113 eyes whose Octopus exams were not affected by pupil size changes of more than 0.5 mm, and/or visual acuity changes of more than 2 lines, and/or more than 25% false answers were selected. A visual field change was considered significant when variation of the mean quadrantic sensitivity was greater than 15% and the initial mean sensitivity was greater than 10 dB. When initial mean sensitivity was less than 10 dB a 40% change in sensitivity was required for the alteration to be considered significant.

A "better" IOP was defined as a decrease of IOP (pre-ALT minus post-ALT) greater than 2 mm Hg. A worse IOP was considered to occur when IOP rose following ALT by more than 2 mmHg. Cases in which the differences between the pre- and post-ALT IOP were less than plus or minus 3 mmHg were considered unchanged.

Mean follow-up was 9 months (min. 3, max. 22); data on patients not last examined at Wills Eye Hospital were supplied by the referring physician.

To be eligible for this study patients had to have phakic primary open angle glaucoma (POAG), exfoliation syndrome glaucoma (ESG) or pigment dispersion syndrome glaucoma (PDSG). Patients with other types of glaucoma or complicating factors were not included. Thus, those in whom an open angle glaucoma developed after a prior uveitis, or young adults with an open glaucoma but an atypical appearance of the angle, etc., were not included.

RESULTS

Tables 1 to 6 summarize the findings. Table 1 shows the average pre- and post-treatment IOP, the mean percentage change from pre-trabeculoplasty values; primary open angle glaucoma cases are separated from eyes with the exfoliation syndrome (ESG) and pigmentary glaucoma (PDSG). In Table 2, linear regression analyses of pre-treatment IOP and percentage change, and of age and percentage change are shown. The variations of hydrodynamic effects among eyes with different amounts of pigment in the 12 o'clock position of the trabecular meshwork are shown in Table 3. The distribution of cases having a percentage IOP change of more than -10% and -19% is shown in Table 4. In Table 5 and 6 are summarized visual field changes as measured with Octopus computerized perimetry.

Table 1. Intraocular Pressure (IOP) changes after Argon Laser Trabeculoplasty (ALT)

Type of glaucoma	No. of eyes	Age in years mean (SD)	Mean IOP (SD)[b]		Mean IOP Δ% (SD)[c]	F.U. (Min.–max.) in months
			pre-ALT[b]	post-ALT[b]		
POAG	186	69 (±12)	21.7 (±7.5)	17.5 (±9)	−19.5 (±19.5)	9 (3–22)
PDSG	20	54 (±10)	22 (±5.5)	15.2 (±4.4)	−30 (±11.4)	10.5 (4–21)
ESG	26	72 (±9)	27.5 (±6.5)	18.4 (+4)	−33.2 (±15.5)	9 (3–22)
Total	232	68 (±13)	22.6 (±7)	17.3 (±6)	−21.6 (±19.2)	9 (3–22)

[a] POAG = Primary Open Angle Glaucoma; PDSG = Pigment Dispersion Syndrome Glaucoma; ESG = Exfoliation Syndrome Glaucoma.
[b] mmHg by Goldmann applanation tonometry paired t-test significant (p < 0.001) for each group.
[c] IOP Δ% = percentage change from pre-treatment intraocular pressure t-test are as follows:

Total vs POAG   p < 0.02
Total vs PDSG   p < 0.01
Total vs ESG   p < 0.001

Table 2.

Effect of age on percentage intraocular pressure change (IOP Δ%) after Argon Laser Trabeculoplasty:

$$(IOP\ \Delta\% = intercept + slope\ x\ age)$$
$$IOP\ \Delta\% = 30.3476 - 0.1283\ x\ age$$
$$r^* = -0.0849 \qquad n = 232$$
$$0.5 > p > 0.1$$

Effect of pre-treatment intraocular pressure (pre-IOP) on percentage intraocular pressure change (IOP Δ%) after Argon Laser Trabeculoplasty:

$$(IOP\ \Delta\% = intercept + slope\ x\ pre\text{-}IOP)$$
$$IOP\ \Delta\% = -1.947 + 1.0313\ x\ pre\text{-}IOP$$
$$r^* = 0.3627791 \qquad n = 232$$
$$p < 0.001$$

*r = correlation coefficient

Table 3. Percentage intraocular pressure change (IOP Δ%) related to amount of pigmentation[a] of the trabecular meshwork

Amount of pigmentation	POAG[b] IOP Δ% (SD)	N	p value[c]	PDSG[b] ESG IOP Δ% (SD)	N	p value[c]
0	−12.3 (± 25)	15	> 0.5	−	0	−
1 +	−23.7 (± 21)	65	> 0.5	−22.5 (± 14)	4	> 0.5
2 +	−18 (± 21)	65	> 0.5	−32 (± 18)	19	> 0.5
3 +	−15 (± 11)	7	> 0.5	−35 (± 12)	14	> 0.5
4 +	−34.4 (± 22)	10	< 0.1	−29.5 (± 9)	9	> 0.5
Total	−19.5 (± 19.5)	186[d]		−31.5 (± 14.4)	46	

[a] As measured at the 12 o'clock position; grading is from 0 (no pigment seen) to 4 + (dark brown or black).
[b] POAG = Primary Open Angle Glaucoma; PDSG = Pigment Dispersion Syndrome Glaucoma; ESG = Exfoliation Syndrome Glaucoma.
[c] p values from student's t-test (observed value vs mean value of each diagnostic group).
[d] 24 eyes of the sample were lacking reliable informations of trabecular pigmentation.

Table 4. Distribution of eyes with IOP improvement greater than 10% or than 19%

Type of glaucoma[a]	N	IOP improvement greater than 10% N (%)	IOP improvement greater than 19% N (%)
POAG	186	47 (25)	107 (58)
ESG + PDSG	46	2 (4.5)	38 (83)
Total	232	49	145

χ^2 test with Yates' correction for continuity = p < 0.01.
[a] POAG = Primary Open Angle Glaucoma; PDSG = Pigment Dispersion Syndrome Glaucoma; ESG = Exfoliation Syndrome Glaucoma.

Table 5. Visual field changes after argon laser trabeculoplasty[a]

	No. of eyes	No. of expected variations (%)	No. of unexpected variations (%)
Worse	32	24 (75)	8 (25)
Unchanged	62	57 (92)	5 (8)
Better	19	18 (95)	1 (5)
Total	113	99 (88)	14 (12)

Mean F.U. 10 months (max. 21; min. 4).
[a]See text for definitions of unchanged, better, worse, expected and unexpected.

Table 6. Visual field changes after argon laser trabeculoplasty related to stage of the disease

	Early + medium	Advanced + far advanced	Total
Worse	7	25	32
Unchanged	35	27	62
Better	6	13	19
Total	48	65	113

x^2: $p < 0.01$.
[a] Mean IOP improvement (percentage) = 19 ($\pm$ 19).
[b] Mean IOP improvement (percentage) = 20 ($\pm$ 18).

DISCUSSION

Since Von Grafe's time, lowering of intraocular pressure has been advocated as treatment for glaucoma. Argon laser trabeculoplasty causes a decrease in intraocular pressure in a significant portion of treated patients (2, 5, 7, 9, 10). Relatively little is known regarding the factors influencing the pressure-lowering effect of ALT. The influence of this procedure on the glaucomatous visual field is also not fully understood.

In our group of patients ALT caused a significant decrease of intraocular pressure: this effect was larger in glaucoma associated with the exfoliation syndrome (ESG) and with the pigment dispersion syndrome (PDSG) than in primary open-angle glaucoma patients (POAG) (Table 1). The possible effect of age or of pre-treatment level of IOP on the result of ALT was analyzed by plotting a linear regression of these two factors (Table 2). This showed a highly significant correlation between pre-treatment IOP and percentage change in IOP, but no correlation with age. This lack of association between age and effect of ALT was found for each individual subgroup as well as for the entire population. This is surprising in view of other studies reporting contrary findings (1, 10). However, other reports may not have selected patients with the degree of diagnostic clarity employed in this study.

Another parameter evaluated was the amount of trabecular pigmentation, measured at the 12 o'clock position in the eye. When examining each diagnostic group separately there was no correlation between amount of pigment

161

and effect of ALT on IOP. The observed variations were statistically significant only for the groups of eyes with 3+ and 4+ pigmentation (P < 0.05) in the third column of Table 3. However, this probably is a factor of the higher incidence of the exfoliation syndrome and pigment dispersion glaucomas in these two groups. Less significant (P < 0.1) was the difference observed in the 4+ pigmented eyes in the primary open-angle glaucoma group.

It seems unlikely that a change in IOP less than 10% represents a biologically significant improvement. On the other hand, an IOP fall of 20% more probably signifies a meaningful change in the hydrodynamics of the eye. As readily seen by inspection of Table 4, the change of obtaining a "poorer" result is greater in POAG and obtaining a "good" result greater (a factor of 10!) in PDSG and ESG. Other studies have shown better results in EGS than POAG (7, 8). Results on PDSG published by other authors are controversial (2, 3, 7, 8). These differences may be due to variations in diagnostic criteria or in length of follow-up.

In order to assess visual field changes after argon laser trabeculoplasty, all patients with sufficient visual acuity underwent pre- and post-laser Octopus computer-assisted perimetry. Quantitative analysis of retinal sensitivity changes was considered in 113 eyes which met the requirements for selection. Since all our cases were losing visual field prior to ALT, one would expect the visual field to get worse in those in whom the IOP was not lowered significantly by ALT. An "expected" result would, therefore, be a result in which 1) IOP and visual field both got "better", or 2) IOP got "better" but visual field remained "unchanged", or 3) IOP was "unchanged" and the visual field was "worse", or 4) IOP was "worse" and visual field was "worse". "Unexpected" results would be those in which 1) IOP was "better" and visual field was "worse", or 2) IOP was "unchanged" and visual field "better", or 3) IOP and visual field were both "unchanged", or 4) IOP was "worse", and visual field was "better", or 5) IOP was "worse" and the visual field was "unchanged". As shown in Table 5, an improvement or a stabilization of the visual field was obtained in more than 2/3 of our cases. The relatively higher amount of unexpected behavior seen in the worsened group is explainable; among those eight cases, five were in "terminal" stages, and one had a temporary acute rise of pressure right after argon laser trabeculoplasty.

Table 6 shows that the result of IOP, in terms of effect on visual field, is directly related to stage of disease, the better results being obtained with those with less advanced disease.

Our data confirm that argon laser trabeculoplasty is effective in lowering intraocular pressure in open angle glaucoma. Patients with pigment dispersion and exfoliation syndrome glaucoma, as well as those with most heavy pigmentation of trabecular meshwork, showed a larger effect on IOP from ALT than those with POAG alone and with less pigment. The better response of ESG and PDSG cases observed in the full spectrum of trabecular pigmentation makes it uncertain whether better absorption of laser energy can be an influential factor. Moreover, in performing ALT the power of the laser was adjusted in order to avoid overheating of the target. This presumably lessened the influence of pigmentation. The correlation between percentage intraocular pressure fall and pre-treatment intraocular pressure level can be a mechanical consequence of the increased outflow facility caused by argon laser trabeculoplasty (4, 8), which might work more efficiently with higher pressure gradients. In this study, patients with more advanced disease had poorer functional response to ALT than patients with less advanced disease; the effect of ALT on IOP was comparable in the two groups. Although visual field changes and intraocular pressure changes did not overlap always as expected, there is a good correspondence between hydrodynamic and functional success. Therefore we can assume that eyes which fit into a category in which larger hydrodynamic effects are expected will have greater chances of having arrested the progression of their glaucoma.

REFERENCES

1. Forbes, M. and Bansal, R. Argon laser goniophoto-coagulation of the trabecular meshwork in open-angle glaucoma. Trans Am. Ophthalmol. Soc. 79:257 (1981).
2. Lunde, M.V. Argon laser trabeculoplasty in pigmentary dispersion syndrome with glaucoma. Am. J. Ophthalmol. 96:721–725 (1983).
3. Liberman, M., Hoskins, H. and Hetherington, J. Laser trabeculoplasty and the glaucomas. Ophthalmology 90:790 (1983).
4. Schwartz, A., Whitten, M., Bleiman, B. and Martin, D. Argon laser trabecular surgery in uncontrolled phakic open angle glaucoma. Ophthalmology 88:203 (1981).
5. Schwartz, A. and Kopelman, J. Four-year experience with argon laser trabecular surgery in uncontrolled open-angle glaucoma. Ophthalmology 90:771 (1983).
6. Schwartz, L.W., Spaeth, G.L., Traverso, C.E. and Greenidge, K.C. Variation of techniques on the results of argon laser trabeculoplasty. Ophthalmology 90:781–784 (1983).
7. Thomas, J., Simmons, R. and Belcher, D. Argon laser trabeculoplasty in the presurgical glaucoma patient. Ophthalmology 89:187 (1982).
8. Wilensky, J.T. and Jampol, L.M. Laser therapy for open angle glaucoma. Ophthalmology 88:213–217 (1981).
9. Wise, J. and Witter, S. Argon laser therapy for open angle glaucoma. A pilot study. Arch. Ophthalmol. 97:319 (1979).
10. Wise, J. Long-term control of adult open angle glaucoma by argon laser trabeculoplasty. Ophthalmology 88:197 (1981).

Authors' address:
Wills Eye Hospital
William and Anna Goldberg
Glaucoma Service and Research Laboratory
Ninth and Walnut Streets
Philadelphia, PA 19107
U.S.A.

ARGON LASER TRABECULOPLASTY. VARIATION OF METHODS AND IMMEDIATE COMPLICATIONS

YOSHIAKI KITAZAWA, SHIROAKI SHIRATO, TETSUYA YAMAMOTO
and SHUICHIRO EGUCHI
(Tokyo, Japan)

ABSTRACT

Argon laser trabeculoplasty (ALT) was performed in 157 eyes with primary open-angle glaucoma or capsular glaucoma. Three different methods of ALT were employed to determine if the variation of methods affects the incidence of immediate intraocular pressure (IOP) rise. Thirty-six eyes received 100 burns for 360° to the posterior trabecular meshwork and were categorized as Group 1. Group 2 comprised 84 eyes given 50 burns for 180° to the posterior meshwork. Group 3 consisted of 37 eyes treated with 50 burns for 180° to the anterior trabecular meshwork. The duration of each burn was set for 0.2 sec in Group 1 and 0.1 sec in Groups 2 and 3. The power of each burn ranged from 700 to 1000 mW in each group. The immediate postlaser IOP rise was defined as the pressure elevation exceeding prelaser value by 5 mmHg or greater. In Group 1 the incidence of IOP rise was 83% and it was 60% after the first session in Group 2. In Group 3 it was only 30%. The sustained, marked pressure rise was most frequently observed in Group 1 as compared with other two groups. Other complications including sustained iritis, peripheral anterior synechiae and hyphema were most frequently seen in Group 1 and least in Group 3. The rate of successful IOP control defined as IOP less than 20 mmHg was achieved in 39% in Group 1, 68% in Group 2 and 49% in Group 3. The follow-up period ranged from 2 to 56 months.

INTRODUCTION

Argon laser trabeculoplasty (ALT) is effective in reducing intraocular pressure (IOP) in open-angle glaucoma patients and eliminates some of the risks of filtering surgery (3, 4, 6, 7). However, ALT is not without complication. Among various complications acute elevation of IOP can be the most disastrous (1, 3–7).

In an attempt to circumvent this potentially most deleterious complication we have investigated the effect of various modifications of ALT on IOP. The purpose of the present paper is to report on the results of the study.

165

E.L. Greve, W. Leydhecker & C. Raitta (eds.), Second European Glaucoma Symposium, Helsinki 1984.
© *1985, Dr. W. Junk Publishers, Dordrecht. ISBN 978-94-010-8934-0*

MATERIALS AND METHODS

ALT was performed in 155 patients (192 eyes) with primary open-angle glaucoma or capsular glaucoma from June 1979 to February 1984. The clinical records of 129 cases (157 eyes) were analysed who met the following criteria: minimum postoperative follow-up period of 2 months, prelaser IOP of no less than 20 mmHg. ALT was indicated in the presence of sustained elevation of IOP and/or the progressive deterioration of visual field while the patients were on their maximum tolerable medication. ALT was performed using a continuous wave argon laser apparatus (Coherent Model 900). Three different methods were employed; 36 eyes received 100 burns for 360 degrees to the posterior trabecular meshwork, i.e. posterior to pigment band and anterior to scleral spur, and were categorized as group 1. Group 2 comprised 84 eyes given 50 burns for 180 degrees to the posterior trabecular meshwork. Group 3 consisted of 37 eyes treated with 50 burns for 180 degrees to the anterior trabecular meshwork, i.e. anterior to pigment band and posterior to Schwalbe's line. A 50-micron spot was used in all cases. The duration of each burn was set at 0.2 sec on Group 1 and 0.1 sec in Groups 2 and 3. The power of each burn ranged from 700 to 1000 mW. The power was selected in each eye which was just sufficient to cause a slight blanching of pigment or the smallest visible bubbles. The type of glaucoma in each treatment group is listed in Table 1. A Goldmann three mirror lens with an anti-reflective coating was used following topical administration of 0.4% benoxinate

Table 1. Type of glaucoma, number of cases (eyes)

Type	Group 1	Group 2	Group 3
Primary open-angle glaucoma	22 (29)	56 (64)	28 (32)
Capsular glaucoma	7 (7)	16 (20)	5 (5)
Total	29 (36)	72 (84)	33 (37)

Follow-up period (mo.) Group 1 – 19–56 (mean: 38)
Group 2 – 2–22 (mean: 13)
Group 3 – 2–10 (mean: 6)

drops. IOP was determined with a Goldmann applanation tonometer prior to and after 30 minutes following the ALT, and for 6 hours at one-hour intervals. The IOP was also measured 24 hours and 1 week after the ALT. When the IOP was adequately reduced, the patients were followed every week for one month. The antiglaucoma medication was kept unchanged at least for a month after the ALT. The medication was reduced, one drug at a time, when the IOP reduction appeared to be adequate. Topical betamethasone ophthalmic drops were administered only when a substantial amount of cells and flare was noted in 24 hours after the ALT. The follow-up period ranged from 2 to 56 months. When the IOP was reduced below 20 mmHg without further deterioration of visual field for at least 6 months the ALT was judged as success.

RESULTS

The initial IOP rise after the ALT

The incidence of the immediate IOP rise is given in Table 2, which was defined as the pressure elevation exceeding the prelaser value by 5 mmHg or greater. In Group 1 the incidence of IOP rise was 83% and it was 60% after the first session in Group 2 eyes. The incidence of the positive pressure rise was only 30% in Group 3, the least among the three treatment groups.

Table 2. Immediate IOP rise; number of eyes (%)

IOP rise	Group 1*	Group 2	Group 3
+	24 (83)	51 (60)	11 (30)
−	5 (17)	33 (40)	26 (70)
Total	9	84	37

*Seven eyes were excluded since the IOP was not measured on laser day.

The maximum IOP after the ALT in Group 1 eyes ranged from 17 to 67 mmHg with an average of 38.6 ± 12.9 mmHg, and it was from 15 to 57 mmHg with an average of 31.8 ± 9.0 mmHg after the first treatment session in Group 2. While the maximum IOP ranged from 16 to 38 mmHg with an average of 27.4 ± 5.3 mmHg after the first session in Group 3. The maximum IOP level was noted to be significantly higher in Group 1 than in Group 2 ($P < 0.01$). Also, it was significantly lower in Group 3 as compared with the other two treatment groups (vs Group 1; $P < 0.001$, vs Group 2; $P < 0.01$). In all three treatment groups the peak of the IOP mostly took place within 6 hours and the distribution of the peak time is given in Table 3. The interval from the ALT to the peak time tended to be shorter in Groups 2 and 3 than in Group 1.

Table 3. Immediate IOP rise; time interval to reach maximum IOP (number of eyes)

Time (hours)	Group 1		Group 2*		Group 3*	
0.5	6		26		10	
1	6		33		16	
2	5	66%	11	86%	7	95%
3	2		2		2	
4	7		5		1	
5	1		5		1	
6	2		2		0	
Total	29		84		37	

*Only the results of the first session are listed

The duration of IOP rise was expressed as the time required for recovery of the IOP to the prelaser level and it was found to vary among the treatment groups considerably. In Group 1, 18 out of 24 eyes (75%) with the positive IOP rise (5 mmHg or greater) showed the IOP recovery within 24 hours, whereas in 47 out of 51 eyes (92%) in Group 2 and all of 11 eyes in Group 3 the IOP recovered within 24 hours. The duration of IOP rise was significantly prolonged in Group 1 as compared with the two other groups (vs Group 2; $P < 0.05$, vs Group 3; $P < 0.025$).

Other complications

Iritis was found in all cases but it tended to be more intense and longer lasting in Group 1 as compared with Group 2 or 3. In Group 1, 11 out of 36 eyes (31%) developed iritis which lasted for more than one week in spite of topical administration of betamethasone. Whereas in Groups 2, 4 among 77 eyes (5%) developed sustained iritis and in Group 3 the inflammatory signs disappeared in all cases except for one (3%) within one week.

A slight anterior chamber hemorrhage was encountered in two eyes (6%) in Group 1, in one eye (1%) in Group 2 and in none of Group 3.

Peripheral anterior synechiae (PAS) tended to develop more frequently in Groups 1 and 2 as compared with Group 3. The incidence of PAS extending over more than half of the treated circumference was 6% in Group 1 or 2 and none in Group 3.

The IOP control

The pretreatment IOP was 23.9 ± 3.2 mmHg in Group 1, 24.4 ± 4.0 mmHg in Group 2 and 23.9 ± 3.1 mmHg in Group 3. Among the total of 36 eyes in Group 1, 14 eyes were successfully controlled over a period of more than 6 months; the rate of successful IOP control was 39%, while in Group 2 consisting of 84 eyes, 76 eyes were followed up over the same period of time and 52 eyes were successfully controlled during that period of time; the rate of successful control was 68%. Among 52 successfully treated eyes in Group 2, 8 eyes required the second ALT in the remainder of the angle. The difference in the rate of successful IOP control is significantly different between Group 1 and 2 ($P < 0.01$). For Group 3 the criteria for the IOP control were not applicable since the follow-up was short. However, among the total of 37 eyes, 18 eyes (49%) were controlled over a period of more than 2 months and among those three were brought under the control after the treatment of the remainder of $180°$ angle. In Groups 1 and 3 the control rate is not significantly different between primary open-angle glaucoma and capsular glaucoma, while in Group 2 the rate of successful IOP control was significantly higher in capsular glaucoma (94%) as compared with primary open-angle glaucoma (60%). The amount of medication could be reduced in six among 14 successfully controlled eyes in Group 1, in 28 among 52 successfully treated eyes in Group 2 and in one among 18 eyes in Group 3 respectively. In none of the eyes, however, could the medication be completely withdrawn.

In the above simple statistics the follow-up periods varied greatly among the cases. In addition, a considerable number of eyes had to undergo filtering surgery (trabeculectomy) and this makes it of extremely limited value to calculate the average IOP after a certain follow-up period. Consequently the

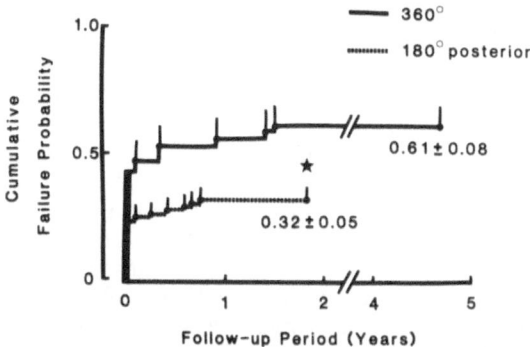

Fig. 1. Cumulative failure probability after the ALT (Kaplan-Meier method). The solid line represents Group 1 and the broken line indicates Group 2.

figure given above may not necessarily indicate the final success or failure rate. Furthermore, it is of interest to find out how the failure takes place after ALT. Therefore, the cases of Group 1 and 2 were analyzed by the life-table method of Kaplan-Meier (2). The results are illustrated in Fig. 1, where the estimated cumulative probability of failure is plotted against time after ALT. In both Groups 1 and 2 about 90% of the failure took place within 6 months. The time process of the failure is, therefore, of the early failure type in these two groups. The eyes of Group 3 were not followed up long enough to allow for this particular method of analysis on a comparable time scale. The final probability of success was calculated to be 39% at the end of 56 months for Group 1 and 68% at the end of 22 months for Group 2 respectively. The difference in the probability of success at the end of 22 months was of statistical significance between two groups (P < 0.05).

COMMENT

The IOP rise immediately after the ALT has been pointed out to be not uncommon at all if the pressure is monitored closely. A considerable IOP rise was noted after the three different methods of ALT. However, treating the whole circumference of the angle in one session (as in the Group 1) was found to induce the more pronounced and more prolonged IOP rise as compared with the treatment of the half circumference (as in the Groups 2 and 3).

A comparison between Groups 2 and 3 revealed that treating the 180° anterior meshwork (Group 3) elicits the least pronounced pressure rise with regard to duration, height and incidence. Although treating the anterior meshwork appears to be safer than the treatment of the posterior meshwork, the hypotensive effects are less favorable as compared with the treatment of posterior meshwork. The results seem to indicate that treatment of posterior trabecular meshwork over 180° in one session at a time (as in the Group 2) may be preferred to the other two methods. This statement seems to be

169

justified since a considerable number of eyes in the Group 2 responded to the treatment of the remaining 180° with a further pressure drop, while both the conventional, statistical and the life-table analyses revealed the rate of successful control and the probability of success in Group 2 to be significantly superior to those of Group 1.

Finally, the analysis of data by means of the life-table method has shown that the therapeutic effect of the ALT is of early failure type. That is, more than 90% of failures take place within 6 months in two groups of patients (Group 1 and 2) treated in accordance with the two different protocols. In other words, the favorable pressure control lasting for the postoperative 6 month-period indicates the sustained IOP control in the patient with primary open-angle glaucoma or capsular glaucoma. However, it should be stressed that the need for long-term follow-up studies remains to determine the duration of the hypotensive effect of the ALT and that the potential for late complications should be kept in mind.

REFERENCES

1. Greenidge, K., Rodrigues, M.M., Spaeth, G.L., Traverso, C.E. and Weinreb, S. Acute intraocular pressure elevation after argon laser trabeculoplasty and iridectomy; A clinicopathologic study. Ophthalm. Surg. 15:105 (1984).
2. Kaplan, E.L. and Meier, P. Non parametric estimation for incomplete observations, J. Am. Stat. Assoc. 53:457 (1958).
3. Kitazawa, Y., Shirato, S. and Yamamoto, T. Japanese study safety and efficacy of laser iridotomy, trabeculectomy, Ophthalmol. Times 6:1 (1981).
4. Shirato, S. and Kitazawa, Y. Laser therapy for open-angle glaucoma. Acta Soc. Ophthalmol. Jpn. 84:2101 (1980).
5. Shirato, S., Yamamoto, T. and Kitwazawa, Y. Argon laser trabeculoplasty in open-angle glaucoma. Jpn. J. Ophthalmol. 26:374 (1982).
6. Thomas, J.V., Simmons, R.J. and Belcher III, C.D. Argon laser trabeculoplasty in the presurgical glaucoma patient, Ophthalmology 89:187 (1982).
7. Wilensky, J.T. and Jampol, L.M. Laser therapy for open-angle glaucoma, Opthalmology 88:213 (1981).

Authors' address:
Dept. of Ophthalmology
University of Tokyo School of Medicine
Tokyo, Japan

Dr. Kitazawa is presently with the
Dept. of Ophthalmology
Gifu University School of Medicine
Gifu, Japan

170

EARLY AND LATE EFFECTS ON INTRAOCULAR PRESSURE OF THE TREATMENT MODE OF LASER TRABECULOPLASTY

M. TERÄSVIRTA, K. NERDRUM and E. TUOVINEN

(Kuopio, Finland)

ABSTRACT

Two hundred and fifty eyes of 188 patients underwent argon laser trabeculoplasty (ALT). One hundred and twenty eyes had primary open-angle glaucoma and 130 eyes had pseudoexfoliation glaucoma. The patients were randomly assigned to four treatment groups. The follow-up periods ranged from 7.1 to 10.2 months. During this period there was no statistically significant difference in the average drop of IOP between the groups. There was a highly significant difference between the two types of glaucoma in the pressure-lowering effect of ALT, pseudoexfoliation glaucoma having the greater reduction of pressure. Furthermore, there was a statistically significant reduction of variation of the average IOP-readings after ALT in all but one group, as judged by diminished standard deviation values of the average IOP-readings.

INTRODUCTION

Intraocular pressure varies somewhat even in non-glaucomatous eyes, and in glaucomatous patients the diurnal variation has been reported to reach values as high as 18 mm of mercury (1).

Argon laser trabeculoplasty, ALT, has been shown to reduce the average IOP significantly (4, 8, 9). ALT has also been reported to moderate the diurnal pressure curve of glaucomatous eyes (2).

The number of burns administered during ALT has been shown to correlate with eventual postoperative rise of IOP (6, 7).

In a study by Schwartz et al. (5), the technique of performing ALT did not influence the magnitude of the fall of average IOP, nor did it have any effect on the frequency of post-laser complications.

According to Wise and Witter (9) IOP does not change significantly within the first week after ALT.

The present study was undertaken to assess the effect of the technique of performing ALT on the mean IOP and on a few other parameters of two types of open-angle glaucoma.

171

E.L. Greve, W. Leydhecker & C. Raitta (eds.), Second European Glaucoma Symposium, Helsinki 1984.
© *1985, Dr. W. Junk Publishers, Dordrecht. ISBN 978-94-010-8934-0*

MATERIALS AND METHODS

Two hundred consecutive patients with either primary open-angle glaucoma (POAG) or pseudoexfoliation glaucoma, treated with ALT between November 1981 and September 1983, were included in the study. Twelve patients were later excluded, seven because of having to undergo trabeculectomy and five because of inadequate follow-up. Follow-up was ruled insufficient if ophthalmological records were not available from the six-month period preceding trabeculoplasty, or if the difference of the number of pre- and post-operative visits exceeded two. The patients were randomly assigned to four treatment groups. The characteristics of the groups are listed in Table 1.

Table 1. Treatment groups

Group	No. of eyes treated		No. of burns	Location of burns	Circum-ference	Average follow-up (months)		Average age of patients	
	r.e.	l.e.				r.e.	l.e.	r.e.	l.e.
I	44	54	100	Post. tm[a]	360°	9.4	10.2	69.8	69.6
II	39	37	50	Post. tm	180°	7.4	7.3	70.1	71.4
III	22	17	100	Ant. tm[b]	360°	7.5	7.1	72.2	67.2
IV	17	20	50	Ant. tm	180°	7.3	7.4	63.4	72.8

[a] Post. tm = posterior trabecular meshwork.
[b] Ant. tm = anterior trabecular meshwork.

The patients were treated as outpatients using the continuous-wave argon-krypton laser by Lasertek. The power settings and the spot size were in accordance with the protocol laid down by Wise (9). The first postlaser visit took place one week after ALT. During the first three months of this study corticosteroids were used locally, but this regime was abandoned as unnecessary after that period.

The following parameters were analyzed: (1) The mean IOP from the six-month period preceding ALT-treatment; (2) the standard deviation of the mean pre-operative IOP; (3) IOP after one week from treatment; (4) the mean IOP during postlaser follow-up; (5) the standard deviation of the post-treatment mean IOP; (6) the glaucoma medication prior to and following ALT; and (7) the effect of the length of the follow-up period on standard deviations.

RESULTS

The pressure responses in each group are listed in Tables 2 and 3, together with data concerning pre- and post-operative medication.

Paired two-tailed T-test was performed to detect any statistically significant changes in standard deviations pre- and post-operatively. In all groups but one (group II) there was a significant to highly significant reduction.

172

Table 2. Pressure response after argon laser trabeculoplasty (right eye)

Group	IOP pre-treatment average mmHg	SD of IOP pre-treatment	Long-term change in IOP		Change in IOP after one week		SD of IOP post-treatment	Medic-ation pre-ALT	Change in medic-ation
			mmHg	%	mmHg	%			
I	25.9	4.9	8.0	30.9	7.7	29.7	2.7***	2.3	0.9
II	25.4	3.8	6.7	26.4	5.0	18.7	3.2	2.2	0.7
III	26.5	5.3	7.1	26.8	6.4	24.2	3.0***	2.2	0.8
IV	25.5	4.0	6.1	23.9	4.7	18.4	2.5*	1.7	0.3

***$p < 0.001$
*$p < 0.05$ paired two-tailed T-test

Table 3. Pressure response after argon laser trabeculoplasty (left eye)

Group	IOP pre-treatment average mmHg	SD of IOP pre-treatment	Long-term change in IOP		Change in IOP after one week		SD of IOP post-treatment	Medic-ation pre-ALT	Change in medic-ation
			mmHg	%	mmHg	%			
I	25.6	4.6	8.5	33.2	7.4	28.9	2.4***	2.4	1.0
II	24.7	4.1	6.7	27.1	4.7	19.0	3.0	2.2	0.6
III	23.8	4.5	5.3	22.3	5.4	22.7	2.4*	2.4	0.7
IV	23.2	3.8	5.6	24.1	6.0	25.9	2.8*	2.3	0.4

***$p < 0.001$
*$p < 0.05$ paired two-tailed T-test

The fall of IOP is significant for each group separately but no significant differences were found between groups on this point.

Table 4 lists some characteristics of the treated eyes when the two glaucoma types and both sexes are considered separately.

Table 4. Characteristics of treated eyes

	Men				Women			
	Primary open-angle glaucoma		Pseudoexf. glaucoma		Primary open-angle glaucoma		Pseudoexf. glaucoma	
	r.e.	l.e.	r.e.	l.e.	r.e.	l.e.	r.e.	l.e.
IOP Pre-ALT mmHg	24.9	24.8	27.4*	23.6	24.5	25.5	26.5	25.5
Change in IOP %	22.9	22.4	33.7**	31.6*	19.5	22.1	29.5**	32.5**
No. of eyes treated	34	30	21	24	25	31	42	43
Average age of patients	65.7	65.1	72.4**	71.2*	68.7	71.7	71.9	72.4

**$p < 0.01$
*$p < 0.05$ two-tailed T-test

The change of IOP is significantly greater in the pseudoexfoliation group for both sexes, as would be expected. The men in the pseudoexfoliation glaucoma group are significantly older than the men in the POAG-group but the same does not hold true for women, for reasons unknown to the authors. The difference of reduction of both IOP and standard deviations is enhanced when both sexes and all treatment groups are considered together (Table 5).

Table 5. Pressure response in twotypes of open-angle glaucoma

	Primary open-angle glaucoma		Pseudoexfoliation glaucoma	
	Right eye N = 59	Left eye N = 61	Right eye N = 63	Left eye N = 67
IOP Pre-treatment average mmHg	24.7	24.7	26.8*	24.8
Long-term change in IOP (%)	21.5	22.3	30.9***	32.2***
SD of IOP pre-ALT	4.3	3.9	4.8	4.4
SD of IOP post-ALT	2.7***	3.0*	3.1***	2.8***

***$p < 0.001$
*$p < 0.05$ two-tailed T-test and paired two-tailed T-test

Because the follow-up periods varied from 3 to 20 months, it seemed feasible — and almost necessary — to test the influence of the length of the follow-up period on the standard deviation figures. Analysis of variance and covariance failed to disclose any statistical significance for the follow-up period (significance of F gt. 5).

DISCUSSION

If standard deviation is accepted as a gauge for measuring the variation of IOP-readings, then this study would point to a moderating effect of ALT on not only the diurnal curve, as shown previously (2), but also on day-to-day variation of IOP in glaucomatous eyes.

The medication offers a point worth considering. Although the differences between pre- and post-operative medication were not dramatic, several patients do well without medication and quite a few do well on just one drop twice a day. It has been shown, although with relatively few data, that glaucoma patients comply better with medication given twice daily than with medication requiring several applications per day (3). This could be a contributing factor, although very hard to prove.

Our results are not entirely in accordance with those of Wise and Witter (9), in that our data show a distinct fall of pressure already at one week level.

Because the first postlaser visit was scheduled one week after ALT, the immediate influence of the number of burns administered can not be accounted for. A one week level, however, there are no significant differences between groups with unequal number of burns.

174

The relatively short follow-up precludes conclusions about possible differences between various techniques of ALT in the distant future, but at the present time it seems reasonable to consider all four treatment modes as equally acceptable.

REFERENCES

1. Drance, S.M. The significance of the diurnal tension variations in normal and glaucomatous eyes. Arch. Ophthalmol. 64:494–501 (1960).
2. Greenidge, K.C., Spaeth, G.L. and Fiol-Silva, Z. Effect of argon laser trabeculoplasty on the glaucomatous diurnal curve. Ophthalmology 90:800–803 (1983).
3. MacKean, J.M. and Elkington, A.R. Compliance with treatment of patients with chronic open-angle glaucoma. Br. J. Ophthalmol. 67:46–49 (1983).
4. Schwartz, A.L. and Kopelman, J. Four year experience with argon laser trabecular surgery in uncontrolled open-angle glaucoma. Ophthalmology 90:771–780 (1983).
5. Schwartz, L.W., Spaeth, G.L., Taverso, C. and Greenidge, K.C. Variation of techniques on the results of argon laser trabeculoplasty. Ophthalmology 90:781–784 (1983).
6. Weinreb, R.N., Ruderman, J., Juster, R. and Zweig, K. Immediate intraocular pressure response to argon laser trabeculoplasty. Am. J. Ophthalmol. 95:279–286 (1983).
7. Weinreb, R.N., Ruderman, J., Juster, R. and Wilensky, J.T. Influence of the number of laser burns administered on the early results of argon laser trabeculoplasty. Am. J. Ophthalmol. 95:287–292 (1983).
8. Wilensky, J.T. and Jampol, L.M. Laser therapy for open angle glaucoma. Ophthalmology 88:213–217 (1981).
9. Wise, J.B. and Witter, S.L. Argon laser therapy for open-angle glaucoma; a pilot study. Arch. Ophthalmol. 97:319–322 (1979).

Authors' address:
Dept. of Ophthalmology
Kuopio University Central Hospital
70210 Kuopio 21
Finland

GONIORETRACTION VS. TRABCULOPLASTY

A. BECHETOILLE and G. JALLET

(Angers, France)

Argon laser trabeculoplasty(ALT) has become within a few years of existence one of the most popular procedures in the treatment of chronic open angle glaucoma (5). Although ALT is quite efficient, there are complications. According to Rodriguez and Spaeth (4) corneal endothelial cell proliferation is induced by the energy of Argon laser beams acting close to the endothelial cells of the cornea.

In 1981, we began exploring a different procedure that we have called Argon laser gonioretraction (ALG), with reference to the Cairns surgical goniospasis (2). While the trabeculum is the target for Argon laser in ALT, the beams in ALG are directed toward the ciliary band in an attempt to get the scar of the burn to pull backward the scleral spur and stretch the trabeculum a bit like pilocarpine does, but permanently.

The procedure was first used from 1981 to 1983 in 43 chronic open angle glaucoma patients with a fairly high rate of success in decreasing intraocular pressure on a one year basis and an acceptable rate of complications of undesirable side effects. (These data are in press (1, 3).)

The aim of the present paper was to compare ALG and ALT in a prospective randomized study. To achieve this goal, 20 eyes were treated on a randomized basis either by ALG (group I/n = 11) or by ALI (group II/n = 9), i.e. by directing the Argon laser beams either toward the ciliary band or the trabeculum. The treatment was applied to primary open angle glaucoma patients (POAG) with intraocular pressure (IOP) controlled by one or most often several medications.

Due to the hazards of randomisation, the two groups of patients were not exactly identical before laser treatment in the sense that ALG was statistically applied to less severe POAG patients than ALT. This prevented us from obtaining statistical comparisons on the post-treatment status by standard tests. However, it appears more than probable from examining the data with the Mann-Whithney test that ALG is at least as effective in lowering IOP as ALT and that this equal efficiency lasts during the first 3 months after laser treatment.

Complications were at a low rate in both groups:
— A questionnaire revealed that the pain level during the laser treatment was comparable.

E.L. Greve, W. Leydhecker & C. Raitta (eds.), Second European Glaucoma Symposium, Helsinki 1984.
© *1985, Dr. W. Junk Publishers, Dordrecht. ISBN 978-94-010-8934-0*

– The IOP elevation during the first 8 hours and the first day post-treatment was in the same range within the two groups: peaking in one hour and returning to the pre-treatment level in about 6 hours and lower than the pretreatment level after 24 hours.

– No visual field changes were observed in any of the treated patients whatever the group.

– There were no angle hemorrhages.

– The rate of peripheral anterior synechias was comparable within the two groups. However, most of the synechias in the ALG were more peripheral involving only once the trabeculum of Schlemm's canal zone versus twice in the ALG group.

In conclusion:

– Both ALG and ALT lowered IOP and/or permitted a reduction in medical treatment during the 3 month follow-up period.

– Due to the fact that the two groups were not homogenous and that the sampling was not large enough, it was not possible to show the superiority of one of the two methods over the other.

– The complication rate of the two groups was similar, especially concerning the amplitude and the duration of the early post-treatment increase in IOP.

– There is a tendency for anterior peripheral synechias to be smaller and more peripheral in ALG than in ALT.

– Finally, there is a need for more sophisticatedly designed studies to discover the advantage of one method over the other. This may be important since ALG may at least theoretically, induce less corneal cell proliferation over the trabeculum.

REFERENCES

1. Béchetoille, A. and Jallet, G. Le gonioretroction au laser à Argon. Journal Français d'Ophtalmologie (in press).
2. Cairns, J.E. Goniospasis, eine Methode die zur Erthlasting der kanalblockage bei primarem Weitwinkelglackom entwickelt wurde. Klin. Mbl. Augenheilk. 165:549–554 (1974).
3. Desormeaux, A. Une méthode de traitement du glaucome chronique à angle ouvert par le laser à argon. Thèse médecine, Angers, 1982.
4. Rodrigues, M.M., Spaeth, G.L. and Donohoo, P. Electron microscopy of argon laser therapy in phakic open-angle glaucoma. Ophthalmology 89:198–210 (1982).
5. Wise, J.B. and Witter, S.L. Argon laser therapy for open angle glaucoma, a pilot study. Arch. Ophthalmol. 97:319–322 (1979).

Authors' address:
Centre Hospitalier et Universitaire d'Angers
Service d'Ophtalmologie
4 rue Lavey
49040 Angers Cedex
France

CYCLOTRABECULOSPASIS – A NEW AND SIMPLE METHOD OF LASER TREATMENT IN GLAUCOMA

M.M. KRASNOV

(Moscow, U.S.S.R.)

ABSTRACT

Different methods of glaucoma treatment by laser have their specific indications, and taken together, can be considered a kind of "system". A new method of the so-called laser cyclotrabeculospasis was developed for use in open-angle simple glaucoma. The anterior surface of the ciliary body (seen gonioscopically) is coagulated by a conventional (argon-gas) laser close to the scleral spur. Tractional pull onto the trabeculum and the inner wall of Schlemm's canal is a probable explanation for hypotensive effect of the procedure and the improved aqueous outflow. There is no risk of serious complications. The laser cyclotrabeculospasis was used clinically to limit the use of surgery, but potentially the method may also have some advantages over therapy by drugs.

INTRODUCTION

Several methods of glaucoma treatment are nowadays used routinely in our clinical practice. These are: 1) laser iridectomy, 2) laser goniopuncture, 3) laser gonioplasty, 4) laser photomydriasis, 5) laser trabeculoplasty (after Wise), and 6) laser cyclotrabeculospasis (after Krasnov). Each has its own specific indications. On the whole more than 2,000 glaucoma patients have been treated in our practice over the past 13 years.

We started to use laser in open-angle glaucoma only for those cases in which surgery appeared unavoidable. Currently, laser is used much more widely, in practice whenever medication is insufficient. This progress is partly due to the development of a new procedure called "laser cyclotrabeculospasis". This paper deals especially with this particular method.

The term "laser cyclotrabeculospasis" originated from the surgical procedure of goniospasis (after J. Cairns) because their ways of action appear to be similar in principle. The treatment is carried out with the aid of conventional (for instance, argon-gas) laser coagulators. The laser beam is directed to the anterior surface of the ciliary body which can be seen by gonioscopy. As is known, the anterior part of the ciliary body is closely linked to the trabecular zone. The pull of its muscle is an important factor, influencing the

179

E.L. Greve, W. Leydhecker & C. Raitta (eds.), Second European Glaucoma Symposium, Helsinki 1984.
© *1985, Dr. W. Junk Publishers, Dordrecht. ISBN 978-94-010-8934-0*

rate of aqueous flow through the filtering region. Coagulation of the anterior portion of the ciliary body is followed by contraction of the tissue, and so a certain pull is, admittedly, transmitted to the trabeculum. The same may also as a force opening Schlemm's canal if it is collapsed. In some of our patients we could see the blood entering Schlemm's canal immediately at the moment of coagulation and corresponding exactly to its place.

The anterior surface of the ciliary body was treated (coagulated) at 90 to 100 points around all its circumference (usually, in 2–3 sessions) close to the scleral spur. The focal spot was usually 50. The intensity of laser beam should be sufficient to produce a visible coagulation spot. A second row of coagulation can be useful at the anterior border of the trabecular band. In some patients this region is not accessible by gonioscopy. If this is the case the procedure of the so-called laser gonioplasty can be very helpful; the iris is coagulated at its root and then it immediately recedes, uncovering the surface of the ciliary body.

A fall in the intraocular pressure is commonly seen in the first days following the procedure. It usually takes two to three weeks before the tension becomes more or less stable at a certain level, and this is the time to assess the immediate effect of the procedure.

RESULTS

The average hypotensive effect was 10.2 ± 4.2 mm Hg. When the initial value of IOP does not exceed 34 mm Hg the probability of tension control is about 65%; when the tension is higher than 35 mm Hg the rate of success ranges from 37 to 50%. The medication could be stopped completely in 31% of patients after the laser cyclotrabeculospasis; in about 42% the intensity of the therapy by drugs could be reduced. The value of "C" (coefficient of outflow) increased at the end of the first month by 76%, at the end of the sixth month by 114%, at the end of one year by 106%.

A randomized study (V.S. Akopian et al,) has been carried out to compare the effect of laser cyclogoniospasis and laser trabeculoplasty (after Wise) in open-angle glaucoma. The laser procedure (trabeculoplasty or cyclotrabeculospasis) has been chosen randomly ("by tossing a coin"). The treatment itself as well as the follow-up have been carried out by different specialists. Ninety-eight patients have been (and still are being) followed to compare the clinical value of laser trabeculoplasty after Wise (52 patients) and laser cyclotrabeculospasis after M.M. Krasnov (48 patients). The results for the moment are as follows:

– Intraocular pressure before and after laser trabeculoplasty after Wise (Maklakov tonometer)

   Before: 34.42 ± 4.18 mm Hg
   After: 21.73 ± 2.33 mm Hg

– Hypotensive effects of laser trabeculoplasty (after Wise) and laser cyclotrabeculospasis (after Krasnov)

   Laser trabeculoplasty: -12.7 ± 3.25 mm Hg
   Laser cyclotrabeculospasis: -10.2 ± 4.2 mm Hg

The changes in the outflow (as detected by tonography) were also very similar.

Laser cyclotrabeculospasis may (at least, theoretically have some advantages over laser trabeculoplasty, because trabeculum itself is not coagulated and there is no danger of its subsequent scarring. Laser cyclotrabeculospasis is preferable when the pigmentation of the trabeculum is slight or absent.

On the whole the laser cyclotrabeculospasis method appears to be quite promising. The injury to the treated eye is almost negligible, and in practice there is no danger of serious complications. Potentially, this kind of treatment has a strong advantage not only over glaucoma surgery, but also over medical treatment, since the hypotensive effect thus produced is more constant (there is no problem of maintaining a sufficient level of drug concentration inside the eye).

Author's address:
Dr. M.M. Krasnov
State University for Eye Diseases
5 Pogodinskaja st.
Moscow 119435
U.S.S.R.

THE IMMEDIATE IOP RESPONSES AFTER NEODYMIUM YAG LASER IRIDOTOMY IN THE HUMAN EYE

W. SCHREMS, O. EICHELBRÖNNER and G.K. KRIEGLSTEIN

ABSTRACT

Acute IOP rises immediately after laser surgery on the anterior segment of the eye are very common in clinical practice. However, very little is known about high-energy, short-pulse lasers like the Neodymium YAG and the hemostasis of IOP. Since the Argon laser causes thermal effects whereas the YAG laser mediates its effects via tissue disruption one could expect essential differences. To elucidate the phenomenon in a qualitative and quantitative manner, YAG laser iridotomy was performed in a series of cataractous eyes prior to surgery. Using an airjet tonometer without anaesthesia careful follow-up of IOP before and after the laser procedure was possible. The IOP levels of the treated eyes were recorded 60, 40, 20 and 5 min before 20, 40, 60, 80, 100 and 120 min after laser surgery. Considerable IOP rises occurred after the iridotomy, which could be influenced in a preventive therapeutic way. Results and cinical implications are discussed in detail.

E.L. Greve, W. Leydhecker & C. Raitta (eds.), Second European Glaucoma Symposium, Helsinki 1984.
© *1985, Dr. W. Junk Publishers, Dordrecht. ISBN 978-94-010-8934-0*

ARGON LASER TRABECULOPLASTY IN CHRONIC OPEN ANGLE GLAUCOMA

V. LJUBOJEVIĆ and Z. KULJAČA
(Belgrade, Yugoslavia)

ABSTRACT

Sixty-three eyes with clinically uncontrolled open angle glaucoma underwent argon laser trabeculoplasty (ALT). Forty-seven of the 63 eyes or 74.6% were clinically controlled with pressures averaging less than 21 mm Hg. The length of the follow-up in these series ranged from 16 to 28 months, with an average of 22 months. ALT provides a safe and effective method in the management of open angle glaucoma prior to filtration surgery.

INTRODUCTION

The use of the laser in an attempt to improve aqueous outflow has been studied in numerous centers around the world since the early 1970's (1, 2, 3, 4, 5, 6, 7).

During the last three years, Wilensky and Weinreb (5) Wise (7) and Kuljača and Ljubojević (8) have reported results confirming Wise's original report (6) of success with 360° ALT.

The purpose of this study was to determine prospectively the effect of the Wise technique of ALT on results and complications.

MATERIALS AND METHODS

Sixty-three eyes with clinically uncontrolled open angle glaucoma underwent argon laser (Rodenstock, LPK — 80) trabeculoplasty (ALT). It should be stressed that all patients had uncontrolled intraocular pressure (IOP), despite maximum tolerated medical therapy and were candidates for filtration surgery.

According to Wise and Witters' treatment protocol (6) a spot size of 50 microns, was used, with a duration of exposure of 0.1 sec and a power setting of 800–1500 mm. 80–120 burns were applied to the pigmented posterior trabecular meshwork, spaced over the 360 degrees of the angle.

The power level used produced coagulation spots and occasional bubbles. Careful attention was given to precise focus with a minimum-sized laser spot.

183

E.L. Greve, W. Leydhecker & C. Raitta (eds.), Second European Glaucoma Symposium, Helsinki 1984.
© *1985, Dr. W. Junk Publishers, Dordrecht. ISBN 978-94-010-8934-0*

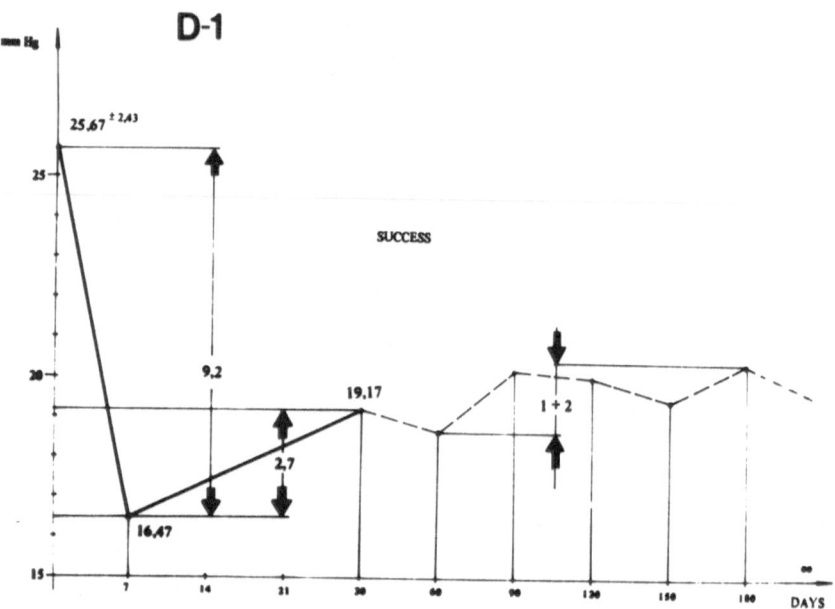

Fig. 1. Graph showing the IOP course in eyes successfully treated with ALT.

RESULTS

1. Among the 63 eyes in this series, 47 eyes or 74.6% have avoided surgery (group I).

    The average reduction of the pressure obtained after ALT was 6.5 mm Hg. (Fig. 1) (25.67 mm Hg–6.5 mm Hg = 19.17 mm Hg, after one month).
2. In the failure group (16 eyes or 25.4% – group II) the mean reduction of pressure after ALT was 2.0 mm Hg (Fig. 2) (26.1 mm Hg–2.0 mm Hg = 24.1 mm Hg, after one month).
3. The greater the decrease of IOP during the first week after ALT, the better the prognosis.

    If the decrease amounts to 25% or more of the original IOP, it is highly likely that ALT will be successful (Fig. 3).
4. No changes in glaucoma medication were made after ALT. In eyes with substantial reduction of IOP (40%) glaucoma medication was reduced (Fig. 4).

DISCUSSION

Our patients responded to ALT in a manner similar to that described by other investigators.

In the present study group of 63 eyes with a mean follow-up of 22 months we found a success rate of 74.6%.

184

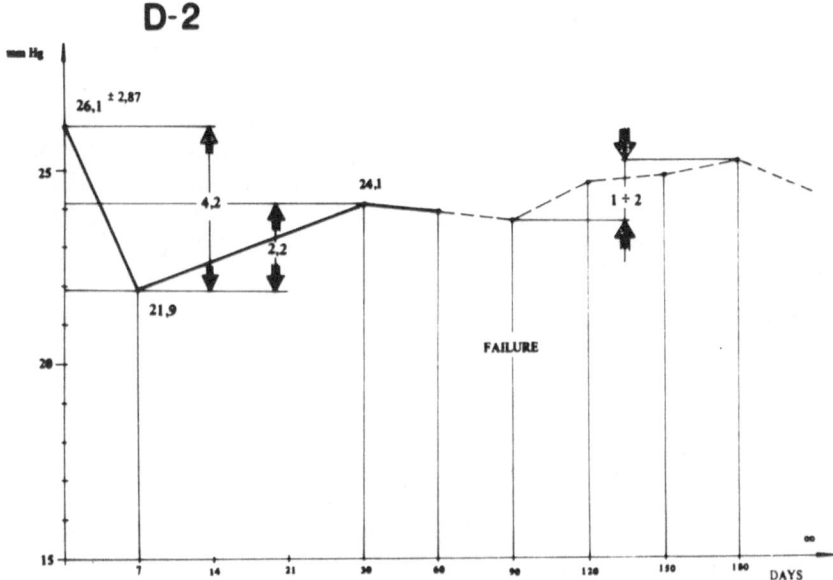

Fig. 2. Graph showing the IOP course in the failure group.

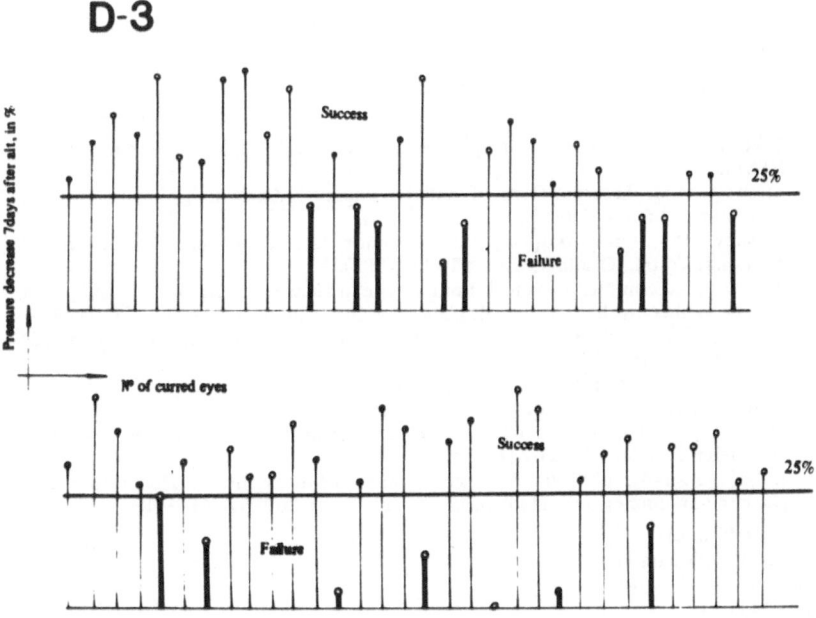

Fig. 3. IOP decrease 7 days after ALT.

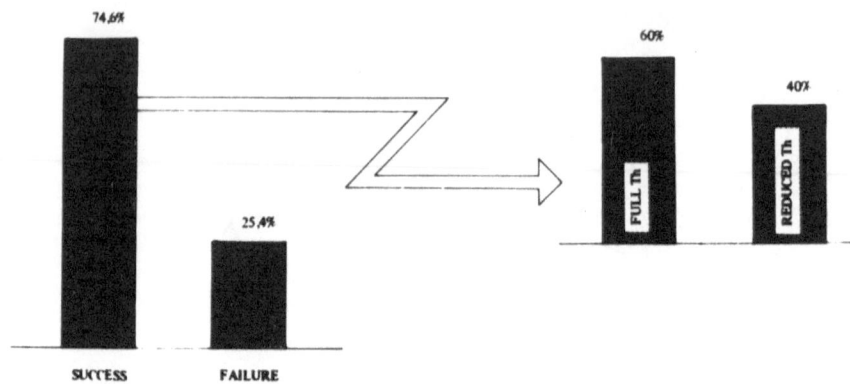

Fig. 4. Changes in glaucoma medication after ALT.

The mean peak pressure in this group fell 25% after treatment. This reduction was beneficial.

Sixty percent of the patients were given maximum medication after ALT; in 40% therapy was reduced.

In the failure group, reduction of pressure were less than 25% of the pre-laser IOP.

Early IOP elevations in five eyes, mild uveitis in two eyes and goniosynechia in three eyes, did not result in any permanent visual loss.

Visual field deteriorations were not obtained.

According to our results, one month is sufficient for evaluation of ALT treatment.

REFERENCES

1. Boyd, F.N. Laser treatment of open angle glaucoma. Highlights Ophthalm. 17:1–9 (1981).
2. Krasnov, M.M. Laserpuncture of anterior chamber Angle in glaucoma. Am. J. Ophthalm. 75:674–678 (1973).
3. Krasnov, M.M. and Akopjan, V.S. Lasernoe lecenie pervicnoj otkritougolnoj glaukomi. Vestnik Oftalmologii 5:18–22 (1982).
4. Schwartz, A.L. and Kopelman, J. Four years experience with Argon-laser trabecular surgery in uncontrolled open angle glaucoma. Ophthalmology 90:771–781 (1983).
5. Wilensky, J.T. and Weinreb, R.N. Low dose trabeculoplasty Am. J. Ophthalm. 95: 423–426 (1983).
6. Wise, J.B. and Witter, S.L. Argon laser trabeculotomy for open angle glaucoma – A pilot study Arch. Ophthalm. 97:319–322 (1979).
7. Wise, J.B. Long term control of adult open angle glaucoma by argon laser treatment. Ophthalmology 88:197–202 (1981).
8. Kuljača, Z. and Ljubojević, V. Argon laser trabekuloplastika mlečenju hroničnog glaukoma otvorenog ugla. Medicinska istraživanja. 16, 1-2, 57–61, 1983.

Authors' addresses:
Institute of Ophthalmology
Clinic – Hospital Center
Baje Sekulića 172
11000 Belgrade
Yugoslavia

LASER-PROPHYLAXIS OF NEOVASCULAR GLAUCOMA

F.M. HONRUBIA, P. GRIJALBO, L. GOMEZ, E. ALBALAD and J. OLIVAN
(Zaragoza, Spain)

ABSTRACT

The clinical histories of 42 patients diagnosed as having ischemic occlusion of the central vein of the retina, have been checked retrospectively between the years 1977 and 1982.

A total of 22 eyes were treated with the panretinian photocoagulation technique, and only 2 eyes (9%) developed neovascular glaucoma. Another group of 20 patients, with the same clinical characteristics, were not photocoagulated, and 11 eyes (55%) developed neovascular glaucoma.

We conclude that prophylactic panretinian photocoagulation in patients with ischemic C.R.V.O. is justified. This is confirmed by the angiofluoresceinic study of the retina and the electrophysiological study by the E.R.G.

INTRODUCTION

In a recent revision of the literature on neovascular glaucoma in C.R.V.O. (4), it has been concluded that the incidence of neovascular glaucoma in ischemic C.R.V.O. is 40–60%, the time of appearance varying from days to weeks after the vascular accident, although in the majority of the cases it appears before 4–5 months have passed. The incidence of simple chronic glaucoma is very high (greater than 50%) in these patients, with an average age of about 65–70 years. It also occurs more frequently in males (67%). The high incidence of cardio-vascular systemic illnesses, particularly hypertensive illness and cardiovascular arteriosclerosis, has also been studied in these patients.

On analyzing the clinical information of the patients included in our study, we see similarities with the information published by other authors (4, 8): more frequent in males, average age of 64 years, high incidence of cardio-vascular systemic illnesses (45%) and high percentage of simple chronic glaucoma (38%).

On analyzing the group of non-photocoagulated patients, the similarities are even greater. The incidence of neovascular glaucoma (55%) is compatible with the figure published by other authors, as is its time of appearance (9 of

187

E.L. Greve, W. Leydhecker & C. Raitta (eds.), Second European Glaucoma Symposium, Helsinki 1984.
© *1985, Dr. W. Junk Publishers, Dordrecht. ISBN 978-94-010-8934-0*

the 11 cases were seen before 6 months of evolution of the retinian occlusive illness had passed).

In conclusion, we think that given the high incidence of neovascular glaucoma in ischemic C.R.V.O., the inefficacy of its treatment once it has developed and the difficulty which arises in establishing an early diagnosis of the ocular neovascularization, prophylactic panretinian photocoagulation in ischemic C.R.V.O. is justified. The diagnosis of this type of occlusion is based on a angio-fluoresceinic study which shows a great extension of retinian ischemia, and in electrophysiological exploration, where a greatly diminished b wave appears in the E.R.G. and even a flat E.R.G., which shows a diffuse ischemia at level of the middle layers of the retina.

Neovascular glaucoma is a serious complication which can develop in eyes which have suffered from the occlusion of the central vein of the retina (C.R.V.O.) (1). Recent studies, both clinical and experimental, have suggested that a correlation exists between the extension of retinian ischemia and the evolutionary development of ocular neovascularization into neovascular glaucoma (2, 13). The differentiation within the clinical pattern of obstruction of the central vein of the retina between the easily prognosticated, non-ischemic type and the more difficult to prognosticate, ischemic type (called haemorrhagic retinopathy by Hayreh (3)) has been important. The development of neovascular glaucoma is more frequent in eyes that have suffered from the occlusion of the central vein of the ischemic type retina, with results of about 40—60% when no prophylactic treatment is carried out (8, 12).

In the same way as panretinian photocoagulation has shown its efficacy in the prevention of the development of the neovascular glaucoma in eyes with diabetic retinopathy with strong ischemic component (5), there is recent evidence that shows the prophylactic efficacy of the retinian photocoagulation in eyes with obstruction of the central vein of the ishemic-type retina (11, 14).

The object of this paper is to present the results obtained in a retrospective study of 42 eyes diagnosed as having ischemic occlusion of the central vein of the retina. The ocular and systemic clinical characteristics of the patients included in the study are analyzed, comparing the incidence of neovascular glaucoma in the group of eyes prophylactally treated with panretinian photocoagulation with the group of non-photocoagulated eyes.

MATERIAL AND METHODS

The clinical histories of 42 patients diagnosed as having ischemic type occlusion of the central vein of the unilateral retina in our Service between 1977 and 1982 were reviewed: 30 were male and 12 female, between 46 and 85 years of age, with an average age of 64 years.

Of the 42 patients, 16 (38%) were diagnosed as having simple chronic glaucoma, or the diagnosis was established on studying the retinian vascular accident. The incidence of cardiovascular systemic illness was also high, and

188

was detected in 19 patients (45%) arterial hypertension being the most common.

Of the 42 patients included in the study, panretinian photocoagulation therapeutics were practiced on 22 patients, according to the technique already published by us (5); on the remaining 20 patients the therapeutics were exclusively of medical pharmacological.

The retrospective review of the clinical histories was carried out to valuate the incidence of neovascular glaucoma in both groups of eyes, determining in the photocoagulated eyes the time which has passed between the presentation of the retinian vascular accident and the panretinian photocoagulation. In eyes which had progressed to neovascular glaucoma, the time between the retinian vascular accident and the development of the neovascular glaucoma was determined with the maximum precision possible.

RESULTS

Of the 42 eyes (72 patients) with ischemic occlusion of the central vein of the retina, 22 eyes (22 patients) were treated by panretinian photocoagulation.

Of the 22 patients, 17 were male and 5 female, with ages ranging between 46 and 79 years, with an average age of 60 years. Cardio-vascular systemic illnesses were diagnosed in 10 patients (45%) and the existence of a simple chronic glaucoma was detected in 5 patients (23%).

The photocoagulation technique was carried out in the majority of the eyes after a month had passed since the diagnosis of retinian vascular accident in 14 eyes; in 4 eyes after 2 months; photocoagulation was only carried out on 4 eyes after 3 months.

In the post-photocoagulation control time of these eyes, which has varied from between a minimum of 1 year and a maximum of 5 years, a neovascular glaucoma has only developed in 2 eyes (9%) (Table 1).

Table 1. Prophylaxis of neovascular glaucoma. Ischemic C.R.V.O.

No. of eyes photocoagulated	22
Average age	60 years
Systemic illnesses	10 patients (45%)
Simple chronic glaucoma.	5 patients (23%)
Time of photocoagulation	
1 month	14 eyes
2 months.	4 eyes
3 months.	4 eyes
No. of eyes neovascular glaucoma.	2 eyes (9%)

The remaining 20 patients were not photocoagulated and the therapeutics administered were exclusively medical, with mainly vasodilating medicines. This group comprised 13 male patients and 7 female patients, with ages ranging between 46 and 85, with an average age of 68 years. Nine of these patients (45%) had cardio-vascular systemic illnesses, and 11 patients (55%) had simple chronic glaucoma.

During the 5 control years of these patients, 11 of the eyes (55%) have developed a neovascular glaucoma, whose appearance has varied from less than 3 months for 5 eyes, from 3 to 6 months for 4 eyes, and 6 months after the retinian vascular accident for the 2 remaining eyes (Table 2).

Table 2. Prophylaxis of neovascular glaucoma. Ischemic C.R.V.O.

No. of eyes not photocoagulated	20
Average age	68 years
Systemic illnesses	9 patients (45%)
Simple chronic glaucoma.	11 patients (55%)
No. of eyes neovascular glaucoma.	11 eyes (55%)
Time of appearance	
Before 3 months	5 eyes
Before 6 months	4 eyes
More than 6 months	2 eyes

COMMENTS

Neovascular glaucoma is very difficult to treat, and once it has developed, it has no efficient medical treatment (10). The most sophisticated surgical techniques manage to keep a blind eye, without pain, and only in rare exceptions can a very limited visual function be maintained (6, 7).

In the opinion of some authors, the only efficient prophylactic therapeutics of the neovascular glaucoma is the panretinian photocoagulation (9, 11, 14), especially in those cases with ischemic C.R.V.O. It has been demonstrated that more than 90% of the neovascular glaucomas, after the C.R.V.O. appear in ischemic occlusions, the risk being in extension of the retinian ischemia and its duration (9).

REFERENCES

1. Gatner, S. and Henkind, P. Neovascularization of the iris. Surv. Ophthalmol. 22: 291 (1978).
2. Glaser, B.M. The demonstration of angiogenic activity from ocular tissues. Ophthalmology 87:440 (1980).
3. Hayreh, S.S. So called "central retinal vein occlusion". Ophthalmologica 172:1 (1976).
4. Hayreh, S.S., Rojas, F. and Podhjsky, P. Ocular neovascularization with retinal occlusion. Ophthalmology 90:488 (1983).
5. Honrubia, F.M., Albalad, E., Oliván, J. Gómez, L. and Grijalbo, P. Profilsaxis del glaucoma neovascular en diabéticos. Arch. Soc. Esp. Oftal. (in press).
6. Honrubia, F.M., Gómez, L., Hernández, A. and Grijalbo, P. Long-term results of silicone tube in filtering surgery for eyes with neovascular glaucome. Am. J. Ophthalmol. (in press).
7. Krupin, T. and Kaufman, P. Long-term results of valve implants in filtering surgery for eyes with neovascular glaucoma. Am. J. Ophthalmol. 95:775 (1983).

8. Magargal, L.E. and Brown, G.C. Neovascular glaucome following central retinal vein obstruction. Ophthalmology 88:1095 (1981).
9. Magargal, L.E. and Brown, G.C. Efficacy of panretinal photocoagulation in preventing neovascular glaucoma. Ophthalmology 89:780 (1982).
10. Pastor, J.C. El glaucoma. Profilaxis y tratamiento. Arch. Soc. Esp. Oftal. 44:1 (1983).
11. Sedney, S.C. Photocoagulation in retinal vein occlusion. Doc. Ophthalmol. 40:1 (1976).
12. Sinclair, S.H. Prognosis for rubeosis iridis in central retinal vein occlusion. Br. J. Ophthalmol. 63:735 (1979).
13. Smith, R. Neovascularization in ocular disease. Trans. Ophthalmol. Soc. U.K. 81: 145 (1961).
14. Tasman, W. and Magargal, L.E. Effects of Argon Laser photocoagulation on rubeosis and angle neovascularization. Ophthalmology 87:400 (1980).

Authors' adress:
Servicio de Oftalmologia
Hospital Miguel Servet
Zaragoza, Spain

OCULAR EFFECT ON NEODYMIUM-YAG LASER*

A.A. KHODADOUST, ARKFELD, J. CAPRIOLI and M.L. SEARS
(New Haven, Connecticut, U.S.A.)

ABSTRACT

To evaluate the effect of the YAG-laser on the anterior segment of the eye we have aimed the neodymium-YAG laser step-wise fashion from air to the anterior portion of the vitreous in experimental animals. The effect on corneal endothelium, the lens, and on the dynamics of intraocular fluid was studied.

Corneal endothelial damage was seen as far as 3.5 mm away from the optical breakdown of laser. The degree of endothelial damage was inversely proportional to the distance from the optical breakdown, and the pattern for a given distance was the same whether the optical breakdown was anterior or posterior to the corneal endothelium.

A single application of four millijoules power of YAG Laser causes disintegration and liquifaction of the lens cortex in a spherical area $300\,\mu$ in diameter and extends posteriorly for a distance of $450\,\mu$. The effect of optical breakdown denatures the surrounding cortical fibers for an area of $50-80\,\mu$.

There was an increase of intraocular pressure in all instances of anterior or posterior capsulotomy. This increase of pressure is probably due to release of liquified cortical material and mechanical obstruction of the chamber angle. There was no elevation of intraocular pressure in other instances as long as the lens capsule remained intact. Based on these observations, we do not recommend YAG-laser anterior capsulotomy, and for posterior capsulotomy we advise using the least possible energy and least number of applications of YAG-laser for each case.

*To be published in the American Journal of Ophthalmology.

E.L. Greve, W. Leydhecker & C. Raitta (eds.), Second European Glaucoma Symposium, Helsinki 1984.
© 1985, *Dr. W. Junk Publishers, Dordrecht. ISBN 978-94-010-8934-0*

ARGON LASER TRABECULOPLASTY AFTER TRABECULECTOMY

F.M. HONRUBIA, P. GRIJALBO and L. GOMEZ

(Zaragoza, Spain)

ABSTRACT

Argon laser trabeculoplasty has been carried out on 13 eyes which have been surgicaly operated on with the trabeculectomy technique and with bad control of their glaucoma in spite of the post-surgical medical antiglaucomatose treatment. All the eyes, candidates for a new filtering operation were photocoagulated without complications. The post-photocoagulation period ranged from 12 to 18 months. The average ocular pressure before the photocoagulation was 24 mm Hg and after the photocoagulation it was 18 mm Hg. A new surgical operation was carried out on one eye and 11 eyes were well controlled, the medical antiglaucomatose therapeutics having been reduced in 7 of the eyes.

INTRODUCTION

Argon laser trabeculoplasty has been used very efficiently during the last few years in the treatment of chronic open angle glaucoma, mainly in phakic eyes in elderly patients (1, 2, 3, 4, 7, 8, 9). More recently, its use has been extended to certain types of secondary glaucoma, although the results published are not as good as in the previous group (10).

In the group of secondary glaucomas, we included eyes with glaucoma unsuccessfully operated on with antiglaucomatose filtering techniques, and where a new kind of surgery would present serious difficulties and more than a few complications. In these eyes the application of the laser could be of therapeutic importance.

The object of this paper is to present the results obtained with laser trabeculoplasty in 13 eyes previously operated on unsuccessfully with the trabeculectomy technique. The tensional results obtained are reviewed at a minimum post-photocoagulation study period of 12 months and a maximum study period of 18 months.

MATERIAL AND METHODS

We include 13 eyes belonging to 13 patients (average age: 63 years) with chronic open angle glaucoma operated on unsuccessfully for trabeculectomy.

193

E.L. Greve, W. Leydhecker & C. Raitta (eds.), Second European Glaucoma Symposium, Helsinki 1984.
© *1985, Dr. W. Junk Publishers, Dordrecht. ISBN 978-94-010-8934-0*

All eyes were submitted to intense antiglaucomatose medical treatment after surgery without achieving an adequate tensional control.

The average ocular pressure of the 13 eyes was 24 mm Hg; ocular pressure was higher than 21 mm Hg in 12 eyes, and there was an average "C" drainage coefficient of 0.11 (Table 1).

Table 1. Trabeculoplasty post-trabeculectomy: Pre-photocoagulation study

No of eyes	13
Average age	63 yrs
Average ocular pressure	24 mm Hg
Average "C"	0.11

Argon laser trabeculoplasty was carried out on all the eyes (1) with 80—100 laser shots of 50 diameter, 300—1,200 mW intensity and 0.1 sec duration. No eye was included in the study which did not have at least 180° of the angle free from synechias, so that photocoagulation could easily be practiced.

After photocoagulation, all patients continued with their medical-antiglaucomatose therapeutics, adding topical corticosteroids or inhibitors of the synthesis of the prostaglandines, which were maintained during the first days according to the inflammatory reaction in the anterior chamber.

In the following controls the antiglaucomatose therapeutics were varied according to the tensional evolution of each eye, and the results obtained with the normal exploratory techniques of the eyes with glaucoma.

RESULTS

The post-photocoagulation control time of all the eyes varied between a minimum of 12 months and a maximum of 18 months.

The average ocular pressure of all the eyes dropped to 18 mm Hg, (as 25% reduction), the ocular pressure being higher than 21 mm Hg in two eyes, one of which due to progressive loss of visual field had to be operated on with another trabeculectomy.

The average "C" drainage coefficient was 0.15, the "C" having increased in 11 of the eyes with regard to the drainage coefficient which existed before the photocoagulation.

It was significant that during the control time, in accordance with the tensional evolution and the exploratory results obtained, it was possible to decrease the medical antiglaucomatose treatment in 7·of the 13 eyes.

In short it can be concluded that the trabeculoplasty has been efficient in the antiglaucomatose control of 11 of the 13 eyes, which means an efficacy higher than 84%. (Table 2).

COMMENTS

At the present time total unanimity exists with regard to the efficacy of the Argon laser trabeculoplasty technique in the treatment of open angle

Table 2. Trabeculoplasty post-trabeculectomy: Post-photocoagulation study

Average ocular pressure	18 mm Hg
Average "C"	0.15
Decreased medical treatment	7 eyes
New trabeculectomy	1 eye
Control time	12–18 months
Efficacy of the trabeculoplasty	11 out of 13 eyes (85%)

glaucomas, in phakic, mainly elderly patients (1, 2, 3, 4, 7, 8, 9). On the contrary, less information and unanimity exists with regard to its efficacy in the treatment of secondary glaucomas (5), and some authors even doubt that trabeculoplasty is indicated in the therapeutics of certain types of secondary glaucoma (10).

The use of the argon laser trabeculoplasty in the therapeutics of badly controlled glaucomas in eyes previously submitted to antiglaucomatose filtering surgery, has not been widely published.

In 1982, Thomas (6) published the results obtained in the treatment of 20 eyes with an average control of 4 months. His results offer a therapeutic efficacy in 70% of the eyes with an average reduction of 8 mm Hg (about 25% of the prephotocoagulation ocular pressure). More recently Robin and Pollack (5) obtained a notable tensional reduction in 6 out of 7 eyes with unsuccessful filtering surgery, and were able to reduce the antiglaucomatose medication in 3 eyes.

In the group of patients included in our study, with a control period ranging from 12 to 18 months, we achieved an average reduction of ocular pressure of 25%, which has meant an adequate control of the glaucoma in 11 of the 13 eyes; only 1 eye has needed a new filtering surgery. According to Moulin and Haux (3) the results obtained with the trabeculoplasty can be considered definitive after 3 months. Thus, in our study, with a much more dilated control period, the results can be taken as stable with more certainty and with 85% therapeutic efficacy.

We can conclude from our study, that in accordance with what has been published by other authors, the trabeculoplasty with Argon laser is the chosen therapeutics in all patients with glaucoma who have been operated on previously and without success with any filtering antiglaucomatose technique, with the provision that at least 180° of the angle of the anterior chamber is open and without synechias to be able to carry out the trabeculoplasty. The trabeculoplasty is a technique which is carried out ambulatorily. It is much less aggressive and has fewer complications than a new trabeculectomy on an eye which has already been surgically operated on.

REFERENCES

1. Honrubia, F.M. Terapéutica Láser de Argón en Oftalmología. Monografía Chivret 2:21 (1983).
2. Honrubia, F.M., Gómez, M.L., Brito, C. and Grijalbo, M.P. Trabeculoplastia Láser de Argón en Glaucoma crónico simple. Arch. Soc. Esp. Oftal. (in press).

3. Moulin, F. and Haut, J. Résultats du traitement au láser l'argon de 100 yeux atteints de glaucome á angle ouvert. J. Franç D'Optalmol. 6:661 (1983).
4. Pollack, I.P. Argon laser trabeculoplasty. Ophthalmic. Surg. 13:637 (1982).
5. Robin, A.L. and Pollack, I.P. Argon laser trabeculoplasty in secondary forms of open-angle glaucoma. Arch. Ophthalmol. 101:382 (1983).
6. Thomas, J.V. Argon laser trabeculoplasty. Ophthalmology 89:187 (1982).
7. Wilensky, J.T. and Jampol, L.M. Laser therapy for open-angle glaucoma. Ophthalmology 88:213 (1981).
8. Wise, J.B. and Witter, L.L. Argon laser therapy for open-angle glaucoma: A pilot study". Arch. Ophthalmol. 97:319 (1979).
9. Wise, J.B. Long-term control of adult open-angle glaucoma by argon laser treatment. Ophthalmology 88:197 (1981).
10. Wise, J.B. Status of Laser treatment of open angle glaucoma. Ann. Ophthalmol. 13:199 (1981).

Authors' address:
Servicio de Oftalmologia
Hospital Miguel Servet
Zaragoza, Spain

THE BLOOD AQUEOUS BARRIER EFFECTS OF NEODYMIUM YAG LASER IRIDOTOMY IN THE HUMAN EYE

W. SCHREMS, O. EICHELBRÖNNER, W. WALLER, G.K. KRIEGLSTEIN

(*Würzburg, W. Germany*)

ABSTRACT

The present clinical study was designed to investigate the immediate disturbances of the blood aqueous barrier after Neodymium-YAG-laser iridotomy. Two groups of 10 patients each were subjected to iridotomy with a Q-switch Nd-YAG laser 100 ($\pm$ 10) min before cataract extraction under standardized conditions. The anterior chamber was tapped with a 27-gauge needle prior to cataract extraction in order to analyse the protein content as well as the albumin and IgG concentrations. The protein assay was performed using a micromethod with a standardized 'Coomassie brilliant blue' solution, albumin and IgG assay was done using a radial immuno-diffusion technique. YAG-laser iridotomy caused a significant barrier dysfunction in the human eye which could be treated in a preventive manner by topically applied indomethacin.

INTRODUCTION

Like any other mechanical or chemical trauma laser surgery of the anterior uvea will cause an immediate disruption of the blood aqueous barrier. The prostaglandins of E-type play a key role in this phenomenon (3–11). With the introduction and the widespread use of high-power, short-pulse Nd-YAG lasers more and more clinical interest is raised in the physiopathologic mechanisms caused by laser surgery. The present study was designed to get more information about the extent of the blood aqueous barrier dysfunction after YAG laser iridotomy in the human eye.

METHODS

The present study comprised 30 eyes of 30 patients with senile cataract excluding patients with other eye diseases. In the control group (including 10 eyes) no laser iridotomy was performed, group 2 was pretreated with topically applied indomethacin (including 10 eyes) before laser surgery,

197

E.L. Greve, W. Leydhecker & C. Raitta (eds.), Second European Glaucoma Symposium, Helsinki 1984.
© *1985, Dr. W. Junk Publishers, Dordrecht. ISBN 978-94-010-8934-0*

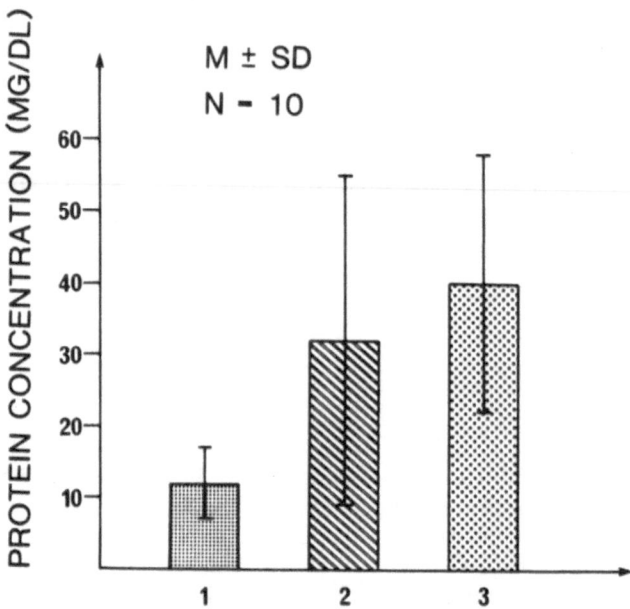

Fig. 1. Mean values and standard deviations of the protein concentration in the aqueous humour in 3 series of 10 eyes each. In the control group (series 1, left column) no laser iridotomy was performed, group 2 was pretreated with topically applied indomethacin, group 3 underwent laser iridotomy without medical pretreatment.

group 3 (including 10 eyes) underwent laser iridotomy without medical pretreatment. Group 2 was pretreated with indomethacin eyedrops (Indoptic®, Chibret Company, Switzerland); on each pretreated eye 30 μl of Indeptic® eyedrops were applied five times before the laser procedure. For iridotomy the eye was anaesthetized with topical application of 0.4% oxybuprocain hydrochloride (Novesine®). The same Nd-YAG-laser was used throughout the study (model Microruptor II/Lasag Co., Thun/Switzerland). The laser iridotomy was done in all patients via a special lens (contact glass CGI_1 of Lasag Co.), in the 12 o'clock position of the peripheral iris. The following laser parameters served throughout the whole study: 1 burst of 4 single shots with an energy of 12–14 mJoule, with a time interval of 20 msec. Exposure time was 12 nsec, the spot size 70 μm. The anterior chamber was tapped 100 ± 10 min after the laser iridotomy under standardized conditions (with a 27-gauge needle) before cataract extraction. The protein concentration was determined with a computerized, bichromatical colorimeter (Protianalyser of Kipp and Zonen Co.) using a stabilized Coomassie brilliant solution. The albumin and IgG concentration was measured with a radial immunodiffusion technique (low concentration plates of Behring Co./FRG). Paired t-test as well as Wilcoxon test was used to decide on the statistical relevance of the results on the basis of a confidence level of 5%.

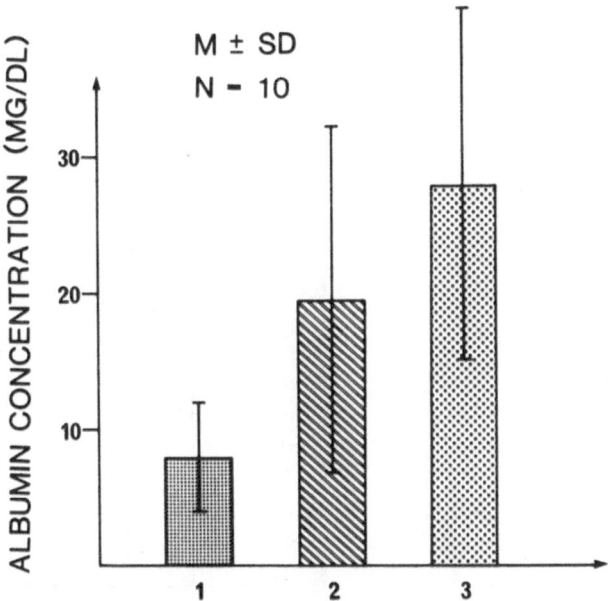

Fig. 2. Mean values and standard deviations of the albumin concentration in the aqueous humour in 3 series of 10 eyes each.

RESULTS

Nd-YAG-laser iridotomy induced a significant increase ($p < 0.05$) of the protein concentration in the aqueous humour as measured 100 ± 10 min after the laser procedure (Fig. 1). The protein concentration was 40 ± 18 mg/dl in the laser-treated group versus 12 ± 5 mg/dl in the control group. Pretreatment with topically applied indomethacin resulted only in a slight decrease of protein leakage as measured in group 2, where the protein concentration was 32 ± 23 mg/dl. A similar tendency was observed regarding the concentration of albumin and immunoglobulin IgG. The albumin concentration was highest in the laser-treated group 3 with a mean of 27.7 ± 12.9 mg/dl and was lowest in the control group 1 with a mean of 7.7 ± 3.9 mg/dl. Again there was a slight, non-significant decrease in the medically pretreated laser group 2 with a mean of 19.4 ± 12.7 mg/dl (Fig. 2). The mean values and standard deviations of IgG are given in Fig. 3. In group 1 it was 1.1 ± 0.5, in group 2 it was 2.3 ± 1.2 and in group 3 it was 2.8 ± 1.4 mg/dl.

DISCUSSION

The mechanism of high power, short-pulsed Nd-YAG-laser is based on a confined microexplosion (1, 2). The time course of Nd-YAG-laser iridotomy with regard to the blood aqueous barrier disruption has been studied in an experimental model recently (10). The protein leakage into the aqueous

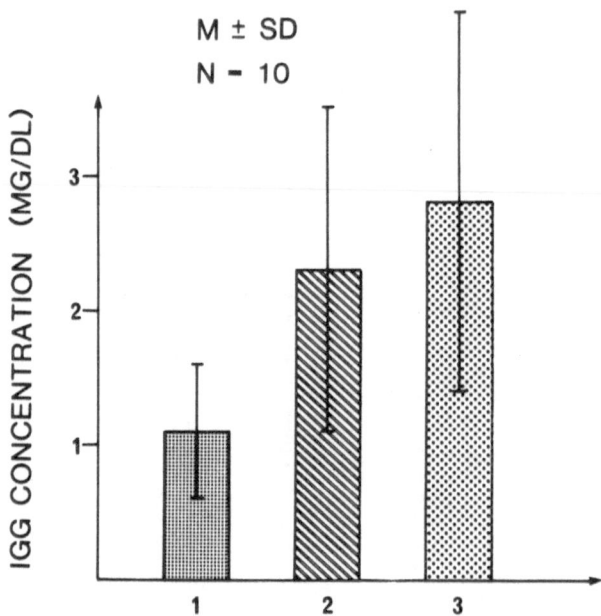

Fig. 3. Mean values and standard deviations of the IgG concentration in the aqueous humour in 3 series of 10 eyes each.

reached a maximum 100 min after laser iridotomy. In the present study 3 parameters of the blood aqueous barrier function were examined: the total protein content, the albumin concentration (molecular weight 69.000 Dalton) and the immunoglobulin IgG concentration (molecular weight 150.000). All three parameters increased significantly after Nd-YAG-laser iridotomy. The favourable effect of prostaglandin inhibitors given prior to surgery (8, 9, 11) confirms that the problem is partially related to a prostaglandin-linked disruption of the blood aqueous barrier (3–7). The intraocular pressure rises after Nd-YAG-laser surgery can also be blocked by indomethacin pretreatment (11). The results of the present study surprisingly show an insignificant effect of indomethacin pretreatment. This phenomenon could be explained as follows: 1) the Nd-YAG-laser iridotomy causes a tissue disruption and a lot of debris and intracellular material as well as heat-denaturated proteins are liberated into the aqueous humour; 2) micro-hemorrhages occur due to the direct laser impact or due to the propagation of shock waves caused by the instant ionisation. These two mechanisms overlap the blood aqueous barrier effects.

REFERENCES

1. Fankhauser, F., Lörtscher, H. P. and Zypen, van der E. Clinical studies on high and low power laser radiation upon some structures of the anterior and posterior segments of the eye. Int. Ophthalmol. 5: 15–32 (1982).

2. Fankhauser, F. and Zypen, van der E. Future of the laser in ophthalmology. Trans. Ophthalmol. Soc. UK 102: 159–163 (1982).
3. Hall, D. W. R. and Bonta, I. L. Prostaglandins and ocular inflammation. Doc. Ophthalmol. 44: 421–434 (1977).
4. Katz, I. M. Indomethacin. Ophthalmology (Rochester) 88: 455–458 (1981).
5. Kremer, M., Baikoff, G. and Charbonnell, B. The release of prostaglandins in human aqueous humour following intraocular surgery. Effect of indomethacin. Prostaglandins 23: 695–702 (1982).
6. Podos, S. M. Prostaglandins, nonsteroidal anti-inflammatory agents and eye disease. Trans. Am. Ophthalmol. Soc. LXXIV: 638–660 (1976).
7. Rich, W. J. C. C. Prevention of postoperative ocular hypertension by prostaglandin inhibitors. Trans. Ophthalmol. Soc. UK 97: 268–271 (1977).
8. Schrems, W., Dorp, van H. P., Mager, S. and Krieglstein, G. K. The effect of prostaglandin inhibitors on the laser induced disruption of the blood aqueous barrier in the rabbit. Graefe's Arch. Clin. Exp. Ophthalmol. 221: 61–64 (1983).
9. Schrems, W., Dorp, van H. P., Mager, S. and Krieglstein, G. K. The effect of topically applied prostaglandin inhibitors on the laser induced disruption of the blood aqueous barrier (in press).
10. Schrems, W., Dorp, van H. P., Wendel, M. and Krieglstein, G. K. The effect of yag laser iridotomy on the blood aqueous barrier in the rabbit. Graefe's Arch. Clin. Exp. Ophthalmol. 221: 179–181 (1984).
11. Schrems, W., Eichelbrönner, O., De Natale, R. and Krieglstein, G. K. The effect of topically applied indomethacin in the prevention of laser induced intraocular pressure rises (in press).

Author's address:
W. Schrems
Univ. Augenklinik
Josef-Schneider-Str. 11
D-8700 Würzburg, Fed. Rep. Germany

EXPERIMENTAL AND CLINICAL LASER IRIDECTOMY WITH ARGON AND Nd YAG Q SWITCHED LASER

M. BRIHAYE, G. VRENSEN, F. VERWORST, G. BELGRADO and
O. PETERS

(Brussels, Belgium/Amsterdam, The Netherlands)

ABSTRACT

Experimental studies on iridectomies demonstrated that the combination of argon laser and Nd YAG Q switched laser resulted in permanent perforating lesions. In first instance, the thermal effect of the argon laser provokes coagulation of blood vessels and prevents hemorrhage; secondly, the mechanical effect of the Nd YAG laser results in perforation of the iris and prevention of cell proliferation which otherwise would have closed the perforation. We carried out this combined treatment on 41 glaucomatous eyes. Long-lasting iridectomies with a favourable effect on intraocular pressure, even after reduction of medical treatment, were obtained.

The first iridectomies with argon laser were performed in 1975 by the groups of Abraham, Anderson and Patti. Since then, a few authors have published good results; others have discarded this technique as ineffective or have described complications.

EXPERIMENTAL

We performed 400 experimental iridectomies on rabbits using the argon laser and the Nd YAG Q switched laser, or both in combination. Histological characteristics of the iridectomy depend on the operation of the laser. The argon laser has a thermal effect and the Nd YAG laser a mechanical one.

The radiation produced by the argon laser is continuous; its maximum power is 3 W and its wavelength is between 388 and 504 nm. The radiation is absorbed by melanin pigment and hemoglobin and is thus effective only for pigmented tissues. Microscopically, we demonstrated that argon laser first produces cellular necrosis followed after 4 days by the appearance of macrophages loaded with pigment. Later on, the proliferation of the fibroblasts and the pigment epithelium cells leads to closure of some iridectomies (6, 7, 8, 45). The frequency of perforations increases with increasing power; with 2,500 mW, perforations were obtained in 95% of the experiments. However, after one week, only 22% of the original perforating iridectomies were

Eye clinic of the University of Brussels (A.Z.V.V.B) and Amsterdam (AM.C.) and Netherlands Ophthalmic Research Institute (IOI).

This work was subsidiated by the belgian foundation for research (N.F.W.O.).

203

E.L. Greve, W. Leydhecker & C. Raitta (eds.), Second European Glaucoma Symposium, Helsinki 1984.
© 1985, Dr. W. Junk Publishers, Dordrecht. ISBN 978-94-010-8934-0

still open. In addition, with such high power, irradiation complications occur, consisting in temporary opacifications of the cornea and persistent local opacifications of the lens.

We therefore performed experimental iridectomies using the quality switched laser with Neodymium and Garnet of Aluminium and Yttrium. This laser can develop tremendous power (8×10^{11} Watts = 8 gigawatts) in extremely short periods of time (pulse duration = 12 nanosec); 1 to 9 pulses might be obtained; the radiation has a wavelength of 1060 nm, which is close to the infrared. The Nd YAG laser induces ionisation in its focal spot which provokes microexplosions. Consequently, it creates an optical strain and plasma formation, followed by a shock wave. The opaque plasma provides a protective screen for the retina. Due to this mechanical action, the final result is total cellular disruption. The Nd YAG laser also works on non pigmented tissues (11, 12, 13, 14, 41).

Microscopically, rupture of all iris layers without secondary pigment reaction is immediately obtained but some vessels are torn off, provoking frequent iris hemorrhage (7, 43).

To prevent the high percentage of iris bleeding which occurs when the Neodymium YAG Laser is used, coagulation of vessels is obtained by treatment with argon laser used at low power (500 to 1000 mW). We performed experimental iridectomies with a combined treatment vis. argon laser followed by Nd YAG laser at various intervals. With an interval of one week, a perforation without bleeding was obtained in 95% of the experiments. There were no corneal and lens complications (44).

CLINICAL IRIDECTOMIES

Material and methods

We performed 41 iridectomies on 30 glaucomatous patients. We always strive for medical control before laser iridectomy: instillation of pilocarpine 2 to 4% and/or timoptol 0.5%; some patients also used 1 to 4 x 250 mg acetazolamide each day and/or oral glycerine.

Indication for a combined laser therapy was a persistent pathological intraocular pressure (IOP) in spite of topical and general medical treatment. Treatment was also indicated when the medical treatment induced a decrease in visual acuity even with a normalised IOP. A third indication was present in patients who violated the protocol of treatment.

Before laser treatment, pilocarpine 2% was instilled in the eye to maintain miosis; it was followed by topical anesthetic. The laser treatment occurred in two steps: argon laser coagulation with a spot size of 200μ, a power of 500 mW and an exposure time of 0.2 sec. The number of argon coagulations needed to treat an area of 1 mm was 20 to 50.

Afterwards, the same area was subjected to Nd YAG laser irradiation, the following parameters being used: a spot size of 50μ, exposure time of 12 nsec, 1 pulse, the minimal energy to provoke a perforation (6 to 30 mJ); the number of applications varied from 5 to 15. More iridectomies were performed near the 10 to 2 o'clock position from the middle to the extreme periphery of the iris.

Post-operatively, topical steroid, 2×50 mg aspirin and 250 mg acetazolamide were added to the antiglaucomatous treatment.

The patients ranged in age between 51 and 87, the mean age being 61. Eighty-five per cent of these patients had a primary glaucoma, 37% had an acute angle closure glaucoma, 49% had a chronic narrow angle glaucoma, and 14% were fellow eye of patients with acute angle closure glaucoma.

Fifteen percent of the patients had a glaucoma secondary to aphakic pupillary block (17%), anterior uveitis (50%) or incomplete surgical iridectomy (33%).

RESULTS

In 74% of the cases, laser iridectomy was successfully performed in one single session, while the remaining 26% required several sessions.

The mean intraocular pressure before laser treatment was 28.9 mm Hg under medical therapy, 18.3 mm Hg one day and 17.8 mm Hg one week after laser iridectomy. The IOP remained beneath 21 mm Hg during the whole follow-up period, which was 2 to 12 months (Table 1). In 92% of the cases,

Table 1. Laser iridotomy: Mean intraocular pressure in 41 eyes (mmHg)

Before laser therapy	
without med. treatment	46.0
with med. treatment	28.9
After laser therapy	
1 day	18.3
1 week	17.8
1 month	17.4
3 months	17.2
6 months	18.7
9 months	19.6
12 months	17.0

no surgery was needed, thanks to the laser therapy: only 3 eyes (7.3%) underwent surgery, because IOP remained uncontrolled in spite of intensive medical therapy. An attempt was made to reduce medical therapy on a prospective way in order to determine the minimum treatment required for keeping the pressure below 21 mm Hg. Six months after laser therapy, 20% of our patients did not require any further medical treatment, 40% of the eyes were controlled without carbonic anhydrase inhibitors and 40% required the same preoperative treatment, but at lower doses (Table 2).

Complications

Complications were minor and temporary: one day after laser iridectomy, we observed light inflammatory reaction (69.1%), local corneal haze (15%), Descemet lesion (7.5%), increase of IOP (5%), and microscopic hemorrhage

Table 2. Laser iridotomy: Mean number of drugs per patient

Medical treatment	General	Local
Pre laser	1.02	2.24
Post laser		
1 day	1.02	2.24
1 week	0.77	2.11
1 month	0.58	2.07
3 months	0.55	1.83
6 months	0.54	2.18
9 months	0.3	1.6

(18%). One week after laser application, these complications were already minimized. Within a few weeks, all keratitis and the only case with hyphema, iris bombe and extensive rubeosis iridis, were cured. Posterior synechiae were the only persistent complication (Table 3).

Table 3. Laser iridotomy

Complications	After 1 day	After 1 week
Hyperhaemia	97.0%	5.0%
Corneal oedema	15.0%	–
Keratitis	5.0%	5.0%
Descemet lesion	7.5%	2.5%
Pig. disp. cornea	7.5%	7.5%
Tyndall +	69.0%	5.0%
Increase IOP	5.0%	–
Pigment on lens	5.0%	5.0%
Post synechiae	5.0%	5.0%
Hemorrhage	18.0%	–
Hyphema	2.5%	2.5%

DISCUSSION

Using a combined treatment with argon and Nd YAG laser, we obtained iris perforations in 100% of our clinical cases. Ninetythree percent of the eyes have a normalised IOP; 7% needed filtering surgery because of remaining uncontrolled IOP after one month (angle closure glaucoma with extensive goniosynechiae). There is no report concerning a combined iris treatment with argon and Nd YAG laser.

Fankhauser (14) observed successful perforations of all iris irradiated with Nd YAG laser. But there is no report available in the literature concerning the evolution of IOP after YAG laser and the complications of this treatment.

Many authors have published different results as regards iris perforation with normalised IOP after argon laser treatment: Quigley (28) reported 100% perforations, Abraham and Miller (2) 98.5%, Karmon 94.5%, Yamamoto et al. (46) 93%, Haut et al. (16) 88%, Hong et al. (19) 71.4%, Pollack (26) 68%, Malthieu and Turut (22) 64.7%.

According to these authors, IOP remained uncontrolled in 6 to 12% of the cases.

Using a pulsed argon laser, Stiegler (37) obtained 100% of iris perforations, Schwartz (34) 75%. We observed during the first day after laser a transitory rise of IOP in 5% of cases. This phenomenon was observed in 92% of the iridotomies by Hong et al. (19) and in 33% by Karmon. According to Yamamoto et al. (46), the rise of IOP reaches a maximum one hour after laser treatment. The low percentage of rise of IOP after our combined laser treatment may be due to the Nd YAG laser, which limits the inflammatory reaction. The administration of antiglaucomatous drug after treatment can also be a factor in reducing the percentage of intraocular hypertension. The percentage of complications is different according to the series published.

We observed transitory Descemet's lesions of the cornea in 7.5% and epithelial reactions (keratitis) in 5%. Yamamoto et al. (46) reported epithelial lesions in 34% and endothelial lesions in 49.3%. Hong et al (19) observed an increase of the endothelial cell size amounting to 19%.

Focal opacities of the lens were described and ranged from 6.25% (22) to 16.6%. We observed small bleedings at the borders of the iridotomy in 18% of our cases and hyphema in 2.5%. Hodes et al. (18) reported about one case of hyphema in a patient having no predisposing pathological condition, which reabsorbed within 5 days, but the iridotomy was not patent. Robin and Pollack (32) described such small hemorrhages in 100% of the eyes treated with a Q-switched ruby laser and an hyphema in 10% of them. The smaller amount of bleeding we observed must be due to the argon laser coagulation of the iris vessels.

A slight inflammatory reaction is present in almost all cases in our series, as in those of Quigley (28), Yamamoto et al. (46) and Karmon, but only in 1.25% according to Malthieu and Turut (22).

Posterior synechiae ranged from 1.9% (22) to 28%. We observed synechiae at the border of the iridectomy in two eyes (5%). According to Haut et al. (16), in case of acute angle closure with pronounced iritis reaction, it is suitable to change the laser treatment in order to prevent an important inflammatory reaction with synechiae and increase of IOP. Closure of the iridotomy occurred within a few weeks after treatment and ranged from 4.9% (46), to 22% (25). An opening of the hole of the iris was obtained after a second or several sessions. In 5% of our cases, a closure of the hole occurred within the first week. It was easily reopened after a second session.

In two cases, macular oedema was observed (5, 10); these lesions resorbed within a few weeks. Superficial retinal burns were described in L'Esperance (21). Balkan et al. (4) reported a case of loss of vision one day after peripheral laser iridotomy. The patient had a glaucoma since several years with bad visual field and an important disk cupping. He was also in a severely unstable cardio-vascular condition.

CONCLUSION

Forty-one eyes were treated with low energy argon laser followed by Q switched Nd YAG laser. The first step with argon laser prevents the iris hemorrhage. Compared with the argon laser iridotomy, the combined treatment with argon and Nd YAG laser prevents pigment dispersion and limits the inflammatory reaction, reducing secondary iris closure. It allows easy treatment of both the pigmented and unpigmented iris.

Long-lasting iridotomies were obtained without bleeding in 93% of the cases. It appears to be a safe and efficient procedure to control IOP in cases of angle closure or suspect angle closure. A number of advantages over surgical iridectomy are obvious; the procedure may be handled in an out-patient department; only instillation of a topical anaesthetic is required; fewer intraocular bleedings are observed; there is no risk of endophtalmitis; wound leakage with intraocular hypotension does not occur; there is no post-operative period of poor vision; and there is no risk of malignant glaucoma.

REFERENCES

1. Abraham, K. and Miller, L. Outpatient argon laser iridectomy for angle closure glaucoma: a two-year study. Trans. Am. Acad. Ophthalmol. Otol. 79:529–538 (1975).
2. Abraham, K. and Miller, L. Outpatient argon laser iridectomy for angle-closure glaucoma: a $3\frac{1}{2}$-year study. Adv. Ophthalmol. 34:186–191 (1977).
3. Anderson, D.R., Forster, R.K. and Lewis, M.L. Laser iridotomy for aphakic pupillary block. Arch. Ophthalmol. 93:343–346 (1975).
4. Balkan, R.J., Zimmerman, T.J., Hesse, R.J. and Steigner, J.B. Loss of central visual acuity after laser peripheral iridectomy. Ann. Ophthalmol. 721–723 (1982).
5. Bass, M.S., Cleary, C.V., Perkins, E.S. and Wheeler, C.B. Single treatment laser iridotomy. Br. J. Ophthalmol. 163:29–30 (1979).
6. Brihaye, M., Vrensen, G., Nieus, C., Braeckman, C. and Willekens, B. Coagulation expérimentale de l'iris au laser à l'argon. Bull. Soc. belge Ophtalmol. 190:33–42 (1980).
7. Brihaye, M., Verworst, F., Verlaeken, L., Schyns, P. and Van Looy, H. Traitement du segment antérieur au laser pulsé au Néodymium YAG. Bull. Soc. belge Ophtalmol. 199–200:27–30 (1982).
8. Brihaye, M., Vrensen, G., Swinnen, M.C., Verworst, F., Peters, O. and Jager, M. Behandlung der Iris mit Argonlaserstrahlen. Experimentelle Studien. Klin. Mbl. Augenheilk. 180:65–67 (1982).
9. Brihaye, M., Herzeel, R., Verworst, F., Tassignon, M.J., Peters, O. and Belgrado, G. Traitement des affections du segment antérieur par le laser pulsé au Néodymium YAG. Sobeveco, 11e International Congress, 1983, 195–200.
10. Choplin, N.T. and Pyene, C. Cytoid macular edema following laser iridotomy. Ann. Ophthalmol. 15:172–173 (1983).
11. Fankhauser, F. Lasertherapie. Die physikalischen und biologischen Wirkungen der Laserstrahlung. Klin. Mbl. Augenheilk. 170:219–227 (1977).
12. Fankhauser, F., Roussel, P., Van Der Zypen, E. Microchirurgie par laser Q switched dans le traitement des segments antérieur et postérieur de l'oeil. Bull. Mém. Soc. fr. Ophtal. 93e année 94 (1982).
13. Fankhauser, F., Roussel, P., Steffen, J., Van Der Zypen, E. and Chrenkova, A. Clinical studies on the efficiency of high power laser radiation upon some structures of the anterior segment of the eye. Int. Ophthalmol. 3:129–139 (1981).
14. Fankhauser, F., Lortscher, H., Van Der Zypen, E. Clinical studies on high and low power laser radiation upon some structures of the anterior and posterior segments of the eye. Survey Ophthalmol. 27:405–406 (1983).
15. Fankhauser, F. in Trockel 1983.
16. Haut, J., Nicaise, A., Monin, Cl. and Sarnikowski, Cl. Technique de l'iridotomie au laser à l'argon. Bull. Soc. Opht. France 82:1351–1352 (1982).

17. Haut, J., Nicaise, A., Van Effenterre, G., Larricart, P. and Sfeir, T. Avantages et inconvénients de l'iridotomie au laser. Bull. Soc. Opht. France 82:1353–1356 (1982).
18. Hodes, B.L., Bentivegna, J.F. and Weyer, N.J. Hyphema complicating laser iridotomy. Arch. Ophthalmol. 100:924–925 (1982).
19. Hong, O., Kitazawa, Y. and Tanishima, T. Influence of argon laser treatment of glaucoma on corneal endothelium. Jpn. J. Ophthalmol. 27:567–574 (1983).
20. Ingram, R.M. and Ennis, J.R. Acute glaucoma: results of treatment of bilateral simultaneous iridotomy, now without admission to hospital. Br. J. Ophthalmol. 67: 367–371 (1983).
21. L'Esperance, F.A. Ophtalmic Laser. Mosby, St Louis, 1983.
22. Malthieu, D. and Turut, P. Iridotomie au laser à argon dans le glaucome à angle fermé. A propos de 160 cas. J. Fr. Ophtalmol. 6:123–128 (1983).
23. March, W.F. Advances in Ophthalmic Laser Therapy. Aesculapius, Birmingham, Alabama, 1983.
24. Patti, J.C. and Cinotti, A.A. Iris photocoagulation therapy of aphakic pupillary block Arch. Ophthalmol. 93:347–348 (1975).
25. Podos, S.M., Kels, B.D., Moss, A.P., Ritch, R. and Anders, M.D. Continuous wave argon laser iridectomy in angle-closure glaucoma. Am. J. Ophthalmol. 88:836–842 (1979).
26. Pollack, I.P. Use of argon laser energy to produce iridotomies. Tr. Am. Ophthalmol. Soc. 77:674–706 (1979).
27. Pollack, I.P. Laser iridotomy in the treatment of angle-closure glaucoma. Ann. Ophthalmol, 13: 549–550 (1981).
28. Quigley, H.A. Long-term follow-up of laser iridotomy. Ophthalmology 88:218–224 (1981).
29. Quigley, H.A. Argon laser peripheral iridotomies in the treatment of primary angle closure glaucoma. Arch. Ophthalmol. 100:919–923 (1983).
30. Ritch, R. Argon laser treatment for medically unresponsive attacks of angle-closure glaucoma. Am. J. Ophthalmol. 94:197–204 (1982).
31. Robin, A.L. Argon laser peripheral iridotomies in the treatment of primary angle closure glaucoma. Arch. Ophthalmol. 100:919–923 (1982).
32. Robin, A.L. and Pollack, I.P. The Q-switched ruby laser in glaucoma. Ophthalmology 91:366–372 (1984).
33. Rodrigues, M.M., Streeten, B., Spaeth, G.L. and Schwartz, L.W. Argon laser iridotomy on primary angle closure or pupillary block glaucoma. Arch. Ophthalmol. 96:2222–2230 (1978).
34. Schwartz, L.W. et al. Argon laser iridotomy in primary angle-closure or pupillary block glaucoma. Tr. Ophthalmol. Soc. U.K. 99:257–263 (1979).
35. Shin, D.H. Argon laser iris photocoagulation to relieve acute angleclosure glaucoma. Am. J. Ophthalmol. 93:348–350 (1982).
36. Snyder, W.B. Laser coagulation of the anterior segment. I. Experimental laser iridotomy. Arch. Ophthalmol. 77:93–98 (1967).
37. Stiegler, G. Laser iridektomie; eine 6-Jahresstudie. Klin. Mbl. Augenheilk. 180: 347–349 (1982).
38. Tessler, H.H., Peyman, G.A., Huamonte, F. and Menachof, I. Argon laser iridotomy in uncomplete peripheral iridectomy. Am. J. Ophthal. 79:1051–1052 (1975).
39. Trockel, S.L. YAG Laser Ophtalmic Microsurgery. A.C.C. Norwalk, Connecticut, 1983.
40. Turut, P. and Malthieu, D. L'iridectomie au laser argon; à propos de 30 cas. Bull. Soc. Opht. France 82:253–256 (1982).
41. Van Der Zypen, E. and Fankhauser, F. Effekte eines neuartigen Lasertyps auf fixiertes Gewebe der Kammerwinkelregion des Affenauges. Klin. Mbl. Augenheilk. 172:436–437 (1978).
42. Van Der Zypen, E., Fankhauser, F. and Bebie, H. On the effects of different laser energy sources upon the iris of the pigmented and the albino rabbit. Int. Ophthalmol. 1:39–48 (1978).

43. Van Der Zypen, E., Fankhauser, F., Bebie, H. and Marshall, J. Changes on the ultra-structure of the iris after irradiation with intense light. A study of long-term effects after irradiation with Argon Ion, Nd: YAG and Q switched Ruby lasers. Adv. Ophthalmol. 39:59–180 (1979).
44. Verworst, F., Brihaye, M., De Jong, P., Vrensen, G. and Peters, O. Traitement de l'iris par le laser à l'argon et le laser pulsé au Néodymium YAG. Note préliminaire. Bull. Soc. belge Ophtal. 203:151–157 (1982).
45. Vrensen, G., Brihaye, M., Willekens, B., Mataw, I. and Swinnen, M.F. Argon laser lesions of the rabbit iris: quantitative aspects. v. Graefes Archiv. Klin. Exp. Ophthalmol. 219:80–91 (1982).
46. Yamamoto, T., Shirato, S. and Kitazawa, Y. Argon laser iridotomy in angle-closure glaucoma: a comparison of two methods. Jpn. J. Ophthalmol. 26:387–396 (1982).
47. Yassur, Y., Melamed, S., Cohen, S. and Ben-Sira, T. Laser iridotomy in closed-angle glaucoma. Arch. Ophthalmol. 97:1920–1921 (1979).

Authors' address:
Academisch Ziekenhuis
Afdeling Oogheelkunde
Vrye Universitait Brussel
Laarbeeklaan 101
1090 Brussel
Belgium

210

SURGERY AND ITS DOCUMENTATION IN GLAUCOMA

W. LEYDHECKER
(Würzburg, F.R.G.)

1. IS GLAUCOMA SURGERY USEFUL?

A discussion of glaucoma surgery makes sense only if the pressure theory of glaucoma is accepted, since the aim of surgery is the normalization of intraocular pressure (IOP). Surgery cannot restore function loss, but normalization of IOP delays or stops further loss, and increased IOP is the main cause of functional damage.

It has been suggested in recent publications that a high IOP does not matter and that normalization of IOP by medical treatment does not prevent further damage. Such statements are often based on insufficient therapy and monitoring. I had a discussion with the authors of a study from Africa, in which they had concluded that normalization of IOP did not prevent further damage, but my questions revealed that the ignorant patients were not informed about the nature of their disease and were not trained in the application of eyedrops. One could not be sure whether the patients had the money to buy new samples of drops once a bottle was empty. IOP was checked once in 6 months, 1–2 hours after the application of miotics, and the field was checked with the I/4 stimulus of Goldmann's perimeter only. It is not astonishing that under these conditions patients with approximately 20 mm Hg did not do better than the group with approximately 24 mm Hg. It does not prove anything against the pressure theory if the instruction of the patient is lacking and monitoring is insufficient.

High IOP without functional loss has been called ocular hypertension, and according to some authors no treatment was given, regardless of the height of the IOP (1, 24). Even with loss of function, the pressure theory was called a tradition based on obsolete ideas and not justified by positive results (2).

I do not share these opinions. Ocular hypertension is, in my opinion, a condition with IOP above 21 but below 26 mm Hg, a normal optic disc upon examination in mydriasis by slit lamp and contact lens, and a normal visual field when tested by computer-assisted age-adapted perimetry. This condition needs no treatment, unless in a risk patient (17). Eyes with 26 mm Hg or more and normal fields should better be called eyes with suspicion of glaucoma, and treatment should be started. High IOP is the main damaging factor in glaucoma and it is the only one to be influenced. My reasons are that high IOP in experimental animals or in secondary glaucoma produces the

211

E.L. Greve, W. Leydhecker & C. Raitta (eds.), Second European Glaucoma Symposium, Helsinki 1984.
© *1985, Dr. W. Junk Publishers, Dordrecht. ISBN 978-94-010-8934-0*

same damage as found in so-called primary glaucoma, and that normalization of the IOP prevents further damage (23).

We observed 236 glaucomatous eyes for an average period of over 10 years after normalization of their IOP below 22 mm Hg. A progression of glaucomatous field decay was found in 5 eyes only (2.1%). It might be argued that even these 5 eyes would not have had further field loss if their IOP had been truly norized, i.e. below 15 mm Hg.

We must therefore not leave out of account the only screw we can turn in order to save sight. When surgery normalizes IOP, it makes sense because it stops a further decay of function.

2. THE PRE-SURGICAL ANALYSIS OF PATIENTS

Surgery is recommended in open angle glaucoma if medical therapy fails to control IOP and to stop the loss of function. The decision for surgery requires in each individual case an exact analysis of the past history. However, the data collected and the monitoring of the patient are very often insufficient. With a well-monitored medical therapy, indications for surgery will be less frequent. The analysis of the present condition comprises the inspection of the optic disc by microscope with the 3-mirror lens with dilated pupils, gonioscopy, automated and threshold-adapted perimetry, and a diurnal tension curve without treatment. The next step is to repeat the diurnal curve with that treatment that showed the best compromise between tension-lowering effect and side-effects. Further tonometries are done every 4 weeks, just before the next application of the drug, which is under miotic therapy 5–6 h after the last drop; the field is checked at least every 6 months, in risk cases more often.

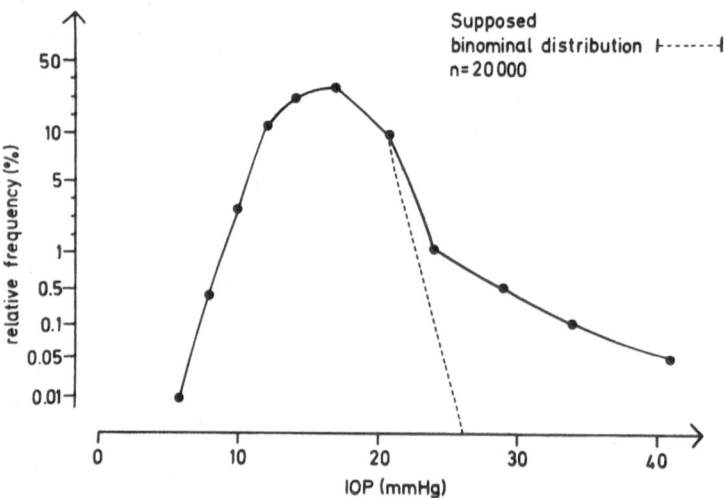

Fig. 1. Drawn-out curve: IOP in 20,000 eyes. Dotted curve: supposed distribution of normal values (Leydhecker 1958). Lower limit 8 mm Hg. Upper limit 25 mm Hg.

In this context, the term normalization must be defined more precisely. Normal IOP ranges statistically between 8 and approximately 21 mm Hg. The upper end of the distribution of normal IOP cannot be defined exactly. It varies with age and sex, but repeated readings of 26 mm Hg or more are definitely not normal. The probability that an IOP over 21 mm Hg is normal decreases strongly with each mm Hg added. The most common IOP in normal eyes is 15 mm Hg (Fig. 1). In treatment, all tonometries must be below 20 mm Hg if normalization is attempted. In patients with constricted fields or general vascular disease (sclerosis, diabetes) or in those who originally had IOPs near 10 mm Hg, the range between 15 and 20 mm Hg is not always good enough. If their fields keep on deteriorating one should attempt to lower IOP below 15 mm Hg. An average IOP of more than 21 mm Hg should not be called "normalized". Of course, any such number does not give a sharp limit separating those who will do well from those with a bad prognosis. Comparison between eyes with 20 mm Hg and others with 24 mm Hg will most probably show not much difference, but a comparison between those below 15 mm Hg and others above 30 mm Hg will do so. All these values refer to the results of diurnal tension curves, not to single tonometries now and then. The success of medical therapy depends furthermore on the compliance of the patient, which can be expected only from informed patients.

3. INFORMATION FOR THE PATIENT

In Germany, the doctor is obliged to discuss the pros and cons of surgery with the patient before intervention, and to mention possible complications. I think that good information for the patient is necessary right from the beginning to obtain his compliance. We have tested the success of step-by-step information. The first step represents the information at the time of diagnosis, consisting of a few simple explanations to the patient, instructions on how to apply the drops, together with a free leaflet (Fig. 2). The second step for patients is the reading of my booklet, which is available in German, English, and Spanish (Fig. 3). The third step is the discussion of indications and risks of surgery, if this was considered.

Five days after surgery, the patient was asked a standard set of questions. These were developed together with psychologists in order to test the effect of the presurgical information on the patient, and also his memory. To our astonishment, it was found that practically all patients gained more confidence in the hospital and the doctor by these open discussions, and that they were not more afraid than before of having surgery, quite a number even less so. They remembered correctly much technical information, for example the approximate limits of normal IOP or the reasons for monitoring by tonometry and perimetry. These tests were also applied to patients with a low educational standard. Those who would understand or remember less were the group of the aged and sclerotic patients. We consider the results of our information a great communicative success and also a necessary legal protection, since most legal suits for malpractice do not claim surgical mistakes but insufficient information (4, 5, 6, 7, 19, 21).

Merkblatt
für Patienten mit Augendrucksteigerung

1.

Die Nachricht hat Sie erschreckt, daß der Arzt bei Ihnen Glaukom (grünen Star) fand. Sie haben vielleicht in älteren Büchern gelesen, daß man am grünen Star erblinden kann. Heutzutage trifft das bei rechtzeitiger Behandlung nicht mehr zu, denn wir haben bessere Medikamente und, falls nötig, auch bessere Operationen als früher. Sie müssen aber den Ratschlägen Ihres Arztes genau folgen und die verordneten Augentropfen regelmäßig anwenden und bei sich tragen. Wenn das Auge rot wird, wenn Sie Schmerzen haben oder das Sehen sich verschlechtert, gehen Sie sofort zu Ihrem Augenarzt. Andernfalls **kommen Sie alle 4 bis 6 Wochen zu ihm.**

2.

Ohne Behandlung schreitet die Krankheit fort. Sie **spüren davon zunächst nichts.** Mit ausreichender Behandlung verschlechtert sich aber der Zustand nicht mehr. **Medikamente** oder Operationen können allerdings Ihr Sehvermögen bei grünem Star nicht bessern, sondern nur **weiteren Schaden verhindern.**

3.

Im Augeninnern wird dauernd eine Flüssigkeit gebildet. Wenn sie schlecht abfließen kann, steigt der Augeninnendruck und der Sehnerv leidet. Der Druck sollte möglichst nicht höher als 20 mm Hg sein. Er schwankt im Laufe des Tages und muß deshalb häufig gemessen werden. Der Augenarzt mißt mit einem feinen Instrument. Mit dem Finger **kann man nicht selbst fühlen, ob der Druck zu hoch ist.**

4.

Wir benutzen Tropfen und Salbe, um den Druck normal zu halten. Welche Tropfen Sie nehmen müssen und wie oft, kann der Arzt nur durch häufige Druckmessungen entscheiden. Falls Medikamente nicht ausreichen, stellt man mit einer Operation einen neuen Abfluß für die Flüssigkeit her. Da das Auge lebendiges Gewebe ist, kann sich manchmal der Abflußkanal wieder schließen, und man muß eine neue Operation vornehmen. Manchmal gewöhnt sich auch das Auge an die Tropfen, so daß sie unwirksam werden. Deshalb sollten Sie **regelmäßig zum Augenarzt** kommen, auch wenn Sie die Medikamente nach Vorschrift nehmen oder wenn eine erfolgreiche Operation vorgenommen worden ist.

5.

Durch manche Tropfen werden die Pupillen kleiner, wodurch manche Menschen einen ziehenden Schmerz und eine Abnahme des Sehvermögens nach dem Eintropfen empfinden. Das geschieht besonders dann, wenn man zum ersten Mal Tropfen benutzt. Fast immer gewöhnt man sich bald daran, es treten dann keine Schmerzen mehr auf.

6.

Wenn Sie einen anderen Augenarzt aufsuchen wollen, bitten Sie den bisher behandelnden Arzt, einen **Bericht** über den Verlauf an den neuen Arzt zu senden.

7.

Sie brauchen Ihre **normale Lebensweise nicht einzuschränken!** 2 Tassen Kaffee oder Tee sind erlaubt. **Mäßiger** Alkoholgenuß ist unschädlich und wirkt bei manchen Menschen sogar drucksenkend. Versuchen Sie seelische Aufregungen zu vermeiden. Tragen Sie keine engen Kragen. Sie sollten nicht rauchen. Sorgen Sie für regelmäßigen Stuhlgang. Verschaffen Sie sich 8 Stunden Nachtruhe und 1/2 Stunde Mittagsruhe. Mittagsruhe.

Aus der Universitätsaugenklinik Würzburg, Direktor Prof. Dr. W. Leydhecker

Before surgery the patient has to sign a printed form which summarizes in short and understandable language the essential information on the disease and on the possibility of post-operative hemorrhages, inflammations, cataract, or cicatrisation. The form also contains the printed consent of the patient to have surgery performed. It must be signed by the patient and by the doctor who gave the additional oral information (Fig. 4).

4. INDICATIONS FOR SURGERY

In a few conditions surgical therapy is my first choice, as in hydrophthalmia, in which I do not try any medical treatment at all, and in acute angle block glaucoma, preferably after drugs have reduced the IOP. In such cases, the second eye usually has a very narrow angle, and I recommend iridectomy in order to prevent an acute angle block of the second eye.

In open angle glaucoma surgery is indicated if the visual field deteriorates with the lowest IOP obtainable with drugs. The decision must be made upon an individual basis and does not only depend upon a certain IOP level, because tension tolerance is very different individually. However, generally I would prefer surgery if the IOP with treatment is often above 30 mm Hg. I would not operate on glaucoma without hypertension, if the IOP is always near or below 15 mm Hg, because the risk of surgery is not well balanced by a possible minimal decrease of IOP. Parameters which have to be evaluated individually are the speed of field decay and the height and stability of IOP. A quick decay of the field calls for surgical action, and so does a high or strongly changing IOP. The decision for surgery is psychologically easier if surgery was successful in the fellow eye, but unsuccessful intervention in one eye would not speak against surgery in the other if there are reasons for it. Further reasons for surgery are poor compliance of the patient in applying the drops or in keeping his appointments, and allergy or intolerance towards drugs.

A large cupping and atrophy would be additional reasons for surgery, and an increase of the cupping during observation time is certainly a good reason for surgery. Due to the development of computerized perimetry, we can rely much more on the results of perimetry, because they are observer-independent and well-repeatable in contrast to kinetic perimetry, which in the past gave only a poor base for the statement that the field had really deteriorated, because any change could also have been influenced by the observer.

It has been claimed that a field defect near the fixation point argues against surgery. In my opinon, the contrary is true: such a condition calls for

---

Fig. 2. Free leaflet as the first step of written information. It explains to the patient that he should have tonometry every 4–6 weeks; drugs cannot improve his condition but keep it as it is; he cannot feel or estimate his IOP for himself; regular checks are required as his condition may not be stable; drugs may have side effects; he should ask for a report for his ophthalmologist should he change doctors; he can lead a normal life without giving up coffee, tea or alcohol.

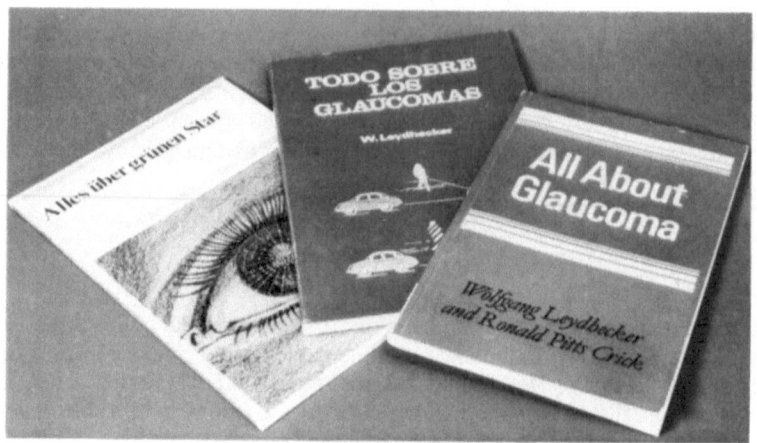

Fig. 3. My booklet on glaucoma is the second step for more comprehensive information.

surgery. I have never observed a sudden decrease of central vision because of surgery, unless there was a hemorrhage or a choroidal detachment or a flat chamber after surgery, complications which are not typical of eyes with narrow fields. There can be a decrease of vision independent of surgery, and this can also occur when surgery is postponed. The sudden decrease of vision in a very constricted field is a psychological and legal problem. This possibility must be discussed with the patient before surgery, preferably in the presence of witnesses, and the information that the sudden decrease is possible after surgery but not because of surgery must be made perfectly clear and documented in the case sheet.

Psychological and social parameters must be regarded. Some patients in developing countries do not appreciate the work involved with medical therapy and monitoring; they will respect a doctor only if he acts surgically, or they are too poor and too uneducated to understand that the disease will not be cured by the first bottle of eye-drops. Working in South India I realized that the choice was to do nothing at all, or to operate on the spot. This decision had to be based mostly on an IOP above 30 mm Hg, since the illiterate patients could not comply with any examination of their visual field and the examination of their optic discs was often prevented by cataracts. This type of unorthodox decision was facilitated by finding one eye already gone blind by glaucoma in a very large number of those patients (18, 25, 26).

5. THE CHOICE OF SURGICAL TECHNIQUES

5.1. External filtration procedures have in common that a round or a rectangular piece of tissue is excised at the limbus and covered by a scleral flap and conjunctiva so that filtration develops. Older techniques were originally called after Elliot's sclerocorneal trephination. Later authors added the lamellar scleral flap, which is a valuable modification, since the anterior

216

PATIENTENINFORMATION UND EINVERSTÄNDNISERKLÄRUNG
GLAUKOMOPERATION

Allgemeines
Es liegt bei Ihnen ein grüner Star (Glaukom) vor. Bei der Krankheit ist der Abfluß des Kammerwassers aus dem Auge behindert. was eine schädliche Steigerung des Augeninnendruckes zur Folge hat. Die Veranlagung zum Entstehen der Krankheit im Alter kann vererbt werden. Ein Glaukom kann auch als Folge anderer Augenerkrankungen entstehen: z. B. Entzündung, Verletzung, Gefäßleiden am Auge. Bei der häufigsten Glaukomform wird der Kammerwasserabfluß mit zunehmendem Alter verlegt, der Augeninnendruck steigt langsam auf höhere Werte an, die Krankheit verläuft schleichend. Der Kranke selbst spürt meist wenig, das zentrale Sehen bleibt jahrelang erhalten und Schädigungen machen sich nur in Ausnahmefällen im Gesichtsfeld bemerkbar. Es gibt aber noch eine ganz andere Glaukomform, den „akuten Glaukom-Anfall". Nur beim akuten Glaukomanfall treten h... übung der Hor... plötzlich auf... er Augeninne... ritt ein allmähl... vs ein, der bis...

General information on glaucoma

Das Gla... te, die den Au... e Operation behandelt, die den Abfluß aus dem Auge wiederherstellt.
Bei einfachem Glaukom wird man möglichst medikamentös behandeln unter laufender Kontrolle des Augeninnendruckes. Zur Operation entschließt man sich nur, wenn Medikamente nicht mehr ausreichen. Bei den meisten Operationen wird für das Wasser aus dem Auge ein neuer Abfluß nach außen geschaffen: das sogenannte Sickerkissen. Hierfür gibt es verschiedene Operationsmethoden, aus denen der Operateur die für Sie geeignete auswählt.
Bei der zweiten wichtigen Glaukomform, dem Glaukomanfall, muß der Augeninnendruck möglichst schnell, innerhalb von Stunden, durch Medikamente gesenkt werden. Die anschließende Operation beugt einem weiteren Glaukomanfall vor.
Bei einfachem Glaukom erwarten wir, daß durch die Operation bei ca. 70% der Augeninnendruck ohne Medikamente und bei weiteren 20% mit Augentropfen normalisiert werden kann. Bei 10% kann eine Nachoperation notwendig werden.

Mögliche Komplikationen
bei oder nach einer Augen-Operation
Bei *allen* C... ...ngen an oder im A...

Possible complications in ocular surgery (general)

...ktionen, ...l (Seide, ...en müs-... ...rübergе-... ...ırzeuges ...alle vor ...ache mit
sowie die Kunststof... sen. Nach... hend die stark bee... Wiederau...
dem behandelnden Augenarzt genommen werden muß.

Operation wegen grünem Star
Nach einer Operation wegen grünem Star werden Sehschärfe und Gesichtsfeld in der Regel nicht besser. Die Operation dient nur zur Drucknormalisierung und dadurch zum Bewahren der noch vorhandenen Funktion (Sehschärfe, Gesichtsfeld). Die Drucknormalisierur... ...ırreicht werden, wes... ...edikamente oder eine... ...:önnen. Linsentrübur...

Surgery of glaucoma

...u niedrigem ...r Linsenver-
Augeninn... ...lern. Selten änderung... ...Abfluß und verlegt di... muß dan... ...ickerkissen, dem neugeschaffenen Abfluß des Kammerwassers unter die Bindehaut, können sich später eine Entzündung oder eine Fistel entwickeln, weshalb eine Operation nötig werden könnte.
Besondere Risikofaktoren, die sich bei mir bei oder nach der Operation auswirken können, wie

sind mir bekannt.

Einverständniserklärung
zu einer Glaukom-Operation
Ich bin mit der bei mir/bei meinem Kind vorgesehenen Operation am grünen Star (Glaukom) einverstanden.
Ich wurde über Notwendigkeit, Zweck und Umfang der Operation, ihre Chancen, Risiken und Nachwirkungen im allgemeinen und in meinem speziellen Fall ausreic... ...ich in die Lage v... ...einflußte Entsch... ...Eingriffs abzuge...

Consent to glaucoma surgery

...ande Behandlu... ...he Komplikatic... ...urde ich umfass... ...äuterungen zu meiner Operation habe ich verstanden. Ich hatte ausreichend Gelegenheit, mich mit dem Arzt über die Operation zu unterhalten; an den Operateur habe ich keine weiteren Fragen. Mir ist bekannt, daß jede Operation ein gewisses Risiko bietet und eine Gewähr für den gewünschten Erfolg der Operation nicht gegeben werden kann. Ich kenne auch die Folgen und Risiken, die ohne Operation auf mich zukommen können.

_____, den _____

_____
Unterschrift des Arztes
(der das Aufklärungsgespräch geführt hat)

_____
Unterschrift des Patienten
(bzw. Sorgeberechtigten)

Nach einem Text der Univ.-Augenklinik Würzburg. Direktor Prof. Dr. Dr. h.c. W. Leydhecker.

Fig. 4. The last step, in case of surgery, summarizes the previous information, explains possible complications of surgery and contains the consent to surgery. This is signed by the patient and his doctor.

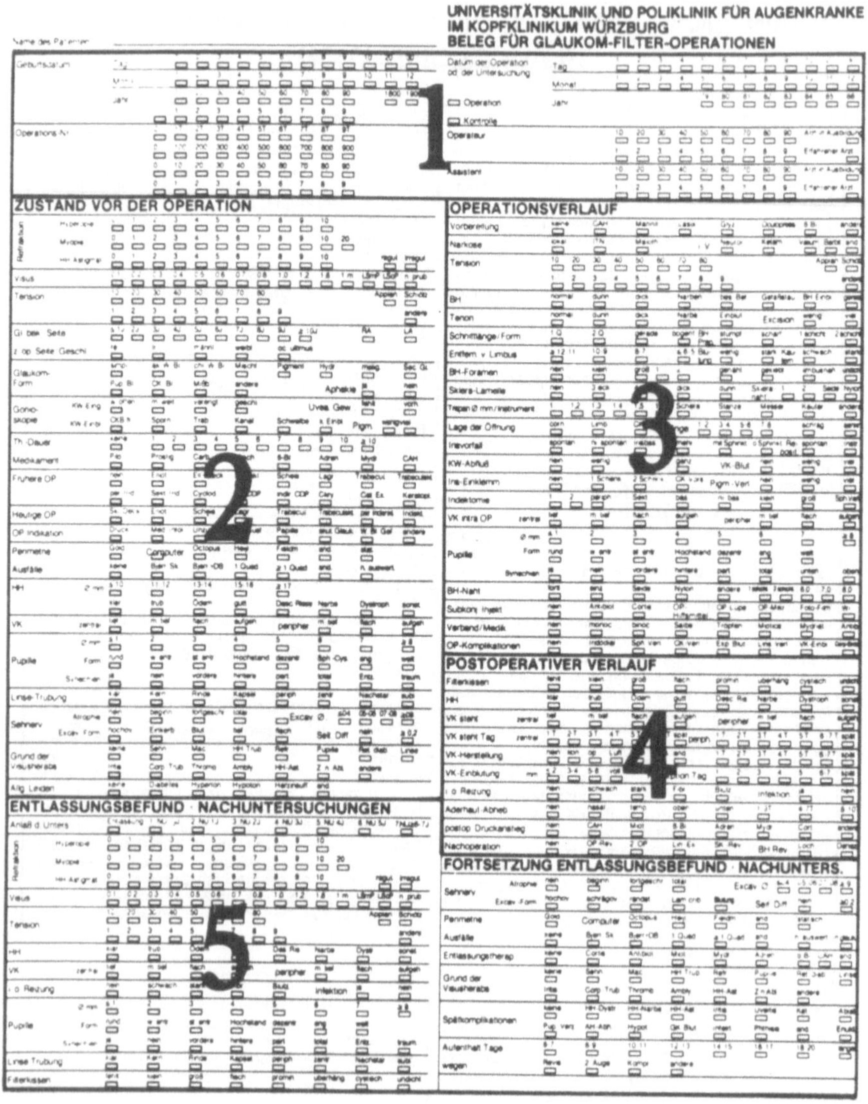

Fig. 5. A documentation form for surgical procedures consists of section (1) the date of the patient, surgeon and assistant, (2) findings before surgery, (3) details of the procedure, (4) the post-surgical condition during the first week and (5) findings at discharge from the hospital or at re-examinations.

chamber usually is reformed by the end of the procedure, and late infections are rare. All other details of modifications and names are less important, for example, whether the excision of tissue is done by a razor blade or a knife or a trephine, whether the excised tissue contains Schlemm's Canal, and whether

218

the excised piece is a bit smaller or larger. External filtration is the cause of pressure normalization in all these procedures. We compared (3) the trephined pieces of tissue as to their anatomical site and to the size of the trephination in 65 eyes in a prospective study. Observation time was 6–39 months. The anatomical localisation of the trephination had no significant influence on pressure normalization, nor was it important whether it contained Schlemm's Canal. The displacement of the trephination more towards the sclera produced more postoperative choroidal detachments. The size of the trephination, which was 1.2 or 1.5 or 1.8 mm in diameter, did not influence the incidence of choroidal detachment or flat anterior chamber (3).

These results were confirmed by d'Epinay et al. (9). No matter how and where the piece of tissue is excised and whether it contains Schlemm's Canal, sufficient external filtration follows after 2 weeks in approximately 80%, but after 2 years only 55% are still normalized; closure of the wound by cicatrisation follows in 10%, and the rest are partial successes, with pressures that can be normalized with miotics which failed before. I therefore prefer to speak of this type of surgery, in honor of its first inventor, as Elliot's operation with scleral flap. I think that modern names like Goniectomy and Trabeculectomy are new names rather than essentially new procedures. The operation is good in wide angle glaucoma and it also works in narrow angle glaucoma.

5.2. Another external filtration can be made by incarceration of a wick of iris. I described a special method of peripheral iridencleisis (12) which has the advantage that the anterior chamber is never lost during surgery. The only disadvantage of iridencleisis is that if later on senile cataract develops, one has to do a corneal section, or else dissect the wick of iris. In this case, I perform a corneoscleral trephination together with the cataract operation. I prefer the peripheral iridencleisis as surgical method for angle block glaucoma, because the incarcerated wick of iris draws the whole iris slightly upwards and thus dilates the rest of the chamber angle. The deepening of the anterior chamber can be observed impressively during surgery. The results of iridencleisis are at least as good as those of trephine operations, and they are permanent. I have under my observation patients whom I operated upon with this type of surgery 18 years ago and who still have normal IOP and a vision of 1.6 in spite of field defects present at the time of operation.

I would not advise doing a simple iridectomy in eyes with angle block glaucoma, because very often a mixed form of glaucoma (chronic simple glaucoma associated with a narrow angle) is present, so that after iridectomy many eyes will need miotics or a second operation, while the combined iridectomy with iridencleisis takes care of the acute attack as well as of the chronic component.

5.3. Goniotomy is the operation of choice for infantile glaucoma, but I also achieved good results with it in persons under 20 years suffering from wide angle glaucoma.

5.4. Iridectomy is indicated for the second eye in patients with acute angle block glaucoma of the fellow eye.

5.5. Cyclodialysis is the operation of choice in aphakia. It should never be done in persons over 45 years of age with phakic eyes, because cataract develops or progresses easily afterwards.

5.6. Cryo-surgery of the ciliary body has replaced diathermy in our hospital. It is essentially a procedure chosen when all other methods have failed or, as in hemorrhagic glaucoma, will probably fail.

5.7. Argon laser treatment of the trabecular meshwork decreases the IOP in open angle glaucoma for approximately 20%, often permanently. It would reserve this treatment for cases with a wide angle and an IOP of 30 mm Hg or less. Research is in progress, and at present the method is overrated so much that I would like to reserve my judgement for later.

6. DOCUMENTATION OF SURGICAL PROCEDURES

We collected at Würzburg over 15 years experiences with different methods of documenting surgical procedures (8, 13, 15).

A very large number of reports on surgery are not based on appropriate documentation and are therefore useless. The usual old method is the free description of the operation in which only major abnormal events are mentioned. The individual terminology of each surgeon results in individual descriptions which cannot be compared with the reports of others (10, 11, 14). Such descriptions are very often incomplete as would be found if one searched later on for the answer to special questions such as: does it matter where exactly the corneolimbal excision is placed? Should it contain a part of Schlemm's Canal? Is it good or bad to excise Tenon's Capsule in the surgical area (20)? Must Tenon's Fascia and the conjunctiva be sutured separately or can this be done by passing the suture through both tissues simultaneously?

Necessary details and the complications are often not mentioned fully in a free description. For evaluation, a student or a younger assistant will usually arrange a table without having appropriate knowledge of surgical methods or of the individual cases. He will try his best to satisfy his instructor by straightening results and completing insufficient reports now and then, and the boss will possibly report at the next congress on these results, giving them a pseudo-mathematical appearance with the help of a statistician.

The next step towards exactness and completeness was to have the surgical procedure split up into smallest steps and to give the surgeon an adequate questionnaire in order to standardize his description of each intervention. The questionnaire itself can be attached to the case sheet by marking the answers to the detailed questions directly on the questionnaire. For an evaluation one has to go through the questionnaire by hand. This is feasible in less than 50 cases. Errors are possible in filling in the case form, in reading it and in transferring it by hand onto a list.

Computer-readable forms are much more reliable. We have developed and constantly improved such forms for cataract surgery (8), performing over

1000 cataract operations per year at Würzburg. The printed form contains more than 500 pieces of information assembled on one single sheet in duplicate. After completion, the original goes to the computer department and the duplicate is attached to the patient's case sheet. Similar forms have been developed for glaucoma surgery. We have approximately 300—400 glaucoma operations per year, including all different types of surgical procedures.

There are five blocks of information (Fig. 5): (1) Data for identification of the patient, surgeon and assistant; (2) pre-operative situation; (3) procedure; (4) immediate postoperative situation; and (5) the patient's discharge examination. Only the procedure section is completed by the surgeon himself, while the other blocks are completed by the resident.

With changing habits of surgical technique, with the development of new procedures or new suture material, alterations of these forms are necessary every 1—3 years. With this type of form, the evaluation of 1 or more years is a very quick procedure and is done entirely by machine. It is possible to give each surgeon at the end of the year his personal statistics and to compare them with the average results of the hospital. In my opinion, only with this type of documentation can reliable statistics be obtained. The main advantages of this method are the filling in of each sheet immediately after each procedure, the necessity to answer a complete set of preformed questions, and the further work-up by the computer. The computer-readable form saves time because there is no need to dictate the whole procedure and have it typed for the case sheet, since the details are already contained in the form which is attached to the case sheet.

However, a documentist is required for checking regularly whether all surgeons fill in the forms completely. There will always be doctors who do not co-operate in documentation and who can be persuaded to do so only by constant nagging. Even with this best method available at present, one can get out of these forms or out of the machine only what has been put in before. It will be easy to tell the number of interventions, or the correlation between age and initial and postoperative IOP, but it will not be possible to answer any questions which occur later, e.g. on the best site of the scleral incision in relation to pressure regulation. Any question one intends to ask must be considered previously. One cannot collect at random as much data as possible, hoping to filter it later on in order to find new ideas or answers to new questions from heaps of data. Any question will first have to be formulated exactly and translated into a computer-readable form. The computer will do the counting for us faster and more precisely than we are able to, but it will still leave the thinking to us.

REFERENCES

1. Anderson, D. Discussions in: Glaucoma Symposium. Trans. New Orleans Acad. Ophthalmol. Mosby, St. Louis, p. 361 (1975).
2. Bengtsson, B. Aspects of the epidemiology of chronic glaucoma. Acta Ophthal. (Kbh.) Suppl. 146: 1—48 (1981).

3. Duzanec, Z. and Krieglstein, G.K. Die Beziehung zwischen Druckregulierung und anatomischer Lokalisation sowie Trepangröße bei der Goniotrepanation. Klin. Mbl. Augenheilk. 178:431–435 (1981).
4. Gramer, E., Leydhecker, W., and Krieglstein, G.K. Erste Erfahrungen mit der schriftlichen Aufklärung des Patienten vor der Operation. Sitzungsbericht 137. Vers. des Vereins Rhein.-Westf. Augenärzte 1979.
5. Gramer, E., Löhr, K., Leydhecker, W. and Krieglstein, G.K. Die Reaktionen des Patienten auf die präoperative Aufklärung über die Staroperation. Zeitschr. f. prakt. Augenheilk. 2:51–57 (1980).
6. Gramer, E., Löhr, K., Leydhecker, W. and Krieglstein, G.K. Erfahrungen mit der umfassenden Aufklärung des Glaukompatienten durch ein Informationsbuch. Zeitschr. f. prakt. Augenheilk. 5:43–49 (1980).
7. Gramer, E., Leydhecker, W. and Krieglstein, G.K. Zur ärztlichen Aufklärungspflicht – juristische Aspekte – Erwartungen der Patienten. Klin. Mbl. Augenheilk. 181:46–53 (1982).
8. Krieglstein, G.K., Duzanec, Z. and Leydhecker: W. Cataract surgery: Types and frequencies of complications. Albr. v. Graefes Arch. Klin. Ophthal. 214:9–13 (1980).
9. Lalive d'Epinay, S., Remé, C. and Witmer, R. Der Einfluß verschiedener Lokalisationen der Trabekulektomie auf die intraokulare Druckregulation beim primären Glaukom. Klin. Mbl. Augenheilk. 182:387–390 (1983).
10. Leydhecker, W. Vorschläge für Veröffentlichungen über Glaukomoperationen. Klin. Mbl. Augenheilk. 136:219–224 (1960).
11. Leydhecker, W. Erfahrungen bei dem Auswerten von Krankenblättern und Vorschläge zur einheitlichen Dokumentation von Befunden. Klin. Nbl. Augenheilk. 149:737–745 (1966).
12. Leydhecker, W. Peripheral iridenkleisis. Trans. Ophthal. Soc. U.K. 86:493–496 (1966).
13. Leydhecker, W. Comparative study of late after-effects of glaucoma operations. Glaucoma Symposium Tutzing 1966, Leydhecker (ed.). Karger Basel, 224–238 (1967).
14. Leydhecker, W. The main difficulties found in the evaluation of case sheets. Glaucoma Symposium Tutzing 1966, Leydhecker (ed.). Karger Basel, 239–240 (1967).
15. Leydhecker, W. and Ricklefs, G. Erfahrungen mit Vordrucken für den Operationsverlauf. Docum. Ophthalmol. 27:64–69 (1969).
16. Leydhecker, W. Alles über grünen Star (2. Aufl.) Thieme-Verlag Stuttgart, 55S. (1984).
17. Leydhecker, W. and Krieglstein, G.K. Ocular hypertension – glaucoma suspect or incipient glaucoma? Res. Clin. Forums 2:122–128 (1980).
18. Leydhecker, Reddy, H.P. and Krieglstein, G.K. The prevalence of glaucoma in South India. A population survey. Bollettino di Oculistica 59:435–445 (1980).
19. Leydhecker, W., Gramer, E. and Krieglstein, G.K. Patient information before cataract surgery. Ophthalmologica, Basel 180:241–246 (1980).
20. Leydhecker, W., Waller, W.K. and Krieglstein, G.K. Untersuchungen über die Tenonexcision bei der Trepanation nach Elliot mit lamellärer Skleradeckung. Vorläufige Ergebnisse. In: Wundheilung des Auges und ihre Komplikationen, G.O.H. Naumann and B.P. Gloor (eds.). J.F. Bergmann, Verlag, München, S. 257–263 (1980).
21. Leydhecker, W., Löhr, K., Gramer, E. and Krieglstein, G.K. Die Aufklärung Glaukomkranker vor der Operation. Zeitschr. f. prakt. Augenheilk. 5:50–56 (1980).
22. Leydhecker, W. and Crick, R.P. All about Glaucoma. Faber and Faber, London & Boston, 76 S. (1981).
23. Leydhecker, W. Is glaucoma therapy useless? In: Glaucoma Update II, G.K. Krieglstein and W. Leydhecker (eds.). Springer-Verlag, Berlin–Heidelberg–New York–Tokyo, S. 95–102 (1983).
24. Podos, S.M. Discussion in: Glaucoma Symposium. Trans. New Orleans Acad. Ophthalmol. Mosby, St. Louis, p. 361 (1975).

25. Reddy, H., Leydhecker, W. and Krieglstein, G.K. Difficulties of an epidemiological study of glaucoma in rural areas in India. Bollettino di Oculistica 59:147–150 (1980).
26. Reddy, H., Leydhecker, W. and Krieglstein, G.K. Glaucoma survey in eye camps. A study of its practicability. Bollettino di Oculistica 59:299–303 (1980).

Author's address:
Prof. Dr.Dr.h.c. W. Leydhecker
Direktor der Univ.-Augenklinik
Josef-Schneider-Str. 11
D-8700 Würzburg
F.R.G.

SCLERAL CHANGES AFTER DIATHERMY AND INCISION
(SCANNING ELECTRON MICROSCOPE STUDY)

P. ROZSÍVAL and S. ŘEHÁK

Hradec Králové, Czechoslovakia)

ABSTRACT

Scleral changes after diathermy and incision (operative approach used in Scheie's anti-glaucoma iridectomy) were evaluated in rabbits by scanning electron microscopy. Immediately after the operation the region of coagulation on the scleral surface and the gap into the anterior chamber can be found. In the course of healing process, the wound is gradually filled with denser and denser collagen meshwork. Six months after diathermy and incision in the wound are irregular new-formed collagen fibres, the sclera is there thinner and on the anterior chamber face collagen fibres are still in direct contact with aqueous. Despite interindividual variations it is possible to conclude that healing of the sclera after diathermy and incision is not even complete six months after the operation.

INTRODUCTION

Scheie was the first who reported a combination of iridectomy and cauterization of the sclera in the literature when he wrote in the Archives of Ophthalmology in 1959: "A fistula is produced by causing the lips of a scleral incision, made as for peripheral iridectomy, to retract by application of a cautery superficially to the wound edges". He explained the positive effect of cauterization by the mechanical retraction of the wound.

The purpose of our experimental work was to evaluate scleral changes after diathermy and incision since, in contrast to Scheie (3), we tend to agree with the opinion of Soll (4) about a complex effect of diathermy where, besides the thermal destruction of the sclera, aqueous filtration through the site of the intevention plays a role.

METHODS

A total of 35 male and female chinchilla grey rabbits were used in our study. After intraperitoneal administration of Pentobarbital, an incision of the sclera 4 to 5 mm long was made under the scleral flap at the limbus. The

225

E.L. Greve, W. Leydhecker & C. Raitta (eds.), Second European Glaucoma Symposium, Helsinki 1984.
© *1985, Dr. W. Junk Publishers, Dordrecht. ISBN 978-94-010-8934-0*

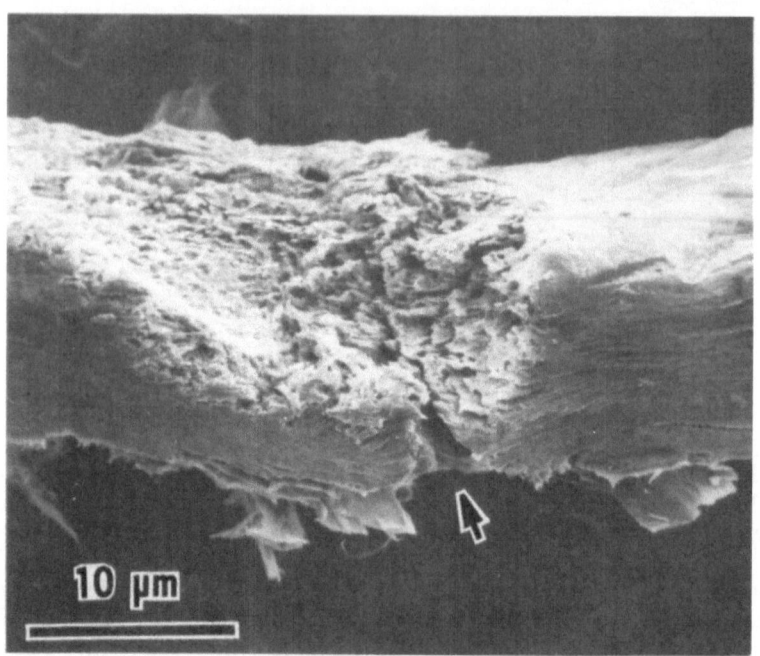

Fig. 1. Sclera immediately after diathermy and incision

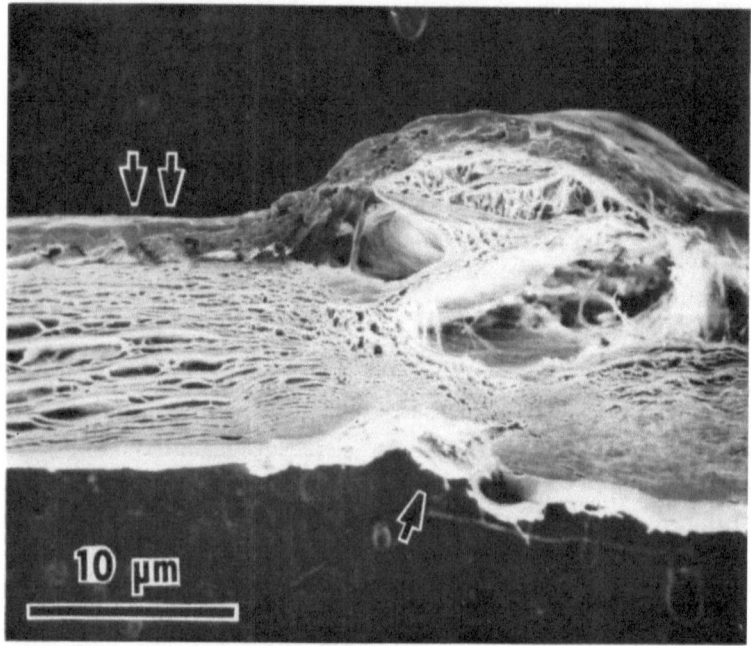

Fig. 2. Sclera two weeks after diathermy and incision

226

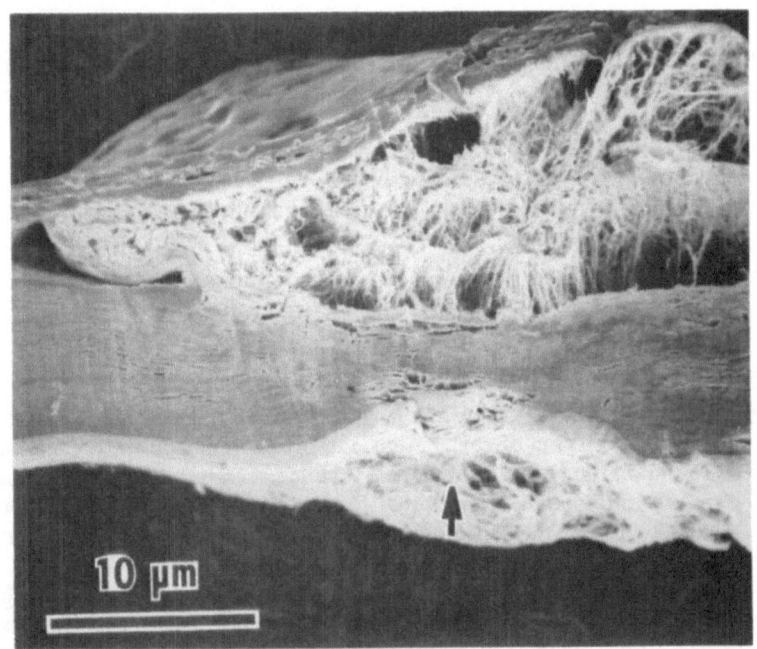

Fig. 3. Sclera three months after diathermy and incision

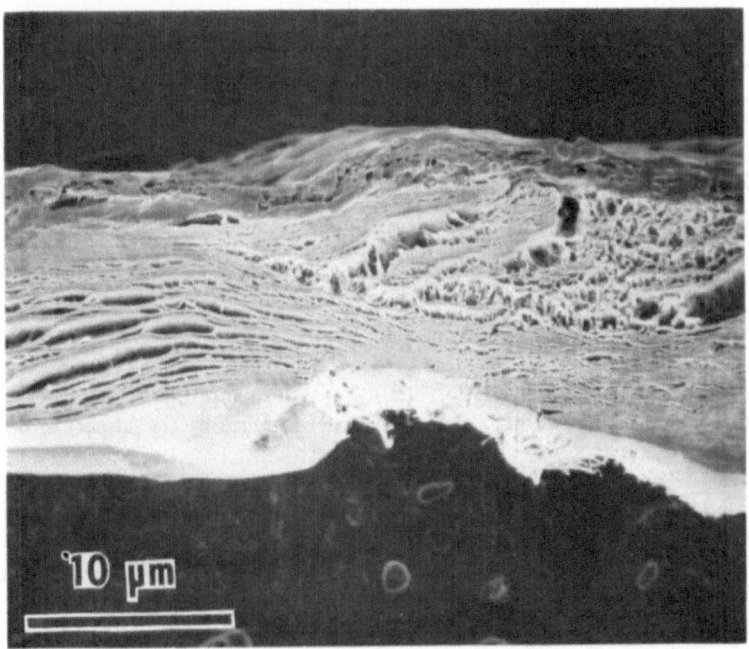

Fig. 4. Sclera six months after diathermy and incision

region of incision was coagulated with a cauter heated above a gas burner and opened into the anterior chamber of the eye with a razor blade. After running suture of the conjunctiva an ointment containing antibiotics and corticoids was applied into the conjunctival sack. The sclera for scanning electron microscopy (JSM 35 R, JEOL, Ltd.) was fixed in the alkalic medium and processed using the technique described in detail by Kuběna et al. (2). In short, the processing consists of gradual cleaning of the collagen skeleton of the sclera from undesirable low-weight proteins and final contrast reaction with chromium salts.

RESULTS

Figure 1 shows the sclera immediately after diathermy and incision (magnification 40x). The region of coagulation, sharply dropping on the corneal side, can be found on the corneal surface, from which thermally denaturated tissue was removed in the preparation process, and thus the extent of the injury can be fully seen. There is an opening into the anterior chamber after the razor blade cut in the lower part of the sclera (arrow).

Figure 2 shows the sclera two weeks after diathermy and incision (magnification 40x). The wound (arrow) is filled with thin collagen fibres. Cystic spaces are formed under the conjunctiva. The sclera was reinforced with adhesive tape before cutting to prevent its deformation (double arrow).

Figure 3 shows the sclera three months after diathermy and incision, (magnification 40x). The preparation is reinforced with an adhesive tape. Cystic spaces can be found under the conjunctiva. Sclera is thinner at the site of operation with a distinct gap in the Descemet membrane with a loose structure of collagen fibres which are in contact with aqueous humour (arrow).

Figure 4 shows the sclera six months after diathermy and incision (magnification 40x). The wound is filled with irregular newly formed collagen fibres; sclera is thinner there and the defect in the Descemet membrane is not closed. Collagen fibres are still in direct contact with aqueous.

DISCUSSION

Histological examination of postoperative experimental material in the time sequence reveals individual stages of changes induced by the surgery and thus enables a reconstruction of their development.

On the basis of our results, it can be suggested that Scheie's original idea (3) about mechanical opening of the wound by diathermy is not sufficient for explaining the long-term effect of the operation. A permanent patency of artificially made aqueous humour outflow channel after the termal cautery of the sclera was very well explained, on the basis of literary reports (1, 5, 6) and his own clinical experience, by Soll in 1973: "The thermal cautery has an immediate effect on the properties of scleral collagen which abets the continued patency of the cleft. The continued filtration of aqueous has permanent effect on the scleral collagen in the area of the cleft, thus helping to insure permanent functioning of the filtering tract". Results obtained in our study are in full agreement with this theory.

REFERENCES

1. Kornbleuth, W. and Tenenbaum, E. The inhibitory effect of aqueous humor on the growth of cells in tissue culture. Am. J. Ophthalmol. 42:70 (1956).
2. Kuběna, K., Krul, Z. and Svoboda, V. Bělima zdravého oka zobrazená řádkovacím elektronovým mikroskopem. Čs. Oftalmol. 38:196 (1982).
3. Scheie, H.G. Peripheral iridectomy with scleral cautery for glaucoma. Arch. Ophthalmol. 61:291 (1959).
4. Soll, D.B. Intrascleral filtering procedure for glaucoma. Am. J. Ophthalmol. 75:390 (1973).
5. Teng, C.C., Chi, H.H. and Katzin, H.M. Histology and mechanism of filtering operations. Am. J. Ophthalmol. 47: (1959).
6. Teng, C.C., Chi, H.H. and Katzin, H.M. Aqueous degenerative effect and protective role of endothelium in eye pathology. Am. J. Ophthalmol. 50:365 (1960).

Authors' address:
Dept. of Ophthalmology
Charles University
500 36 Hradec Králové
Czechoslovakia

LONG-TERM OBSERVATIONS ON GONIOTREPHINATION

N.G. LAMBROU and C.N. CHRISTAKIS

(Athens, Greece)

ABSTRACT

Goniotrephination is a surgical procedure applied by many ophthalmologists in glaucoma with good results. Its favourable assessment has been based on observations covering no more than a five-year postoperative period. The evaluation, however, of any surgical procedure can be more strictly tested and thus better validated by a more prolonged period of observation. 108 eyes operated on were followed-up closely for ten or more years. The following information retrieved from the patients' records were studied: indication to operate, preoperative IOP, postoperative IOP after ten or more years, need of conservative treatment postoperatively, bleb morphology and its relation to the IOP values, fate of the visual function, etc. These observations did not substantially change the early statisfactory assessment of the results that have been published to date.

INTRODUCTION

Goniotrephination is a surgical procedure applied by many ophthalmologists in glaucoma with good results. The favorable assessment of this technique so far has been based on observations covering no more than a five-year post-operative period. The evaluation, however, of any surgical procedure, can be more strictly tested and thus better validated by a more prolonged period of observation.

We have been applying goniotrephination as our method of choice in dealing with open angle glaucoma cases for 15 years now, contributing to its formation and standardisation, as collaborators of Fronimopoulos. We believe that a review of the results obtained over a ten-year period permits us to contribute to a sounder evaluation of the procedure.

MATERIAL AND METHOD

From 1968 until September 1983 goniotrephination was carried out on 1258 eyes with open angle glaucoma. The study does not include operations carried

231

E.L. Greve, W. Leydhecker & C. Raitta (eds.), Second European Glaucoma Symposium, Helsinki 1984.
© *1985, Dr. W. Junk Publishers, Dordrecht. ISBN 978-94-010-8934-0*

out after 1973 but is limited to 493 operations performed 10 or more years previously. From the 493 eyes operated on between 1968 and 1973 (about 82 per year) we have excluded from this study those that for a variety of reasons could not be followed up continuously to date or those that showed structural and functional changes in the course of time. Thus, the cases eliminated from the study consist of patients that moved to another town, died in the interim, underwent a cataract operation or showed structural and functional changes postoperatively.

Thus, 108 of the eyes operated on have been followed up closely for ten or more years. These eyes belong to 69 patients, 28 men and 41 women. Operation was bilateral in 39 and unilateral in 30 cases. The mean patient age at the time of the operation was 58 years, with 40 and 72 years at the extremes.

The following information has been retrieved from the records of these patients: (a) indication to operate, (b) preoperative IOP value under maximal therapy, (c) postoperative IOP every year following the operation, (d) need to continue conservative treatment postoperatively, (e) bleb morphology, (g) IOP in relation to bleb morphlogy, (h) visual functions and their fate in the course of time and (i) later complications that were eventually observed.

OBSERVATIONS

The following observations were made:

(a) The indication to operate. Of the 108 eyes, 80 were operated on because of visual defects, while the IOP could not be brought under control with drugs. Seventeen eyes were operated on because conservative treatment had completely failed to control the IOP despite the absence of any visual defects. Five eyes showed drug intolerance while in six cases conservative treatment had been erratic (Fig. 1).

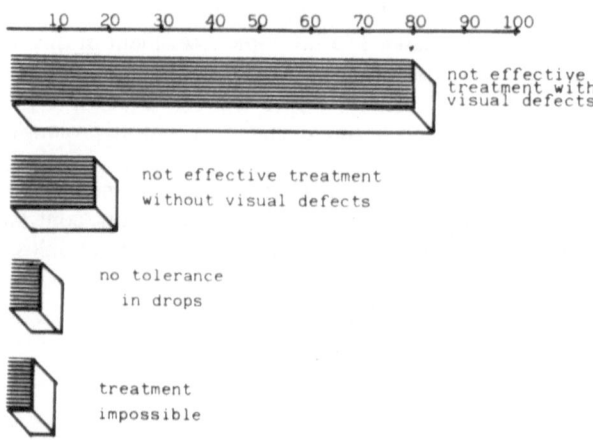

Fig. 1. Indications to operate.

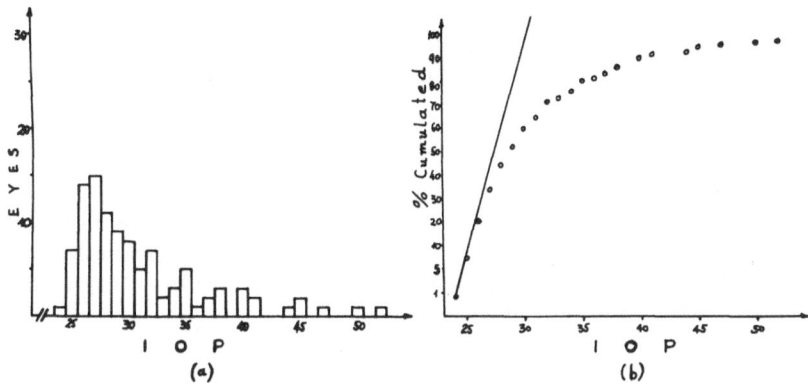

Fig. 2. (a) The non-symmetrical distribution of preoperative IOP values identical to glaucomatous population. (b) The trace of cumulated percentages of the same frequencies obviously deviated in high IOP values.

(b) The preoperative IOP, under maximal therapy (87 eyes) or faulty treatment (11 eyes), ranged between 24 mmHg and 52 mmHg with an average value of 29.1 mmHg. The distribution curve of the preoperative IOP values is shown in Fig. 2a and their cumulative percentage histogramme in Fig. 2b.

(c) The mean value of the postoperative IOP in each postoperative year has been as follows: at the end of the first year 14.2 mmHg; the second, 14.0 mmHg; the third, 14.2 mmHg; the fourth, 14.8 mmHg; the fifth, 15.2 mmHg; the sixth, 15.6 mmHg; the seventh, 16.2 mmHg; the eigth, 16.2 mmHg; the ninth, 16.0 mmHg; the tenth, 16.2 mmHg and over the tenth year (less than 108 eyes) 17.2 mmHg.

The distribution of the IOP values in the tenth postoperative year is shown in Fig. 3a and their cumulative percentage histogramme in Fig. 3b.

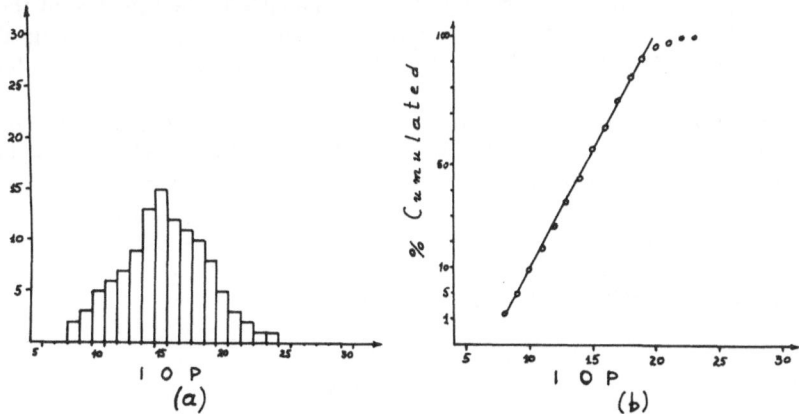

Fig. 3. (a) The symmetrical distribution ten years after the operation identical to normal population. (b) The trace of cumulated percentages of the same frequencies. It shows the restoration of the preoperative histogramme to the Gaussian straight line after the operation.

233

(d) Conservative treatment to control the IOP postoperatively had to be instituted: in 3 eyes (2.8%) during the first year, in 5 eyes (4.6%) during the third year, in 11 eyes (10.2%) during the fifth year and in 13 eyes (12%) during the tenth year.

(e) The morphology of the goniotrephination site presented three patterns: in the majority of cases it was flat and in a small percentage either a circumscribed elevation or cystic degeneration. The latter two patterns showed characteristics identical to those of the bleb formed with the older filtration procedures, while the first pattern showed a configuration identical to an almost normal scleral area with good vascular supply. The frequency of the three patterns is shown in Table 1.

Table 1.

Bleb morphology	1st month	1st year	3rd year	5th year	10th year
Flat	74 (68.5%)	94 (87.0%)	92 (85.2%)	no change	no change
Circumscribed elevation	27 (25.0%)	7 (6.5%)	7 (6.5%)	no change	no change
Cystic degeneration	7 (6.5%)	7 (6.5%)	9 (8.3%)	no change	no change

(f) The mean IOP values in relation to the three patterns of the bleb just described varied widely and could not be accounted for in every single case. Thus the IOP in the presence of a flat and well-vascularised trephination site was: 10.5 mmHg in the first month, 12.5 mmHg in the first year and 13.5 mmHg after the third year. In the presence of a circumscribed elevation the IOP was: 20.5 mmHg in the first month, 19 mmHg in the first year, 18.6 mmHg in the third, 17 mmHg in the fifth and 16.6 mmHg after the tenth year. In the presence of cystic degeneration the IOP was in the first month 5 mmHg, in the first year 6.5 mmHg, in the third year 13.5 mmHg, in the fifth 12.2 mmHg and 12.5 mmHg after the tenth.

If we examine collectively the mean IOP value in relation to the final bleb configuration at the operative site, it was: 14 mmHg in the presence of the flat, well-vascularised conjuctiva pattern, 18.6 mmHg with the circumscribed conjuctival elevation and 9.5 mmHg in the presence of cystic avascular degeneration of the area.

(g) Visual functions were not impressively modified: visual acuity remained unchanged in 101 of the 108 eyes (93.5%), while a slight decrease in visual acuity was noted in the remaining eyes due to a non-progressive lens opacification. The visual fields also remained more or less unchanged except for three cases (2.8%) that showed definite deterioration probably attributable to circulatory disturbances of the optic nerve head.

(h) No long-term complications were observed.

CONCLUSION

The results obtained with goniotrephination beyond a ten-year period should be considered satisfactory for the cases included in this study. The following observations support this conclusion:

1. The majority of the eyes were operated on because of visual defects and the inability to control the IOP by conservative treatment. The correlation of the indication to operate with observed reduction of the visual defects in almost all the cases studied, over a period of ten or more years testifies to the achievement of our main goal.

2. Normalisation of the postoperative IOP values is clearly seen from the comparison between Fig. 2a–3a and Fig. 2b–3b. Preoperative IOP distribution follows the pattern set in a glaucoma population and is, quite clearly, permanently postoperatively to that of a normal population. This is seen beyond doubt in the restoration of the deflected cumulative percentage histogramme of the frequency of the preoperative IOP values to the Gaussian straight line after the operation. It is exactly this finding that we consider of major significance since it is preserved beyond the decade despite the slightly ascending trend of the mean values.

3. In only 8% of these case does the pattern of aqueous outflow in the goniotrephination site take the configuration of an old bleb with an avascular cystic degeneration accompanied by great hypotony. The great majority of cases seem to settle down to more normal structural and functional conditions. This fact lends support to our views already published, namely that the scleral flap opens the way to the formation of the so-called "parathalamos". This is a fine intrascleral space that creates conditions favouring a new outflow function, through which we avoid hypotony on the one hand and on the other establish a more normal relation between aqueous production and drainage, resulting in a permanent retention of the IOP at values close to those of normal people.

4. Finally, observations of the goniotrephination fate for more than a decade do not substantially change the early satisfactory assessment of the results that have been published to date.

REFERENCES

1. Cvetkovic, D., Blagojevic, M. and Dodic, V. Experience with trepanotrabeculectomy. Acta Ophthalmol. 56:150 (1978).
2. Doden, W. and Hosch, W. Zur Operation des primären Glaukoms nach Elliot-Fronimopoulos (Goniotrepanation mit Scleradeckel). Klin. Mbl. Augenheilk. 165:209 (1974).
3. Evers, V. Methodik der Goniotrepanation. Klin. Mbl. Augenheilk. 164:842 (1974).
4. Fisher-Grüner. Goniotrepanation. Klin. Mbl. Augenheilk. 167:630 (1975).
5. Fronimopoulos, J. Die Goniotrepanation mit Skleradeckel in der heutigen Chirurgie des Glaukoms. Klin. Mbl. Augenheilk. 178:159 (1981).
6. Fronimopoulos, J. and Lambrou, N. Goniotrephination with screral flap. In: Bellows (ed.), Glaucoma: Contemporary international concepts, pp. 390–400.
7. Fronimopoulos, J., Lambrou, N., Pelekis, N. and Christakis, Ch. Elliot'sche Trepanation mit Skleradeckel. Klin. Mbl. Augenheilk. 156:1–8 (1970).
8. Fronimopoulos, J., Lambrou, N. and Christakis, Ch. Goniotrepanation mit Skleradeckel. Klin. Mbl. Augenheilk. 159:565–573 (1971).
9. Fronimopoulos, J. and Christakis, Ch. Goniotrepanation (Gotrep) and further observations on this operation for chronic glaucoma. Albrecht von Graefes Arch. klin. exper. Ophthal. 193:135–143 (1975).

10. Hollwich, F., Fronimopoulos, J., Jünemann, G., Christakis, Ch. and Lambrou, N. Indication, technique et résultats de la goniotpepanation avec couvercle scléral dans le glaucome chronique simple. Arch. d'Ophtal. (Paris) 34:283 (1974).
11. Hollwich, F., Jünemann, G. and Kinne, J. Klinische Ergebnisse der Goniotrepanation mit Skleradeckel. Klin. Mbl. Augenheilk. 171:735–743 (1977).
12. Lambrou, N. and Fronimopoulos, J. Die Bedeutung des Skleralappens für die Chirurgie des Glaukoms. Klin. Mbl. Augenheilk. 173:599–606 (1978).
13. Lambrou, N.: The "Parathalamos". A late observation on Goniotrephination. Arch. Arch. North. Greece Ophthalmol. Soc. 28:75–80 (1979).
14. Papst, W., Evers, V. and Kienast, J. Erfahrungen mit der Goniotrepanation. Ber. dtsch. ophthal. Ges. 73:337 (1973).
15. Rahäuser, H. Uber Erfahrungen mit der Goniotrepanation (Elliot–Fronimopoulos) Klin. Mbl. Augenheilk. 173:607 (1978).
16. Riss, B. and Binder, S. Retrospektive auf 402 Goniotrepanationen. Klin. Mbl. Augenheilk. 176:286 (1980).
17. Schnaudigel, O-E. Landzeitergebnisse nach gedeckter Goniotrepanation (Elliot-Fronimopoulos). Klin. Mbl. Augenheilk. 184:202–203 (1984).

Authors' address:
Eye Clinic "Pammakaristos Hospital"
Patriach Joakim 30
Athens 315
Greece

TEN YEAR PROSPECTIVE FOLLOW-UP OF A GLAUCOMA OPERATION

The Double Flap Scheie in primary open angle glaucoma

E.L. GREVE, C.L. DAKE, J.H.J. KLAVER and E.M.G. MUTSAERTS

(Amsterdam, The Netherlands)

ABSTRACT

The results of a long-term prospective follow-up study after the "Double Flap" Scheie filtering operation are presented. Fifty-two eyes of 47 patients with primary open angle glaucoma (POAG) were operated; after ten years 29 eyes of 24 patients could be examined. Twenty patients (43%) had died; in three follow-up was incomplete.

The two and four years results have been published earlier. In the 29 eyes the mean intraocular pressure (IOP) without medical therapy rose from 15.8 mmHg at five years to 16.3 mmHg at ten years (not significant). Additional medical or surgical treatment was necessary in 35% of the eyes. Diurnal variation and outflow facility remained stable. During the ten years 13 eyes showed some deterioration of visual fields. Nearly all clinically important deterioration occurred within five years after the operation.

Cataract progression was noticed in 45% (13 of 29); four times a lens extraction was performed (13%).

Complete success of the operation, as judged by stable visual fields and IOP levels at or under 21 mmHg without additional medical or surgical therapy, was reached in 13 of 20 eyes (45%). Based on IOP alone the success rate was 62% without and 93% with additional treatment.

INTRODUCTION

Data on prospective long-term follow-up results after filtering operations for POAG are sparse in the literature (1, 4, 19). Most studies are retrospective (5, 6, 7, 11, 12, 13, 14, 15, 16, 17, 18, 20) and do not provide evaluation of glaucomatous visual field loss by means of sufficiently exact techniques such as static perimetry. Interpretation and comparison of these data are therefore very difficult.

In 1971 we started a study in which a group of POAG patients was followed prospectively after a filtering operation, the Double Flap Scheie. Pre- and postoperative evaluation was similar in all patients and included yearly diurnal IOP curves, static perimetry, visual acuity determinations, and investigation in mydriasis of lens and optic disc. The present report gives the

237

E.L. Greve, W. Leydhecker & C. Raitta (eds.), Second European Glaucoma Symposium, Helsinki 1984.
© 1985, Dr. W. Junk Publishers, Dordrecht. ISBN 978-94-010-8934-0

ten year follow-up results of this study. The two and four year results have been published before (2, 9, 10).

This report is different from other reports in the following respects: prospective study; all patients similar follow-up period of 10 years; rigorous protocol; control examination by the same ophthalmologist; visual field examination with static perimetry differentiating glaucomatous deterioration from cataract; all IOP measurements in diurnal curves.

PATIENTS AND METHODS

The study was started with 52 operated eyes in 47 patients, representing all those who, during a predetermined period (1-1-1972 up to 31-12-1973) fulfilled the following criteria:

1. An anterior chamber angle in which, in mydriasis, the trabeculum had to be visible over its entire width, covering more than one-half of the angle.
2. Patients previously subjected to operations were excluded.
3. Patients with myopia of more than six diopters were excluded from the study.
4. Only primary open angle glaucoma was included. All other forms of open-angle glaucoma (pigment glaucoma, heterochromic glaucoma, other secondary glaucomas etc.) were excluded from the investigation. Two patients had the pseudoexfoliation syndrome.
5. Other severe corneal or retinal pathology (keratitis parenchymatosa sanata, retinopathia pigmentosa, central-vein thrombosis, etc.) led to exclusion.
6. The patients in principle had to be willing and able to appear for follow-up examination at regular intervals.

The indication for operation was deterioration of the visual field under maximum tolerated medical treatment.

This report describes only those patients who had a complete follow-up of ten years. All patients that died within ten years of the operation or that were lost for follow-up are listed in Table 1.

The technique of the Double Flap Scheie has been described elsewhere (2). In short, a limbus-based conjunctival flap and a scleral flap are prepared; a perforating limbal incision is cauterized and a peripheral iridectomy is made.

Follow-up results are based on yearly examinations including: general opthalmological examination, gonioscopy, lens and disc evaluation in mydriasis (all carried out by one of the authors E.L.G.), diurnal curves (5 measurements) with and without medical therapy and static perimetry. Stereo photographs of the fundus were taken in most cases. Visual acuity was tested with the best optical correction at a Snellen chart. Decrease in visual acuity is expressed as number of Snellen lines lost. Tonometry was done with a Goldmann applanation tonometer. The Tübingen Perimeter and the Visual Field Analyser were used for static perimetry. Judgement of regression or progression of defects was based primarily on the results of static meridional perimetry using the Tübingen instrument. Care was taken to separate the general reduction of sensitivity caused by cataract from local reductions of

Table 1. Survey of patients followed for less than ten years

Patient	Age at last examination (years)	Follow-up (years)	Preop. IOP* (mmHg)	. Last IOP* (mmHg)	Visual field
1. BOE[†]	76	2	28/33	10/12	=
2. CAT[†]	69	5	24/28	19/24	↓
3. END[L]	71	5	42/48	25/28	= th.
4. FOL[†]	76	1	20/30	11/17	=
5. GER[L]	77	7	44/48	16/18	↓
6. HER[†]	78	½	24/32	16/22	=
7. HEU[†]	84	7	36/40	18/22	↓ th.
8. KAT[†]	86	9	34/40	10/14	↓ reop. + th.
9. KEY[†]	76	½	22–26	13/18	↓ ?
10. KON[†]	73	½	27/42	16/21	= th.
11. KOO[L]	71	8	24/27	16	=
12. LAN[†]	73	. 6	34/40	24/26	= th.
13. MON[†]	84	4	28/34	14/17	↓ th.
14. MOS[†]	73	½	22/26	6	=
15. MUL[†]	77	2½	16/28	5/9	=
16. PLU[†]	68	3	25/36	17/22	=
17. SON[†]	70	8	32/41	16/18	= th.
18. STA[†]	68	0.2	35/46	12/15	X
19. VEL[†]	68	5	21/29	15/18	=
20. VIS[†]	77	2½	26/35	7/10	↓
21. WAL[†]	88	6	20/26	18/19	= th.
22. WIT 1[†]	73	9	28/38	11/13	=
23. WIT 2[†]	76	4	26/30	9/11	=

[†]: deceased
[L]: lost to follow-up
*: given are a lowest and highest value in a day curve.

sensitivity caused by glaucoma. Local changes were considered significant if they were more than 0.5 log. units (in general if they exceeded the physiological variation); if they occurred at several positions; and if they did not occur at the edge of defects for maximal luminance.

RESULTS

Ten years after the operation 29 eyes of 24 patients could still be examined. Drop-outs were due to death in 20 cases and to inability to participate in the examination program in three cases. Of the patients left 12 were male and 12 were female. Their mean age was 75 years.

Intraocular pressures

Preoperative and yearly postoperative IOP values of all patients are plotted in Figs. 1–6. The values are based on means of diurnal curves. If the patients received additional medical therapy the IOP values given are those with therapy.

To estimate the results of the operation with regard to reduction in IOP

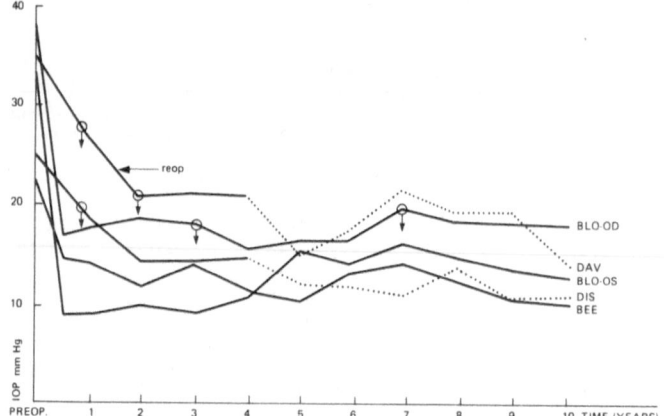

Fig. 1.

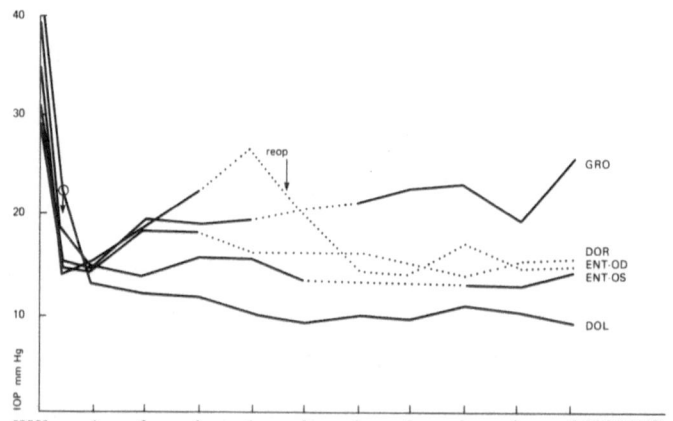

Fig. 2.

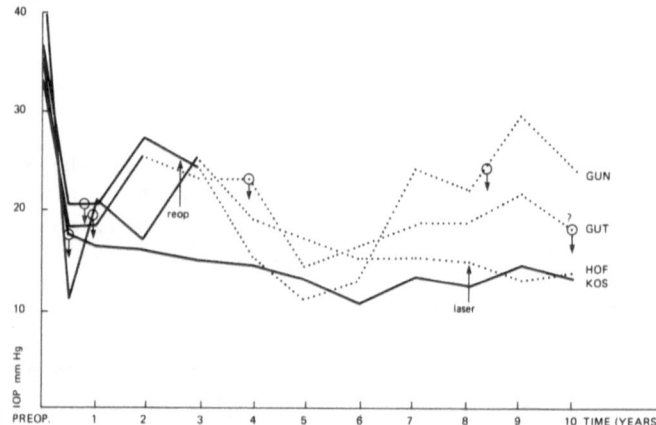

Fig. 3.

240

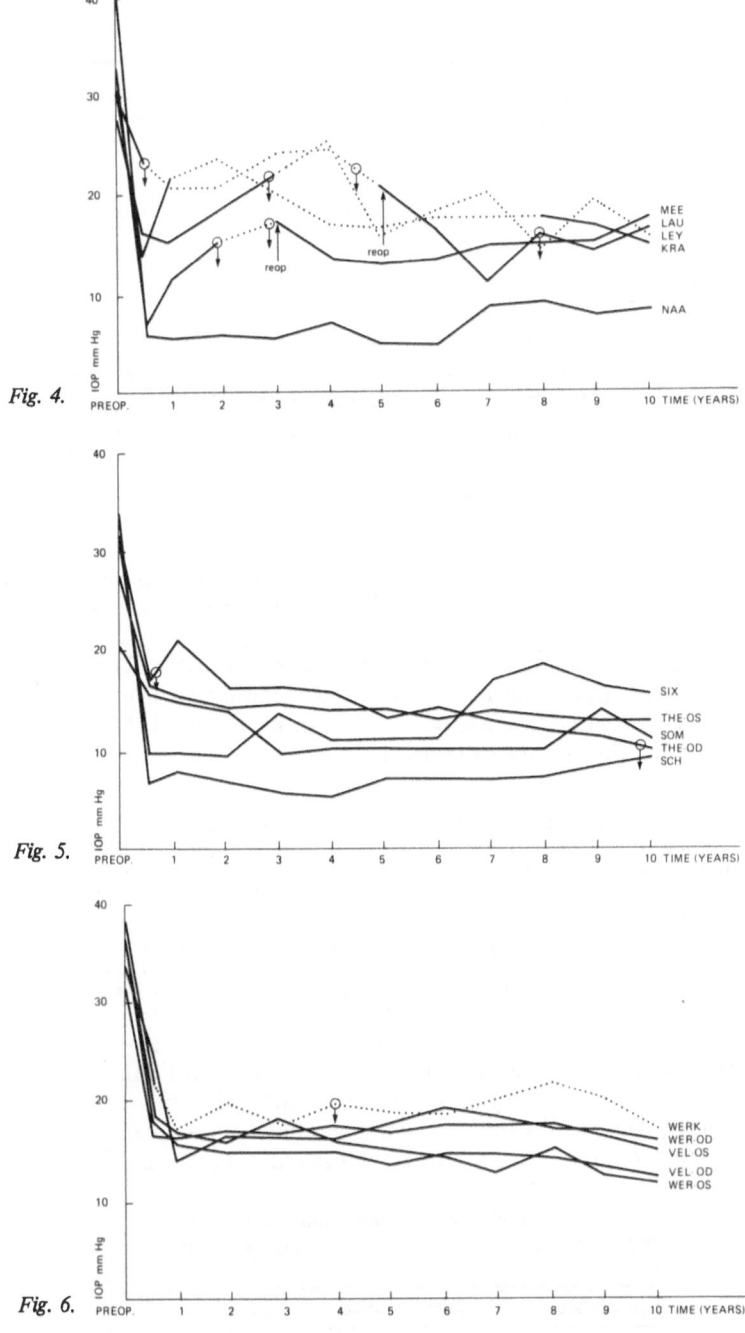

Figs. 1–6. Preoperative and yearly IOP of all patients that could be examined after ten years. Values are means of five measurements in a day curve. ——— with, and - - - - without additional medical therapy. reop = reoperation. Arrows indicate time of detection of visual field deterioration.

241

Table 2. Mean IOP, reduction of IOP and percentage reduction in IOP after each control period

	Preop.	1 yr.	5 yrs.	6 yrs.	7 yrs.	10 yrs.
Mean IOP (mmHg)	34.4	15.9	15.8	15.8	16.0	16.3
Reduction		18.5	18.6	18.6	18.4	18.1
% reduction		53.7	54.1	54.1	53.5	52.6

we made diurnal curves without medical therapy in all patients. The results are given in Table 2. Six cases in which reoperation (5) or laser (1) trabeculoplasty was done are included in these figures. Although a slight rising trend might be concluded from the values, the differences between the means are not significant (t-test). However, in three patients (GRO, GUN and MEE) significant rises did occur despite additional medical and surgical treatment in two of them.

In all, 10 patients (10 eyes) needed additional therapy somewhere during the ten years because of an IOP above 21 mmHg or because of visual field deterioration: 5 reoperations were performed, 1 laser trabeculoplasty was done, and 4 patients had additional medical therapy only. This means that 14 of 24 patients, 60% (19 of 29 eyes), had their IOP adequately regulated during ten years by one filtering operation only.

At ten years 22 patients (27 eyes) had a mean IOP below 21 mmHg, a percentage of 92% (including reoperations and medical treatment). Diurnal variations of IOP in a diurnal curve of 5 measurements remained stable during the ten years after the operation (Table 3).

Table 3. Pre- and postoperative diurnal variations in IOP (mmHg). Mean and standard deviation in a day curve (5 measurements) without additional medical therapy.

Preoperative	Postoperative		
	1 yr.	5 yrs.	10 yrs.
6.8 ± 3.1	4.0 ± 1.6	4.0 ± 2.0	3.2 ± 2.0

Results of tonography are given in Table 4. Of five eyes either no preoperative or no ten year postoperative values are available: the results of 24 eyes are shown. Tonography was carried out without medical therapy. Differences between one and ten year results are not significant (t-test).

Table 4. Tonography results: Mean and standard deviation of preoperative coefficients of ɔutflow facility (C_{0-4})

Preoperative	Postoperative	
	1 yr.	10 yrs.
n = 28	n = 29	n = 24
0.13 ± 0.06	0.34 ± 0.10	0.28 ± 0.11

Visual acuity and cataract

Ten years after the operation visual acuity was decreased more than one line on the Snellen chart in 15 of 29 eyes (52%). Increase of an existing cataract was the chief factor in 13 eyes (45%). In one case the deterioration was due to diabetic retinopathy and in another to premacular fibrosis. Progression of cataract was detected by biomicroscopy in mydriasis and assessment of general reduction of sensitivity in static perimetry. In four cases a cataract operation was performed.

Visual fields

Patients in which progression of visual field defects not due to cataract occurred are listed in Table 5.

Table 5. Patients who showed visual field deterioration*

Patient	0−5 yrs.	5−10 yrs.	Comment
1. BLO (OD)	+	+	temporal island disappearing
2. DAV	+	−	
3. DIS	+	−	
4. DOL	+	−	
5. GUN	+	+	
6. GUT	+	+ ?	cataract?
7. HOF	+	−	
8. KOS	+	−	
9. LAU	+	+	diabetes mellitus + cataract .
10. LEY	+	−	
11. MEE	+	−	
12. THE (OD)	+	+	central island disappearing after 10 yrs.
13. WER	−	+	small temporal island

* For relation of visual field deterioration and IOP see Figs. 1−6.

In seven eyes the visual field deterioration took place within five years postoperatively after which the visual fields remained stable. In six eyes deterioration was seen between five and ten years after the operation. In most cases this late deterioration was of minor degree (reduction in a peripheral island) or some complicating condition (diabetic retinopathy, cataract) was present that prevented clear discrimination of causative factors. In one case a central island disappeared after ten years following a cataract extraction. In Figs. 1−6 the time of deterioration is shown in relation to IOP. A total number of 21 episodes of visual field deterioration in 13 patients occurred. In 9 episodes the IOP was between 18 and 21 mmHg, and in 5 cases there was deterioration despite IOP lower than 18 mmHg.

Comparison of medical and surgical therapy

In most patients deterioration of visual field in the eye not operated on originally urged operation on that eye as well. Only five cases remain in which

243

IOP in the eye not participating in the study has been regulated satisfactorily by eye drops only and in which a valid comparison can be made of operation and medical therapy. In two of these five cases a considerable difference in visual field deterioration was observed in favour of the operated eye, whereas in the other three cases no difference was seen

DISCUSSION

For the evaluation of the results of this type of filtering operation we have chosen a prospective study-design to assure uniform criteria for inclusion into the study and comparable quality of the follow-up examinations. In this way a relatively small group of POAG patients (24 patients, 29 eyes) could be followed for a period of ten years, with all the examinations except visual field testing carried out only by one of the authors. It should be stressed that our group consisted of patients with high preoperative IOP and with progressive visual field defects in all but two cases. Although it proved possible to keep the drop-out due to other causes than death fairly small (6%), 20 of the original number of 47 patients (43%) died within ten years after the operation. This large number reflects the age distribution of the population studied, with an average "ocular age" at the start of the study of 66.2 years. According to Dutch figures of mortality by age and sex, 15 of our patients would be expected to die by chance.

Are there any long-term trends evident from this study? Mean IOP in 29 eyes, measured without medical therapy but including reoperations, rose from 15.8 mmHg after five years to 16.1 mmHg after ten years. In concert with this slight rising tendency is the fact that between five and 10 years two reoperations and one laser treatment were necessary and one eye needed reinstitution of medical therapy after five years. A similar rise in IOP is suggested in another study five years after trabeculectomy (13). On the other hand, tonography results and diurnal variations in IOP do not show a rising trend. Diurnal variations seemed to diminish after five years, although the differences were not statistically significant. The final aim of any treatment for glaucoma is to stop deterioration of visual fields as judged by perimetry. Consequently, any evaluation of the results of a filtering operation should include not only data on pressure reduction but also on performance at visual field examinaton. The visual fields showed little changes between five and ten years: only five of 29 eyes showed definite deterioration in static perimetry, but in all except one case the worsening was of minor clinical significance. Somewhere during the ten years in 13 of 29 eyes (45%) visual field deterioration was detected. It is difficult to compare these figures with those in the literature, because it is seldom clear whether the progression is due to glaucoma or to cataract. Dannheim and Westenberg (3) reported suspected or confirmed postoperative visual field deterioration in 50% of 86 operated patients (follow-up 1 month to 12 years, mean 15 months). Werner and Drance (21) investigated 24 visual fields after trabeculectomy with a follow-up of 18 months to 6 years. Ten eyes (42%) showed postoperative progression. In neither of these two studies was the proportion of glaucomatous visual field loss differentiated from loss due to cataract. In Jerndal and Lundström's series (13) 17 of 102 eyes (17%) with a follow-up of five years after trabeculectomy had glaucomatous progressive visual field loss, but the method of perimetry and the definition of "progressive visual field loss" are not described. In this study it cannot be concluded that central islands are more vulnerable to the effects of filtering operation than the earlier stages of the disease.

Early postoperative complications are dealt with in an earlier report (2). The most important long-term complication cited in the literature is progression of cataract. In the present study progression of lens opacities, as judged by visual acuity loss and findings at the slit lamp, were seen in 45% of the eyes at ten years. At two and four years percentages of 13 and 38 respectively were reported. In 14% of 29 eyes a cataract extraction was performed. The percentages for the development of cataract after filtering operations given in the literature show considerable variation. They range from 9% in a study of POAG patients followed up for 1 to 3 years after trabeculectomy (17), to 66% of 98 eyes 3 months to 5 years after the same procedure or thermosclerotomy (1). Clearly other factors, such as the age of the patients and the use of cataractogenic medication should be considered. It is difficult to ascertain whether the cataract formation in our study was accelerated by the operation or not. All patients in which progression occurred were 65 years of age or older at the time of operation: in none of the six patients who were under 60 was any progression seen, suggesting that the normal ageing process played a considerable role. In six patients a valid comparison between operated and non-operated eyes can be made (in all other patients the eye not participating in the study needed operation later on). In four patients no difference in cataract progression between the operated and the not operated eye was seen; in one cataract progression was worse in the operated eye and in another the reverse was the case. These findings give no firm indication that cataract progression is accelerated by our filtering operation.

The rate of success attributed to a glaucoma operation is dependent upon

Table 6. Rate of success of therapy according to various definitions

	With VF* ↓	With VF ↓	Total
IOP ≤ 21 mmHg regulated by:			
DFS* only	5	13[a]	18[b]
DFS + additional medication	3	1	4[e]
DFS + reoperation	1	0	1
DFS + reoperation + additional medication	2	1	3
DFS + laser + additional medication	1	0	1
	12	15	27
IOP > 21 mmHg	1	1	2
	13	16[d]	29

* see text for further discussion.

the criteria applied. In a strict sense complete success is attained only if IOP is controlled adequately ($\leqslant 21$ mmHg) without further medical or surgical therapy and if no visual field deterioration occurred (Table 6, definition a). According to these criteria the Double Flap Scheie was completely successful in 13 of 29 eyes (45%). Nowhere in the literature is this definition used. If the requirement of absence of visual field deterioration would be dropped, this figure would rise to 18 (62%) (definition b). This definition is used widely in the literature. Both higher and lower findings have been recorded in other long-term studies: Jerndal and Lündström (13): 57% (5 year follow-up, n = 102); D'Ermo et al. (5): 65% (follow-up 1—5 years, n = 48); Mills (16): 73.4% (mean follow-up ± 3 years, n = 220); Shirato (19): 34% (follow-up $\frac{1}{2}$—2 years, n = 67).

With additional medical and/or surgical therapy 27 eyes (93%) had a mean IOP at or under 21 mmHg (definition c), 15 of which had no evidence of visual field deterioration (definition d). In the above mentioned studies the percentages according to definition c range from 65 to 86.9%. It will be clear that any comparison of these figures is problematic due to differences in criteria, patient population and length of follow-up.

In conclusion the results of this study once more underline the unpredictable course of postoperative glaucoma and the importance of long-term postoperative visual field examination. In the light of the good pressure reducing potency of modern medical and laser treatment and the high death-rate in the study population, it can be stated that although this type of filtering procedure appears to be an effective (50% reduction of IOP) and relatively safe procedure it should be performed in patients of such high age as in our group only after other forms of treatment have failed.

REFERENCES

1. Blondeau, P. and Phelps, C.D. Trabeculectomy vs thermosclerotomy. A randomized prospective clinical trial. Arch. Ophthalmol. 99:810 (1981).
2. Dake, C.L. and Greve, E.L. Double flap Scheie (a prospective study of an external filtering operation in glaucoma simplex). Docum. Ophthalmol. 42:353 (1977).
3. Dannheim, R. and Westenberger, W. Ursachen der postoperativen Gesichtsfeldverschlechterung bei fortgeschrittenem primären Glaukom mit offenem Kammerwinkel. Klin. Mbl. Augenheilk. 178:65 (1981).
4. Duzanec, Z. and Krieglstein, G.K. Die Beziehung zwischen Druckregulierung und anatomischer Lokalisation sowie Trepangrosse bei der Goniotrepanation. Eine prospektive Studie. Klin. Mbl. Augenheilk. 178:431 (1981).
5. D'Ermo, F., Bonomi, L. and Boro, D. A critical analysis of the long-term results of trabeculectomy. Am. J. Ophthalmol. 88:822 (1979).
6. Freedman, J., Shen, E. and Ahrens, M. Trabeculectomy in a Black American glaucoma population. Br. J. Ophthalmol. 60:573 (1976).
7. Gliem, H. and Pedal, W. Erfahrungen mit der Trepanotrabekulektomie. Klin. Mbl. Augenheilk. 166:598 (1975).
8. Gloor, B., Niederer, W. and Daicker, B. Trabekulektomie: Operationstechnik, Resultate, Indikationsstellung. Klin. Mbl. Augenheilk. 170:241 (1977).
9. Greve, E.L. and Dake, C.L. Four year follow-up of a glaucoma operation. Prospective study of the Double Flap Scheie. Int. Ophthalmol. 1:139 (1978).
10. Greve, E.L., Dake, C.L. and Verduin, W.M. Pre- and postoperative results of static perimetry in patients with glaucoma simplex. Docum. Ophthalmol. 42:335 (1977).

11. Hollwich, F., Junemann, G. and Kinne, J. Klinische Ergebnisse der Goniotrepanation mit skleradeckel. Klin. Mbl. Augenheilk. 171:735 (1977).
12. Jerndal, T. and Lundström, H. 330 Trabeculectomies. A follow-up study through $\frac{1}{2}$–3 years. Acta Ophthalmol. 55:52 (1977).
13. Jerndal, T. & Lundström, H. 330 Trabeculectomies. A long time study (3–5 years). Acta Ophthal. 58:947 (1980).
14. Loewenthal, L.M. Trabeculectomy as treatment for glaucoma: a preliminary report. Ann. Ophthalmol. 9:1179 (1977).
15. Merritt, J.C. Filtering procedures in American blacks. Ophthalmol. Surg. 88:829 (1979).
16. Mills, K.B. Trabeculectomy: a retrospective long-term follow-up of 144 cases. Br. J. Ophthalmol. 65:790 (1981).
17. Ridgway, A.E.A. Trabeculectomy. A follow-up study. Br. J. Ophthalmol. 58: 680–686 (1974).
18. Riss, B. and Binder, S. Retrospektive auf 402 Goniotrepanationen. Klin. Mol. Augenheilk. 176:286 (1980).
19. Shirato, S., Kitazawa, Y. and Hishima, S. A critical analysis of the trabeculectomy results by a prospective follow-up design. Jpn. J. Ophthalmol. 26:468 (1982).
20. Sugar, H.S. Course of successfully filtering blebs. A follow-up study. Ann. Ophthalmol. 3:485 (1971).
21. Werner, E.B., Drance, S.M. and Schulzer, M. Trabeculectomy and the progression of glaucomatous visual field loss. Arch. Ophthalmol. 95:1374 (1977).

Authors' address:
Eye Clinic of the University of Amsterdam
Glaucoma and Visual Field Dept.
Academic Medical Center
Meibergdreef 9
1105 AZ Amsterdam
The Netherlands

LONG-TERM OBSERVATIONS AFTER TREPHINATION WITH SCLERAL FLAP IN GLAUCOMA WITH THREATENED POINT OF FIXATION

J. VOSSEN and H. NEUBAUER

(Cologne, F.R.G.)

ABSTRACT

Follow-up examinations two months to nine years after filter operation with scleral flap with successful pressure regulation could be carried out in 29 eyes in which a threat to the point of fixation due to glaucoma was present. In the majority of the cases, it was possible to stabilize the visual acuity and visual field by the operation. In the remaining cases, there was a slow melting away of the residual visual field without correlation with lens or macular changes or underlying internal conditions. The cause is taken to be a deficient perfusion in the retrolaminar part of the optic nerve.

The value of surgical therapy of glaucoma has been undisputed for decades. Especially in recent years, microsurgical techniques with increasing efforts to arrive at individual dosage of the "filtering throttle" have led to reduction of bad results of surgery due to overfiltration. For a long time, cases with far advanced visual field defects were exempted from surgical pressure regulation. In the latter cases, medication was given preference in most patients. Becker and Shaffer (1) summarize the literature data in two theses:

1. After filter operation, the central visual field island does usually not get lost.
2. Even in complete postoperative pressure regulation, the decay of a tiny central visual field can progress.

We were interested in ascertaining the late functional deficits which occur after successful filter operations with scleral flap, and whether a typology can be discerned amongst such cases.

We carried out follow-up examinations of all patients in whom a threat of the point of fixation was present preoperatively and who were operated on by one of us (H.N.) with a trephenation with scleral flap at the Department of Ophthalmology, University of Cologne between 1975 and 1983.

We defined paracentral scotomas which reached nearer than 10° to the center as an "endangerment of the point of fixation" when the outer boundary of the test mark I/2 on the Goldmann perimeter was less than 5° from the center in at least two quadrants. The degrees of severity II–IV resulted from

249

E.L. Greve, W. Leydhecker & C. Raitta (eds.), Second European Glaucoma Symposium, Helsinki 1984.
© *1985, Dr. W. Junk Publishers, Dordrecht. ISBN 978-94-010-8934-0*

the number of quadrants in which the scotoma approached the point of fixation over the 10° line.

These conditions were met in 41 out of a total of 301 patients. A scarred filter zone with insufficient regulation of pressure or pressure regulation which could only be achieved by medication was found at the follow-up examination in seven cases. Five patients could not be followed up (death or change of address). In three cases, a cataract or an incomplete central venous thrombosis did not allow a comparison. The present investigation hence takes into account 26 patients with a total of 29 operated eyes in whom the desired pressure regulation was achieved by the operation without additional medication. The preoperative pressure values under therapy were between 14 and 50 mmHg with an average of 31.2 mmHg. The lowering of pressure achieved was between 2 and 35 mmHg with an average of 17.5 mmHg. The postoperative pressure values (without medical treatment) were 21 mmHg in one case, and otherwise between 10 and 18 mmHg with an average of 13.7 mmHg. The period of postoperative observation was between 2 months and nine years with an average of 3.5 years.

The most important criterion of the papillary finding was deliberately not included.

An acute loss of visual acuity did not occur in any case after the operation.

The distant vision improved in two patients, and there was no alteration in ten eyes. A deterioration of more than two lines only occurred in one case (Fig. 1). Lens alterations influenced the postoperative course only in particular cases. Macular changes could not be discerned.

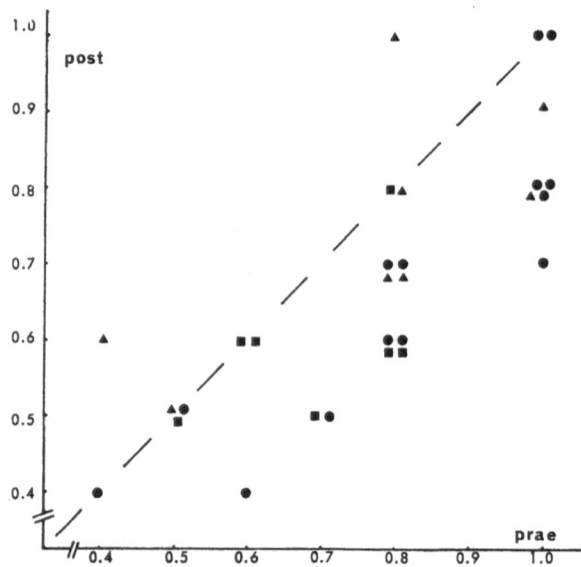

Fig. 1. Visual acuity before and after the operation. Stage II: •; III: ▲; IV: ■.

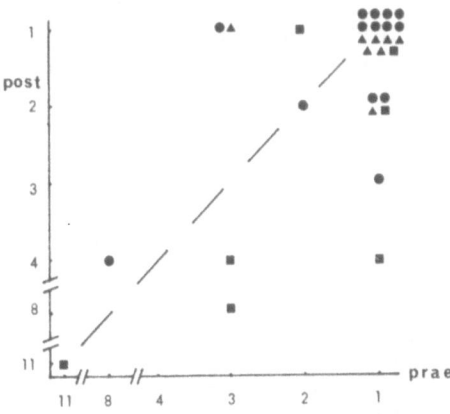

Fig. 2. Near vision before and after the operation (Nieden). Stage II: •; II: ▲; IV: ■.

Near vision improved in four eyes, remained stable in 16 cases, and deteriorated in a total of nine cases (Fig. 2). The higher incidence of deterioration of distant visual acuity is related to the fact that a decrease of two lines from a visual acuity of 0.8–1.0 in the distance does not influence the near vision.

When a preoperative static perimetry had been carried out, the check was performed with the same method. Otherwise the visual fields were compared on the Goldmann perimeter. The results obtained on the Goldmann perimeter were stable with critical consideration of usual fluctuations and of the pupillary changes due to absent medication in 11 cases. There was a more or less distinct improvement in eight cases, and a deterioration in three cases. In static perimetry, which was present in seven patients with deficits splitting the point of fixation, a stable or slightly improved result was found in four cases, and there was a more or less distinct reduction in profile in three cases.

Preexisting vascular diseases (diabetes, hypertension or hypotension, myocardial infarction, myocardial insufficiency) did not have a discernible influence on the postoperative course.

There is agreement in the literature (1, 2, 3, 6) that a slow progression of the visual field defects can occur even after surgical regulation of intraocular pressure irrespective of an increasing lens opacity or macular damage. However, if there is development of a maculopathy, a cataract or an ischemia in the region of the prelaminar optic nerve in the first three postoperative months (4, 5, 7), then as a rule we regard these as resulting from the operation. Vascular factors which mostly cannot be detected by ophthalmoscopy or by examination of an internist are likely to be responsible for the increase of the scotomas. Accordingly, despite stabilization of the result in most cases, there was a deterioration in a total of six cases amongst our patients. A typology could not be discerned. The slowly progressive alterations concerned areas outside the center and also the progress of the scotoma towards the centre. Lens and macular factors played only a subordinate role here.

251

The following statements can be made on the basis of the findings:

1. Apart from deficits of the center due to complications, trephination with scleral flap thus appears to be advisable even in far advanced decay of the pericenter.

2. However, in such situations, postoperative pericentral deteriorations occur even after years. These have often such a slow course that the patient is not necessarily aware of them. According to our impressions so far, they occur very much more slowly than the preoperative deteriorations of the pericenter.

3. There is hope of improvement of the central visual field when an isolated pericentral scotoma is involved. As soon as the progression of such a scotoma is confirmed, one should intervene.

4. Amongst the majority of the visual fields to be designated as "stable", slight pericentral fluctuations in both directions can be detected over a long period. A causal correlation cannot be discerned so far. The more extensive the excavation of the optic nerve, the more meticulous should be the perimetric controls.

Summarizing the results we would recommend an operation even in cases with far advanced visual field defects due to glaucoma.

REFERENCES

1. Becker-Shaffer. Diagnosis and therapy of the glaucomas. Mosby, St. Louis, 1976.
2. Dannheim, R. and Westenberger, W. Ursachen der postoperativen Gesichtesfeldverschlechterungen bei fortgeschrittenem primären Glaukom mit offenem Kammerwinkel. Klin. Mbl. Augenheilk. 178:65–67, 1981.
3. Fanta, H. and Herold, I. Das Verhalten der Restgesichtsfelder nach fistulierenden Operationen. Klin. Mbl. Augenheilk. 148:834–845, 1966.
4. Lawrence, G.A. Surgical treatment of patients with advanced glaucomatous field defects. Arch. Ophthalmol. 81:804–807, 1969.
5. Lichter, P.R. and Ravin, J.G. Risks of sudden visual loss after glaucoma surgery. Am. J. Ophthalmol. 78: 1009–1013, 1974.
6. Nemetz, U.R. and Papanos, G. Zur Frage der Operation beim Glaukom mit hochgradiger Gesichtsfeldeinengung. Klin. Mbl. Augenheilk. 134:83–88, 1959.
7. O'Connel, E.J. and Karseras, A.G. Intraocular surgery in advanced glaucoma. Br. J. Ophthalmol. 60:124–131, 1976.

Authors' address:
Dept. of Ophthalmology
University of Cologne
Cologne, F.R.G.

VALVE TRABECULOTOMY AND FILTERING
IRIDOCYCLRETRACTION IN GLAUCOMA

A.P. NESTEROV, E.A. EGOROV and L.N. KOLESNIKOVA

(Moscow, U.S.S.R.)

ABSTRACT

Surgical techniques of valve trabeculotomy (VT) and filtering iridocyclo-retraction (FICR) are described. The VT was used mostly in open-angle glaucoma. In all, 226 eyes of 169 patients were operated and 146 of them followed for 12 to 39 months. The intraocular pressure was controlled in 125 eyes (85.6%) by surgery alone and in 7 eyes (4.85) by surgery and medication.

The FICR was performed in 91 eyes of 80 patients with either closed-angle or combined glaucoma. Seventy eyes were followed for 12 to 25 months. The IOP was controlled in 61 eyes (87.1%) by surgery alone and in 3 eyes by surgery and medication.

INTRODUCTION

During last decade we have studied several surgical techniques (3–5) in an attempt to find optimal approach to glaucoma surgery. Here we describe two new techniques and analyse the preliminary results.

VALVE TRABECULOTOMY (VT)

Technique

The technique of the VT is shown in Fig. 1. After a conjunctival-tenon incision 8 mm from the corneal limbus, a limbal-based scleral flap is marked out and laminated at the level of about one third of the scleral thickness. The flap may be triangular or rectangular and the length of each of its sides is 4 to 5 mm. One or two preplaced sutures are inserted. Then a middle scleral lamina over the canal of Schlemm and adjacent area (3 mm wide) is excised. A 4 mm incision is made through the deep scleral lamina 1.5 mm behind and parallel to the limbus Two radial incisions are then extended forward 2 mm apart from each other to form an inner scleral flap or 'trabecular valve'. It contains the trabecular meshwork and the limbal tissue. After peripheral

253

E.L. Greve, W. Leydhecker & C. Raitta (eds.), Second European Glaucoma Symposium, Helsinki 1984.
© *1985, Dr. W. Junk Publishers, Dordrecht. ISBN 978-94-010-8934-0*

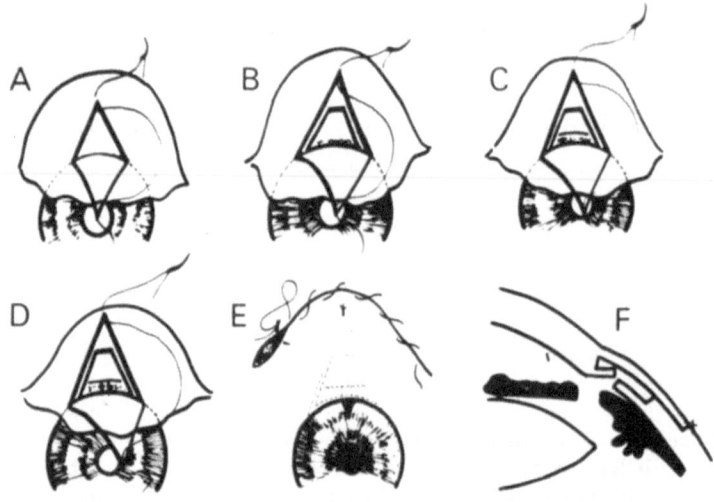

Fig. 1. Valve trabeculotomy. A) Conjunctival and scleral flaps are prepared. B) A middle scleral lamina is excised. C) A 4 mm incision parallel to the corneal limbus is made through the deep scleral layers. D) Two short radial cuttings are made and an inner limboscleral flap (a trabecular valve) is formed. E) After peripheral iridectomy the outer scleral flap and the conjunctival wound are sutured. F) The new formed outflow pathways are shown schematically.

iridectomy the external scleral flap is reapproximated and the preplaced suture is tied up. The conjunctival wound is closed with a running suture.

Results

In all 226 eyes of 169 patients were operated including 198 eyes with open-angle glaucoma, 10 eyes with chronic closed-angle glaucoma, and 18 eyes with combined glaucoma.

The postoperative period was rather quiet in most cases. Hyphaema occurred in 14 eyes (6.2%), mild uveitis in 10 cases (4.4%) and choroidal detachment in 13 eyes (5.8%).

Three to 4 weeks after surgery the intraocular pressure (IOP) was controlled (21 mm Hg or less) in 217 eyes by surgery alone and in 5 eyes by surgery and medication.

At present we have under observation 146 eyes of 113 patients. The duration of the follow-up period varied from 12 to 39 months (mean 25 months). The IOP is controlled in 125 eyes (85,6%) by surgery alone and in other 7 eyes by surgery and medication. The mean IOP and standard deviation were 33.71 ± 5.13 mm Hg before surgery and 17.22 ± 3.18 mm Hg 12 to 39 months after surgery. The C-values were 0.082 ± 0.038 and 0.226 ± 0.065 ci mm/min/mm Hg before and after surgery successively.

Comment

The VT differs from trabeculoectomy after Cairns (1) by two features. The first is the removal of the scleral middle lamina over Schlemm's canal and the adjacent area. The aim of this procedure is to make an intrascleral space filled with the aqueous humour. This seems to facilitate the aqueous humour absorption, to maintain the patency of the new formed outflow pathways and to diminish the regenerative capacity of the scleral tissue, thus preventing scarring of the pathways. The preparation of the inner limbo-scleral flap (trabecular valve) is the second distinctive feature of this operation. One can suggest that this flap serves as a valve during a few postoperative days before its position becomes stable. In case of hypotonia the valve decreases the aqueous outflow but it moves outwardly increasing the outflow if the IOP begins to rise.

The success rate after the VT is about the same as after filtering operations but the rate of complication seems to be lower. Certainly, we have only preliminary results and more time is needed for final evaluation of the operation.

FILTERING IRIDOCYCLORECTRACTION (FICR)

Technique

An 8 mm conjunctival-tenon flap is prepared. Two limbal-based scleral strips are marked out (Fig. 2). The distance between the strips is about 4 mm at the level of the corneal limbus. Each strip is 6 mm long and 1.5 mm wide. It is laminated to the corneal limbus at the level of one-half to two-thirds of the scleral thickness.

After separating the strips, two grooves are formed in the sclera. In each of them a 2 mm incision is made through the deep layers of the sclera at the

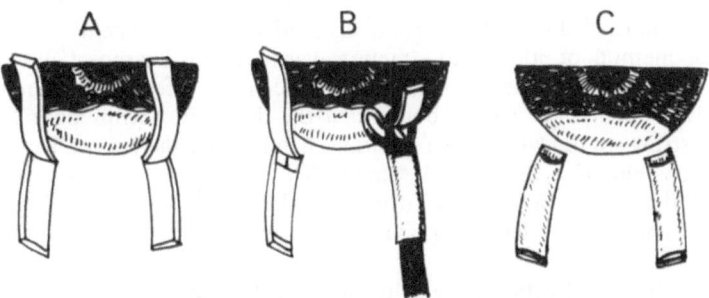

Fig. 2. Filtering iridocycloretraction. A) Two scleral strips are separated to the corneal limbus and two grooves appear in the sclera. B) Two incisions (a posterior and an anterior) are made in each scleral groove. A fenestrated spatula is introduced through the posterior incision into the supraciliary space and projected out of the anterior incision. The end of the scleral strip is threaded through the opening at the end of the spatula. C) Both scleral strips are placed into the supraciliary space.

distance of 5 mm from the limbus. Then the second 2 mm incision is made in each scleral groove. It is situated 1.5 mm behind the limbus and penetrates into the anterior chamber. From the midpoint of this incision a 1.5 mm long radial section of the corneoscleral tissue is extended forward. Thus, a T-form cutting appears at the limbal end of each scleral groove. Then two peripheral iridectomies are performed through the T-form cuttings.

A spatula with an opening at its end is introduced through one of the posterior incisions and after cyclodialisis its end is projected out of the anterior T-form incision. The end of the corresponding scleral strip is threaded through the opening at the end of the spatula. The spatula is then removed, thus drawing the strip into the supraciliare space. The same procedure is repeated with the other scleral strip. The conjunctival-tenon wound is closed with a running suture.

Results

The operation was performed in 91 eyes of 80 patients including 59 eyes with closed-angle glaucoma and 32 eyes with combined glaucoma.

Complications were small and manageable. Hyphaema occurred in 11 eyes (12%), uveitis in 3 eyes (3.3%) and choroidal detachment in 7 eyes (7.7%).

Three to 4 weeks after surgery the IOP was controlled in 88 eyes by surgery alone and in one eye by surgery and medication. In 12 to 25 months (mean 16 months) 70 eyes of 62 patients were examined. The IOP was controlled in 61 eyes without medication (87.1%) and in 3 other eyes with the help of pilocarpine and/or timolol (4.3%).

The mean IOP and standard deviation were 39.51 ± 6.41 mm Hg before surgery and 17.20 ± 4.11 mm Hg 12 to 25 months after surgery. The C-values were 0.053 ± 0.045 and 0.219 ± 0.058 cu mm/min/mm Hg before and after surgery successively.

Comment

Our technique of the FICR has some distinctive features as compared to the original method of iridocycloretraction developed by Krasnov (2). (1) We prepare limbal-based scleral strips. They provide more effective pressure upon the iris root and the ciliary body than the limbal-free strips do. (2) The scleral strips are drawn into the anterior chamber and the supraciliary space with the help of a fenestrated spatula. This facilitates the most difficult part of the operation. (3) The T-form limbal cuttings serve as artificial outflow channels. The scleral strips introduced into the cuttings prevent their closure.

Thus, several effects can be achieved with the help of the FICR: elimination of the pupillary block, widening of the anterior chamber angle, creating the direct communications between the anterior chamber and both the subconjunctival and the supraciliary spaces.

Simplicity of the techniques, low rate of complications and good control of the IOP in the majority of our cases allow us to recommend the new operations for use in clinical practice. The VT is indicated in cases of uncontrolled open-angle glaucoma and the FICR is especially useful in cases of chronic closed-angle glaucoma.

REFERENCES

1. Cairns, J.E. Trabeculoectomy: preliminary report of a new method. Am. J. Ophthalmol. 66:673–679 (1968).
2. Krasnov, M.M. Iridocycloretraction. Vestn. Oftalmol. 6:54–57 (1969).
3. Nesterov, A.P. and Egorov, E.A. Transconjunctival penetrating cyclodiathermy in glaucoma. J. Ocular Ther. Surg. 2:216–218 (1983).
4. Nesterov, A.P., Egorov, E.A. and Batmanov, Y.E. Sinusotomy and trabeculodilatation in glaucoma. Glaucoma 3:253–255 (1981).
5. Nesterov, A.P. and Kolesnikova, L.N. Implanatation of a scleral strip into the supraciliary space and cyclodialisis in glaucoma. Acta Ophthalmol. 56:697–704 (1978).

Authors' address:
Dept. of Eye Diseases
2nd Moscow Medical Institute
1 Ostrovitjanova Street
Moscow 117437
U.S.S.R.

A NEW APPROACH FOR CHAMBER ANGLE SURGERY

J. DRAEGER and H. WIRT

(Hamburg, F.R.G.)

ABSTRACT

Following former recommendations of Barkan (2) and Bietti (3) a new microsurgical technique for cyclodialysis is described. Using an approach as for
goniotomy, the dissection of the ciliary body takes place under visual control.
The substantial advantage of this modification in comparison to the classical
cyclodialysis of Heine (6) is to be seen in the visual control during the entire
operation. Additionally, by injection of hyaluronic acid the dissected cleft
can be enlarged and kept open during the first postoperative phase. This
seems to improve the results. Indications, problems and results are discussed.

INTRODUCTION

The basic principle of chamber angle surgery is to reconstruct the natural
outflow pathway. Already in 1893 De Vicentiis (4) described a new method,
by operating on the trabecular meshwork itself. Today, this operation,
goniotomy, is the surgical procedure of choice in congenital glaucoma. This
was mainly thanks to Barkan. The introduction of his contact lens (1) allowed
the direct view of the mesenchymal tissue which obstructs the normal outflow pathway.

Using the operation-microscope with a direct magnified view in goniotomy
it is now possible to control the microsurgical procedure even better and
more precisely (Fig. 1).

In 1905 Heine (6) established cyclodialysis to achieve pressure regulation
in chronic glaucoma. This method, primarily designed to lead to a reduced
aqueous secretion rate also affects the chamber angle, but it failed as a
standard procedure for primary open angle glaucoma. In spite of its relatively
high complication rate it is still used in secondary glaucomas, especially with
aphakia. Clinical complications are haemorrhages, and in some cases hypotony.

METHODS

Following former recommendations of Barkan (2) and Bietti (3), we tried to
combine the effect of goniotomy and cyclodialysis ab externo, performing

259

E.L. Greve, W. Leydhecker & C. Raitta (eds.), Second European Glaucoma Symposium, Helsinki 1984.
© *1985, Dr. W. Junk Publishers, Dordrecht. ISBN 978-94-010-8934-0*

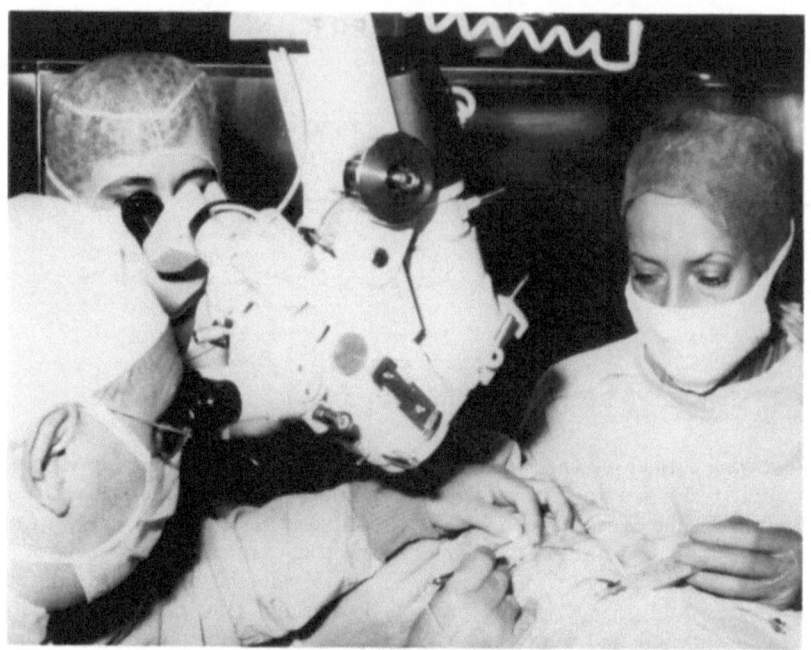

Fig. 1. Microsurgical goniotomy-group.

the dissection of the ciliary body from the sclera using the goniotomy technique. This new approach "cyclodialysis ab interno" is indicated in cases of congenital glaucoma. This is mainly true for advanced cases not responding even to repeated goniotomies, showing destruction or even aplasia of Schlemm's canal. Barkan and Bietti tried to apply this combined procedure for primary chronic glaucoma and secondary glaucoma, but they failed because of the intolerably high complication rate. Now, thanks to advanced microsurgical methods, this new procedure is indicated not only in congenital glaucoma but also in special cases of primary chronic glaucoma or secondary glaucoma, where we already successfully performed a "cyclodialysis ab interno".

The following short review of our surgical procedure is given to demonstrate the advantages compared to classical cyclodialysis. The microscope is set in an oblique position with coaxial illumination and the special Barkan-silicon-lens is placed on the cornea. This lens is light in weight, has more adhesive power at its edges and is even cheaper than lenses made of metacrylate. The convex-concave shape of the lens magnifies by a factor of two. This enables us to use a lower magnification at the microscope leading to a greater depth of field. A cannulated goniotomy-knife after Worst with rounded blade is advanced into the operation site under direct observation. The anterior chamber is maintained by irrigation with an aqueous substitute.

Since 1982, instead of BSS (balanced salt solution) we used hyaluronic acid. This highly viscous substance is rinsed into the operation site during the cutting procedure, keeping intraocular pressure nearly constant, dilating the angle and protecting cornea, iris and lens.

Postoperatively hyaluronic acid keeps dissected tissue separated longer and fills the new created space. The adhesive forces between the layers are nearly eliminated. Thus, early postoperative scar-formation is minimized. Under direct magnified view the dissection of the ciliary body is eased, great vessels can be avoided and the complication rate is diminished.

At the end of the procedure the cyclodialysis cleft is filled up with hyaluronic acid, the goniotomy-knife is withdrawn and a small air bubble is placed into the anterior chamber sealing the entrance to avoid hypotony and bleeding (Fig. 2).

Separation of the dissected structures by hyaluronic acid is maintained for about two days, until it is replaced by aqueous. There are two advantages of this new procedure compared to the classical cyclodialysis: (1) The size of the cleft can be perfectly formed under direct visual control; (2) Complications, especially extensive bleeding, can be minimized by avoiding larger vessels.

RESULTS

Comparing the complications between cyclodialysis ab externo with cyclodialysis ab interno we see that the risk for intraoperative bleeding is nearly the same, but postoperatively haemorrhages are more frequent in classical cyclodialysis (41%) than in cyclodialysis ab interno (25.1%) (Table 1).

Table 1. Complications compared between cyclodialysis ab externo and ab interno

Complications	Cyclodialysis ab externo n = 78		Cyclodialysis ab interno n = 72	
intraop bleeding				
no	35 (44.9%)		32 (44.4%)	
minimal	43 (55.1%)		37 (51.4%)	
severe	–		3 (4.2%)	
postop. bleeding				
no	46 (59.0%)		56 (77.7%)	
minimal	23 (29.5%)		12 (16.7%)	
severe	6 (7.7%)	41%	3 (4.2%)	25.1%
repeated	3 (3.8%)		3 (4.2%)	
shallow anterior chamber	4 (5.1%)		5 (6.9%)	
collapsed anterior	5 (6.4%)		–	
hypotony	5 (6.4%)		6 (8.3%)	
cataract	3 (3.8%)		1 (1.4%)	
vitreous haemorrhage	4 (5.1%)		–	
amotio retinae	3 (3.8%)		–	

n = number of operations

On the other hand, we find a slightly higher percentage of hypotony (8.3% vs. 6.4%) after this new procedure. Probably the size of the cyclodialysis cleft can be reduced in the future, especially when using hyaluronic acid which diminishes the risk of early closure.

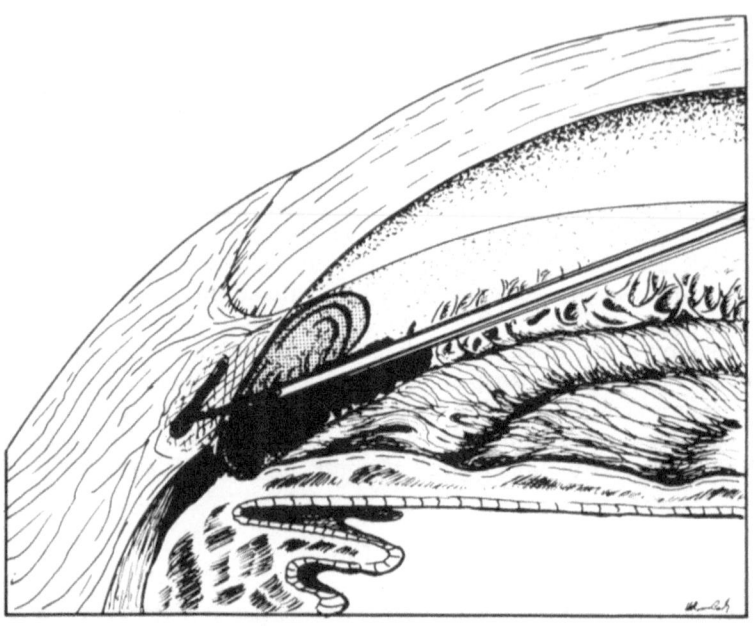

Fig. 2. Schematic drawing, cyclodialysis ab interno with hyaluronic acid injection.

Cataract and in three cases retinal detachment are additional complications we encountered with the classical method. After a follow-up of three months to three years we achieved pressure regulation with cyclodialysis ab externo in 36% for each single operation. In the other group we found pressure regulation in nearly 45% for each single procedure with the follow-up time of 3 to 18 months. The first group consisted of 69 evaluated operations and the second one of 67 (Table 2).

Table 2. Comparison of results between classical cyclodialysis and cyclodialysis ab interno

Technique of operation	Regulated	Unregulated
cyclodialysis ab externo n = 69	25 (36.2%)	44 (63.7%)
cyclodialysis ab interno n = 67	30 (44.8%)	37 (55.2%)

Follow-up time: cyclodialysis ab externo 3 months to 3 years
cyclodialysis ab interno 3 months to 18 months

One main difference between both groups must be considered. The indication for cyclodialysis ab externo was in most cases (81%) secondary glaucoma from aphakia or primary chronic glaucoma. In the other group the main indication was (79.2%) congenital or juvenile glaucoma.

CONCLUSION

There are indications for a combination of goniotomy with "cyclodialysis ab interno". The precise visual control of this microsurgical procedure might extend indication to special cases of secondary or even primary glaucoma. Further experience is needed for more precise adjustment of the extent of the dissected area to the desired reduction of pressure.

REFERENCES

1. Barkan, O. New operation for chronic glaucoma. Am. J. Ophthalmol. 19:951–966 (1936).
2. Barkan, O. Cyclo-goniotomy. A new operation for chronic simple glaucoma. Preliminary report. Bull. Ophthalmol. Soc. Egypt. 49:65–71 (1956).
3. Bietti, G.B. Sui risultati di interventi goniolitici nell'idrophthalmo. Ateneo parmense 23:1–8 (1952).
4. De Vincentiis, C. Incisione del'angelo irideo nel glaucoma. Ann. Ottal. 22:540–541 (1893).
5. Draeger, J. Eine neue mikrochirurgische Operationseinheit. Fortschr. a. d. Gebiet der Neurochirurgie 92–96 (1969).
6. Heine, L. Die Zyklodialyse: Eine neue Glaukomoperation. Dtsch. Med. Wochenschr. 31:824–826 (1905).

Authors' address:
Dept. of Ophthalmology
Hamburg University
Hamburg, F.R.G.

GONIOSCOPIC TRABECULOTOMY. FIRST RESULTS

MANUEL QUINTANA

(Barcelona, Spain)

ABSTRACT

We describe a surgical method of goniotrabeculotomy which achieves a section of the trabecular meshwork without damage to the external wall of Schlemm's canal. Complications are minimal. A one year follow-up shows a fall of intraocular pressure in almost all cases. However, this effect is non-lasting and a slow rise in pressure occurs in most cases. Yet, medical therapy, if reinstituted, achieves a better control than before the operation and usually can be less intense.

INTRODUCTION

Increased resistance to the outflow of aqueous through the trabecular meshwork is the most accepted pathogenic mechanism in the majority of open-angle glaucomas ("trabecular glaucomas"). Thus, the rational treatment of the trabecular glaucomas should consist in opening the trabecular meshwork (TM). This has been attempted since the last century (11, 12, 13) and many times later on (1, 2, 4, 5, 8, 9), but all the techniques described so far have failed (3, 10) despite the in vitro evidence (6, 7) of the effectiveness of trabeculotomy.

MATERIAL AND METHODS

A technique of trabeculotomy has been devised, which eliminates most of the presumed causes of failure of previous methods. The patient is operated under general anaesthesia; both eyes can be done at the same time. Pupils should be miotic. A coaxial operating microscope is necessary, with magnification of x 10. We favour the Swann lens for angle visualisation. Our trabeculotome is a 0.4 x 15 mm needle, or an insuline-type needle; we bend the tip 20–30° with a needle-holder; a factory-made needle (Morie, France) is even better. The needle is inserted into a syringe filled with "healon". "Modus operandi" is as in classical goniotomy (surgeon in the temporal side of the patient, patient's head rotated away from the surgeon, assistant holding

265

E.L. Greve, W. Leydhecker & C. Raitta (eds.), Second European Glaucoma Symposium, Helsinki 1984.
© *1985, Dr. W. Junk Publishers, Dordrecht. ISBN 978-94-010-8934-0*

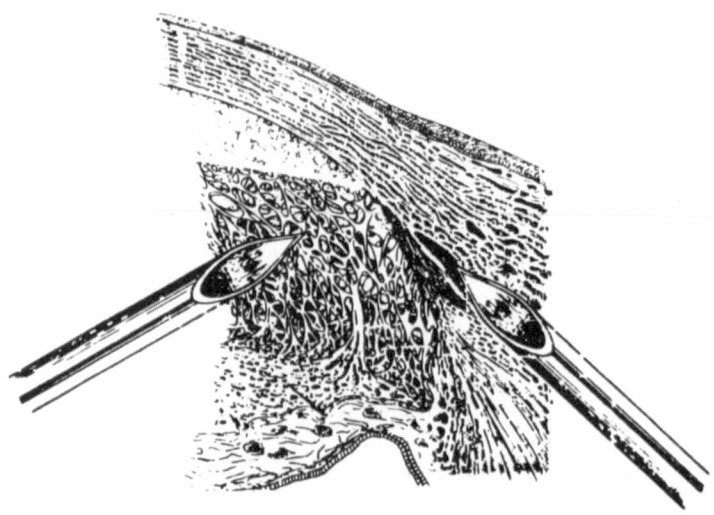

Fig. 1. Schematic drawing comparing the tangential approach to the perpendicular approach as in classic goniotomy or goniotrabeculotomy.

the vertical recti). The needle penetrates the anterior chamber at 6 hours (right eye) or 12 hours (left eye) through the *scleral* side of the limbus; this is in order to run parallel to Schlemm's canal. Penetration at 6 or 12 hours allows a *tangential* approach (Fig. 1) to the angle; this avoids the pupillary field and the convexity of the lens. Penetration is carried on under direct control, to avoid the prismatic effect of the goniolens. Once the needle is in the anterior chamber, the goniolens is inserted, held with the surgeon's left hand. A drop of "healon" is a good wetting agent between cornea and goniolens. The TM is incised with the tip of the needle. From now on, and with the concavity of the tip *towards* the surgeon, the trabeculotome is progressively introduced in the angle. Only the tip of the instrument is introduced into Schlemm's canal, and the TM is stripped slowly, gently and easily from the canal's lumen towards the anterior chamber as the needle progresses in the angle (Fig. 2). Since the convexity of the tip is facing the external wall of the canal, this structure is not damaged. This is why we bend the tip and we point it towards the anterior chamber.

As in goniotomy, the assistant will rotate the globe clockwise as the surgeon introduces the trabeculotome counter-clockwise. A 100–120° trabeculotomy can be achieved. Healon can be injected at will at any time if the surgeon wants to deepen the angle. There is usually no chamber loss, but if this is the case, healon is injected.

Once trabeculotomy is completed, the trabeculotome is withdrawn, taking care of injecting some healon before leaving the anterior chamber (internal "tamponnade"); this avoids any loss of aqueous and the chamber remains full. The goniolens and rectus forceps are also withdrawn. A steroid-antibiotic ointment is applied, as well as a mild mydriatic. The eyes are patched for 24 hours.

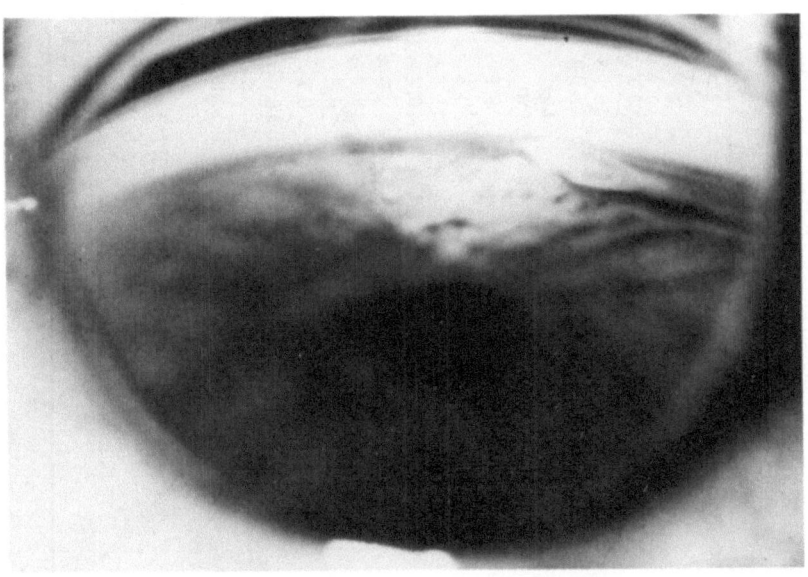

Fig. 2. Goniophotography at operation. The tip of the needle stripping the trabecular meshwork.

Twenty-one eyes of 12 patients have been operated with this technique, with a follow-up period of one year (mean). There are 13 eyes with chronic open-angle glaucoma, 3 with pigmentary glaucoma, 4 disgenetic and 1 steroid-induced. Details are summarized in Table 1.

RESULTS

Complications

There are no operative complications, not even hyphema, provided there is no chamber loss ("ex vacuum" hyphema).

Postoperative complications are hypherma, moderate, in 6 cases; and atropy of the iris in three cases. Iris atrophy does not occur since we give steroids and we dilate the pupils (see discussion).

Clinical results

The behaviour of the ocular pressures over one year is represented in Table 1 and Fig. 3. They can be summarized as follows: fall of pressure below 20 mm Hg in almost all cases in the first postoperative weeks, followed by a progressive rise in the second month (mean). From the second month, medical therapy must be reinstituted in most cases, although less intensively in regard to the preoperative treatment. At one year, most cases are controlled,

267

Table 1. Patient data: age, sex, type of glaucoma, ocular pressures, complications and treatment (P = pilocarpine 2% 3/day; T = timolol 0.50% 2/day; A = acetazolamide, number after A indicates mgrs. per day; COAG = chronic open angle glaucoma).

Patient	Age	Glaucoma	Po Preop./mmHg	Po 15 d.	Complications	Po 2 Months	Po 1 Year
Mrs. C.	60	C.O.A.G.	40 P-T-A 750	17 –	hyphema +	30 –	15 P-T
			40 P-T-A 750	18 –	–	23 –	13 T
Mr. N.	75	C.O.A.G.	20 P-T-A 750	15 –	Iris atrophy	24 –	15 T-A 125
			20 P-T-A 750	17 –	–	23 –	17 T-A 125
Mr. Z.	61	disgenetic	21 P-T	14 –	–	14 –	10 –
			30 P-T	14 –	–	34 –	17 P-T
Mr. B.	66	C.O.A.G.	34 P-T-A 375	18 –	–	26 –	lost
			30 P-T-A 375	38 –	hyphema ++	27 –	lost
Mr. V.	24	disgenetic	25 T-A 250	6 –	hyphema +	22 –	19 T
			23 T-A-250	19 –	hyphema +	25 –	16 T
Mrs. S.	80	C.O.A.G.	30 P-T-A 500	16 –	Iris atrophy	28 –	21 T-A 125
			30 P-T-A 500	18 –	Iris atrophy	23 –	20 T-A 125
Mr. C.	76	C.O.A.G	45 T-A 500	19 –	–	38 –	18 T-A 250
			40 T-A 500	28 –	hyphema +	48 –	19 T-A 250
Mr. V.	62	C.O.A.G.	21 P-T-A 500	14 –	–	23 –	20 –
			39 P-T-A 500	18 –	–	30 –	20 T
Mrs. N.	41	pigmentary	32 P-T	18 –	–	30 –	18 P-T
			24 P-T NO OP.	–	–	–	–
Miss O.	13	C.O.A.G.	46 –	10 –	–	34 –	19 P-T
			24 – NO OP.	–	–	–	–
Mr. V.	45	pigmentary + disgenetic	20 P-T	14 –	–	24 –	24 –
			20 P-T	14 –	–	20 –	22 –
Mr. C.	16	cortisonic (R.E.)	38 P-T	30 –	–	18 P-T	18 P-T
			14				

Dash (–) after Po figures indicates no treatment.
Upper half of each patient: right eye; lower half: left eye

268

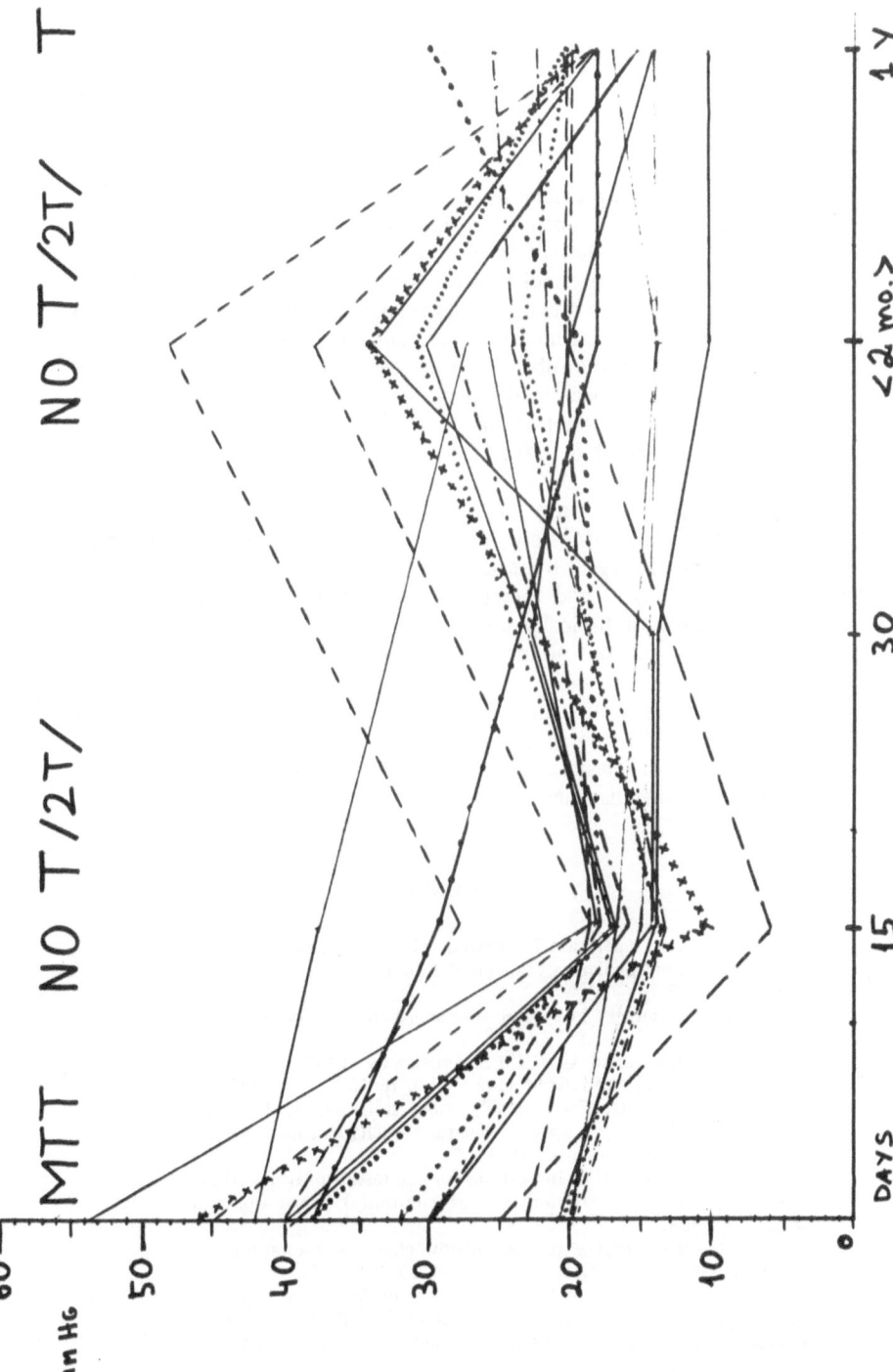

Fig. 3. Graphic showing the behaviour of ocular pressures in the one year period. (MTT = maximum tolerated medical treatment; no T = no treatment; T = treatment – indicated in Table 1).

but very few without treatment. Treatment is always weaker than preoperatively.

DISCUSSION

The fall of pressure was predictable and is a clinical proof of the pathogenic mechanism of the TM in open-angle glaucomas. The rise in pressure after a few months indicates that there is some kind of repair in the surgically damaged area. Yet, the trabecular meshwork cells are known not to reproduce; moreover, with this technique the scleral wall of Schlemm's canal is not damaged. But the remaining cells can enlarge, as do the corneal endothelial cells, and this is the subject of our present research; complete repair does not seem to take place in the majority of cases, since in almost all of them the medical control is better than before the operation.

Hyphema is attributed to reflux from the open Schlemm's canal and is always transient.

Iritis with secondary atrophy, similar to the "Urrets syndrome" described after some cases of keratoplasty, is attributed to the liberation of prostaglandins by the damaged trabecular cells. Avoiding postoperative miosis (since the angle is open) and therapy with topical steroids and antiprostaglandins systemically or topically avoids iritis; this complication occurred in some of our first cases, but no more after we instituted the above-mentioned postoperative care.

In conclusion, our results show that goniotrabeculotomy, although highly successful in the first postoperative month, is in the end a partially successful procedure. Further studies are necessary to disclose the "in vivo" behaviour of the sectioned trabecular meshwork.

REFERENCES

1. Barkan, O. A new operation for chronic glaucoma. Restoration of physiological function by opening Schlemm's canal under direct magnification. Am. J. Opthalmol. 19:951–966, 1936.
2. Barkan, O. Microsurgery in chronic simple glaucoma. Arch. Ophthalmol. 21:403–405, 1938.
3. Becker, B., Podos, S. and Assef, C.F. Microsurgery of the outflow channels. Clinical research. Trans. Am. Acad. Ophthalmol. Otol. 76:405–410, 1972.
4. Bietti, G.B., Quaranta, C.A. Considerazioni sulla terapia di particolari forme di "glaucoma cortisone" con speziali riguardi a quella chirurgia mediane goniotomia. Documenta Ophthal. 20:257–271, 1966.
5. Bietti, G.B., Quaranta, C.A. Indications for and results of iridocorneal angle incision (goniotomy, goniotrabeculotomy or trabeculotomy). Trans. ophthalmol. Soc. N.Z. 20:20–42, 1968.
6. Grant, W.M. Microsurgery of the outflow channels. Laboratory research. Trans. Am. Acad. Ophthalmol. Otol. 76:398–404, 1972.
7. Johnstone, M.A., Grant, W.M. Microsurgery of Schlemm's canal and the human aquaeous outflow system. Am. J. Ophthalmol. 76:906–917, 1973.
8. Quintana, M. Variantes en microcirugía del glaucoma. Arch. Soc. Esp. Oftal. 33:929–932, 1973.

9. Quintana, M. Trabeculotomia ab interno. Arch. Soc. Esp. Oftal. 37:193–200, 1977.
10. Spencer, W.H. Histological evaluation of microsurgical glaucoma techniques. Trans. Am. Acad. Ophthalmol. Otol. 76:389–397, 1972.
11. Tailor, U. Sulla incisione del'angolo irideo (contributo a la cura del glaucoma). Ann. Ottal. e Clin. Oculistica 20:117–127, 1891.
12. Vincentiis, C. and Tailor, U. Incisione del'angolo irideo nel glaucoma. Ann. Ottal. e Clin. Oculistica 22:540–542, 1983.
13. de Wecker, L. La sclérotomie interne. Ann. D'Oculistique 113:95–109, 1985.

Author's address:
Departament d'Oftalmologia
Hospital de Bellvitge
"Princeps d'Espanya"
C/. Feixa Llarga, S/N
Barcelona
Spain

EXPERIMENTAL AND CLINICAL CONSIDERATION OF DIRECT CYCLODIATHERMY

Dj. KONTIĆ, D. CVETKOVIĆ and V. DODIĆ-STEPANOVIĆ

(Belgrade, Yugoslavia)

ABSTRACT

The effect of direct cyclodiathermy was studied in adult chinchilla rabbits over a period of three months. The tonometric, biomicroscopic and histopathologic findings suggested that direct cyclodiathermy acts by inhibition of aqueous humour production secondary to damage to the stroma and the epithelium of the ciliary processus. In various forms of glaucoma with an unfavorable prognosis, especially in cases of haemmorrhagic and aphakic glaucoma, direct cyclodiathermy has been performed. The technical details of this procedure are described. Our paper presents results obtained in the strictly controlled group of patients treated with this procedure. Indications, postoperative care and complications are discussed.

INTRODUCTION

Numerous clinical procedures have been devised to induce partial destruction of ciliary body in an effort to decrease aqueous humor secretion in cases of glaucoma resistent to medical therapy and filtering operations. These procedures are limited to haemorrhagic glaucoma and to glaucoma uncontrollable by other types of surgery. Nonperforating cyclodiathermy was first reported by Weve in 1932 (13) and in 1936. Vogt described the use of perforating cyclodiathermy in glaucoma (11). Initial reports were optimistic and it was widely felt that cyclodiathermy represented a new and valuable operation in the treatment of refractory or advanced cases of glaucoma.

Many complications of cyclodiathermy have been reported, including scleral necrosis, intraocular hemorrhage cyclitis, endophtalmitis, symphatetic ophtalmia, phtisis bulbi (2,5,7,8,9,12). These complications, together with the frequent failure to maintain intraocular pressure at the normal level have encouraged attempts to find other surgical means of decreasing aqueous secretion.

Even in the most resistant cases of glaucoma, severe damage of ciliary body by cryotherapy or application of electric current of high frequency directly onto the ciliary body, may lead to improvement. Thus, Harms,

273

E.L. Greve, W. Leydhecker & C. Raitta (eds.), Second European Glaucoma Symposium, Helsinki 1984.
© *1985, Dr. W. Junk Publishers, Dordrecht. ISBN 978-94-010-8934-0*

Bendikt, Böke and others reported their experiences with application of direct cyclodiathermy in the treatment of glaucoma (1,3,6,10).

In order to establish mode of action of direct diathermy on the ciliary body and its effect on IOP, we carried out our investigation both in clinical and experimental conditions.

MATERIALS AND METHODS

The effect of application of high frequency electric current on the ciliary body was recorded in chinchilla rabbits weighing 2750–3000 g. The intraocular pressure was measured by aplanation pneumotonometer (Digilab, model R.) The apparatus was calibrated every day prior to measuring.

In order to establish normal values of IOP, we measured it in the rabbits 3 days before the operation. The control measuring of IOP was performed at approximately the same time using local anaesthetic.

All the animals were operated with total anaesthesia. As a premedication we used 0.2 ml/kg B.W. "Rompun" – xylazine chloride, an analgetic, sedative and muscle relaxant. We injection 2% xylazin hydrochloride i.m., and 15 min later 0.5 ml/kg of Nembutal – osdium pentobarbital into the auricular vein.

The anterior chamber control was conducted by focal light and biomicroscope. Goldmann's gonioscope was used for monitoring changes in the chamber angle.

The IOP of all the animals was controlled daily in the course of the first week, and afterwards once a week. The animals were observed for a period of 12 weeks. The effect of direct cyclodiathermy was examined with the experimental animals by histologic examination of the enucleated eyes. The enucleations were accompanied in intervals of 1 day to 3 months.

Direct effect of application high frequency electric current on the ciliary body and changes in IOP were investigated in 8 animals.

SURGICAL TECHNIQUE

Incision of bulbar conjunctiva 5 mm of the limbus in the upper half of the globe. The sclera exposed. Haemostasis. The scleral flap 2 mm wide marked with the basis on the limbus from 10 to 1 h. The scleral flap preparated in its full thickness and the ciliary body uncovered. On the ciliary body we applied 20 diathermic applications lasting 1 sec each. Bleeding occurring during preparation discontinuated after the application. The scleral flap was sutured by nonresponsive, single stitches. Continuous suture of the conjunctiva. After the operation, the biomicroscopic control showed prominent hemosis of the conjunctiva.

During the first week in one animal the fibrinous exudation in the anterior chamber was detacted while at all other animals the serous exudation was seen.

Corneas of all the animals showed signs of mild edema, which, together with the serous exudation into the anterior chamber, completely disappeared

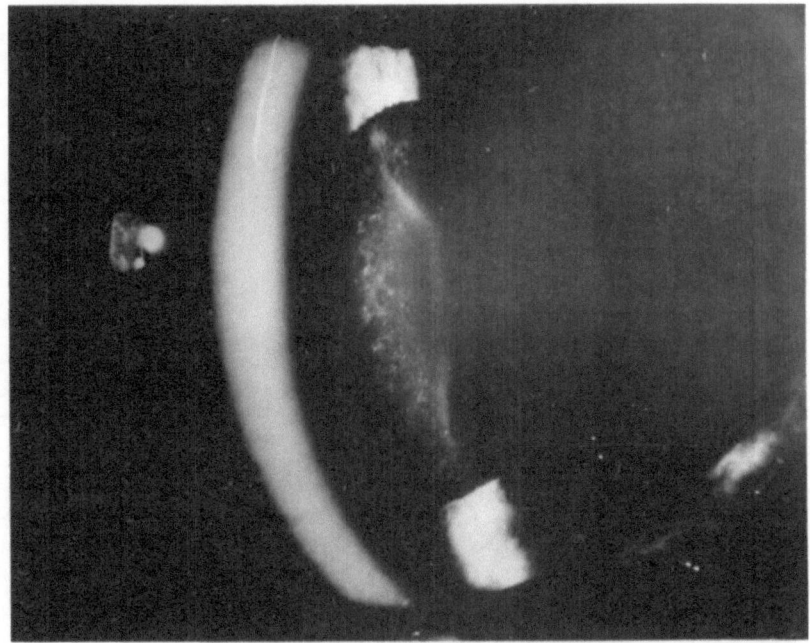

Fig. 1. Lens opacity in rabbit eye 4 weeks after direct cyclodiathermy.

in two weeks. The fibrinous exudation into the anterior chamber also stopped, leaving gonioand posterior synechiae.

The biomicroscopic examination of lenses showed mild opacity of the capsule, which remained during the whole period of recording (Fig. 1). In two animals we found partial atrophy at the roots of the irises (Fig. 2).

CONTROL MEASURINGS OF INTRAOCULAR PRESSURES (IOP)

Immediately after the operation no increase in the IOP was recorded in any of the animals (Fig. 3).

In the postoperative period, the pressure decrease was very prominent, reaching approximate values of 1.28 kPa (SD 0.20) on the first day. Further monitoring showed gradual decrease of IOP. Thus, at the end of the first week, the average IOP was 0.8 kPa–1.5 kPa ($\bar{X}$ = 1.22 kPa, SD 0.20). Even after two weeks no significant changes in IOP values were recorded (Mid. value 1.21 kPa, SD 0.33, interval of variations 0.8–1.9 kPa).

Further control showed gradual increase of IOP; however, at the end of the observation period the mid values remained at 1.48 kPa (SD 0.29 kPa), varying from 1.1 kPa to 1.9 kPa.

Histologic analysis of the ciliary body a day after the application of direct diathermy showed necrosis of the epithelium of the ciliary processus with hemorrhage in the strome, and elements of ciliary processes where damaged both in the epithelium and in stroma.

275

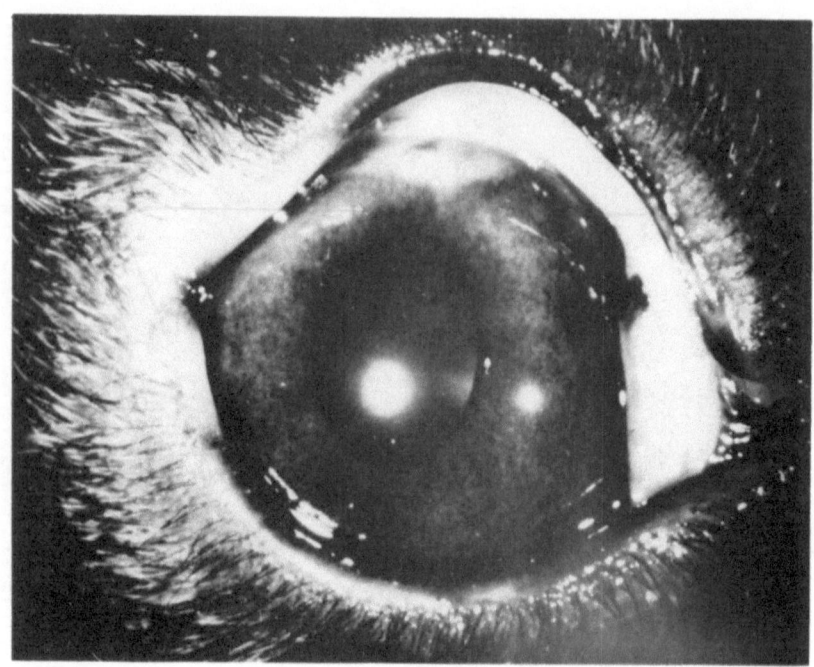

Fig. 2. Slit lamp photograph of rabbit eye with partial atrophy of the iris after direct cyclodiathermy.

The examination of the enucleated bulbus after 12 weeks showed changes indicating development of ciliary body atrophy in the region where the thermic noxa was applied (Fig. 4). The atrophic ciliary processes with proliferous connecting tissue and lymphoplasmocytous infiltrate dominated in histologic findings. The chamber angle examination did not show any further changes except for the mild lymphoplasmocytous infiltration and occasional goniosynechiae.

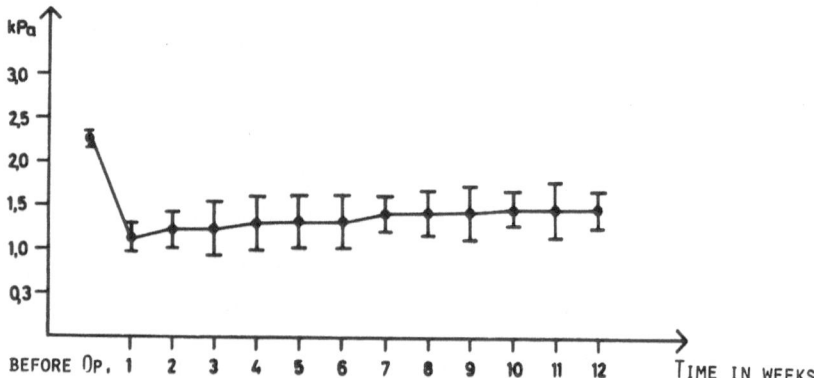

Fig. 3. Intraocular pressure (in kPa) before and after direct cyclodiathermy in 8 rabbit eyes. Arithmetic means and the standard deviations of the means are presented.

276

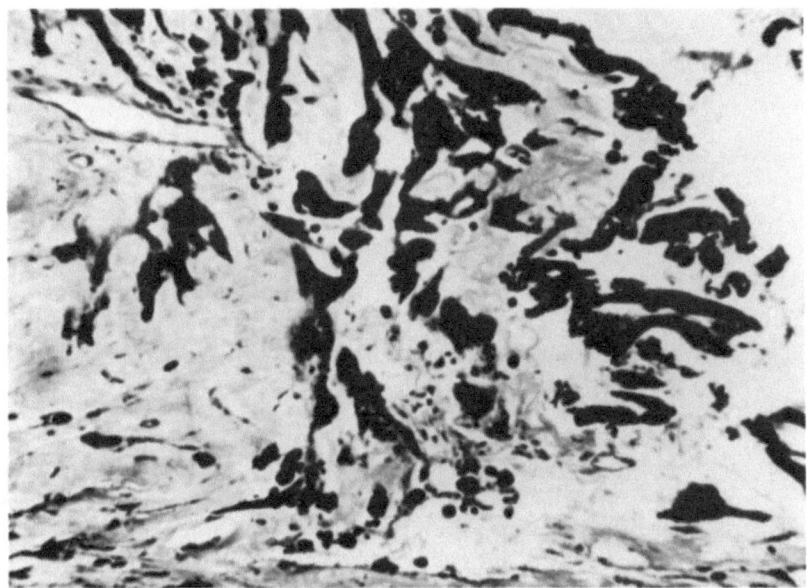

Fig. 4. Photomicrograph showing atrophic area of ciliary body 12 weeks after direct cyclodiathermy.

DIRECT CYCLODIATHERMY – CLINICAL RESULTS

We tried to avoid the temporary effect of transscleral diathermy by direct application of diathermy on the part of the uncovered ciliary body.

The patients selected for this operation were those for whom none of the other methods had a chance for success. They were previously unsuccessfully operated patients, or had prominent changes in the angle of the anterior chamber which made it impossible to apply any of the filtering operations. With the majority of the patients (10) this was the last attempt to avoid enucleation as the only method for relieving pain, while in others prominent degree of changes in the angle of the anterior chamber (neovascularization) made this method the last chance for salvation of the remaining isles of visual fields.

We applied direct cyclodiathermy in 18 patients, mostly in those suffering from hemorrhagic neovascular glaucoma (8). The average IOP of the selected patients after the local therapy was approx. 7 kPa (Table 1).

In the course of operation no complication occurred except for the slight bleeding during the preparation of the scleral flap. These bleedings discontinuated immediately after diathermy.

Measuring of IOP immediately after operation showed that the pressure did not increase in any of the patients. As a reaction of the anterior segment of the eye was usually recorded serous exudation, and in two cases respectively, fibrinous and hemorrhagic. A large staphyloma in the zone of the scleral flap was recorded with one patient.

277

Table 1. Type of glaucoma treated with direct cyclodiathermy

Type of glaucoma	No. of eyes
1. Hemorrhagic	10
2. Posttraumatic	3
3. Aphakic	4
4. Secondary with essential iris atrophy	1
5. Total	18

Table 2. Postoperative results of direct cyclodiathermy

1. Tension controlled without miotics (under 3.0 kPa)	1
2. Tension controlled with miotics and beta blocker (topical medication)	9
3. Uncontrolled	8
4. Total	18

Two years of permanent observation of these patients showed improvement of subjective problems. Normalization of IOP was achieved only in 10 cases, while in 2 patients the eye globe became atrophied (Table 2).

DISCUSSION

Assuming that only necrosis of the ciliary epithelium prevents its regeneration and leads to permanent decrease of IOP, we applied high frequency electric current directly onto the exposed ciliary body.

The high degree of damage of the ciliary epithelium was histologically confirmed as destruction of both layers — pigmented and non pigmented, and by damage of basement membrane and stroma of ciliary processes. This led to decrease of IOP already in the first postoperative days. The reaction on the necrotic epithelium was exhibited as a non-specific inflammation with prominent infiltration of polymerpho-nuclears into the ciliary body. In the course of postoperative observation of 12 weeks, the signs of inflammation decreased and discontinued leaving atrophy of a part of the ciliary body on which high temperature had been applied.

We wanted to induce atrophy of a part of the ciliary body, decreasing in this way the output of aqueous humor. Creation of new ways of drainage across the supraciliary zone and possibly by intrascelerar and subconjunctival filtration through the margins of the sutured scleral flap, helped to significantly decrease IOP, which was showed by occasional filtering bulb.

Clinical application of direct cyclodiathermy gives satisfactory results even in the most severe cases of glaucoma, first of all hemorrhagic and aphakic, relieving subjective problems and regulating IOP for longer periods in relatively high percentage (55.5%).

Direct cyclodiathermy should be reserved for those eyes in which filtering or other operations are contraindicated or have failed to reduce the IOP. The high percentage (11%) of atrophies after direct diathermy suggests that this operation should be used with caution.

REFERENCES

1. Benedikt, O. and Hiti, H. Ziliarkörperfreilegung. Klin. Mbl. Augenheilk. 169:711, 1976.
2. Berens, C. Glaucoma surgery: an evaluation of cycloelectrolysis and cyclodiathermy. Am. J. Ophthalmol. 59:599, 1960.
3. Böke, W., Winter, R. and Pülhorn, G. Ergebnisse der Ziliarkörperfreilegung bei sekundären Winkelblockglaukom. 1. Klinische Befune. Klin. Mbl. Augenheilk. 173:618, 1978.
4. Edmonds, C., de Roetth, A. and Howard, G. H.: Histopathologic changes following cryosurgery and diathermy of the rabbit ciliary body. Am. J. Ophthalmol. 69:65, 1970.
5. Gasteiger, N. Uber die Zyklodiathermiepunktur von Vogt Klin. Mbl. Augenheilk. 107:52, 1941.
6. Harms, H. Die direkte Ziliarkörperkauterisation. Symposium der Öserr. Ophthalm. Ges. 15–16:10, 1976.
7. Leydhecker, W. Spätergebnisse nach Zyklodiathermiepunktur. Klin. Mbl. Augenheilk. 151:35, 1967.
8. Leydhecker, W. Glaukom. Ein Handbuch. 2. Aufl. Springer, Berlin, 1973.
9. Reiser, K. A. Skleradiathermiepunktur, eine einfache Glaukom-operation, Klin. Mbl. Augenheilk. 115:491, 1949.
10. Steinbach, P. D. and Nover, A.: Die direkte Zeliarkörperkoagulation als Therapie bei verschiedenen Glaukomformen. Klin. Mbl. Augenheilk. 172:39, 1978.
11. Vogt, A. Versuche zur intraocularen Druckherabsetzung mittelst Diathermieschädigung des Corpus ciliare. (Zyklodiathermiestichlung.) Schweiz. med. Wchnschr. 66:593, 1936.
12. Vogt, A. Zyklodiathermiepunktur gegen Glaukom. Klin. Mbl. Augenheilk. 103: 591, 1939.
13. Weve, H. J. M. Clinischea Lessen, Nederl. tijdschr. v. geneesk. 76:5335, 1932.

Authors' address:
Clinic for Eye Diseases
"Dr Djordje Nešić" Clinical Center
Medical Faculty
Pasterova St.
Belgrade 2
Yugoslavia

RESEARCH ON THE MECHANISM OF TRABECULECTOMY: THE MAIN PATHWAY OF THE AQUEOUS HUMOR

C.D. BRODEIANU

(Ploiesti, Romania)

ABSTRACT

A wide (120°) trabeculectomy was performed in 10 open angle glaucomas starting from the cornea, without interfering with the post-schlemm draining system. Success was noted only in 6 cases with operatory incidents (sub-conjunctival perforations, incomplete suture of scleral wounds), the filtration blebs having an ephemeral existence in 5 out of 6 cases. These facts prove that:

— the main aqueous flow takes place through the scleral wound even when the macroscopic signs of filtration are lacking.

— the intact or slightly surgically damaged subconjunctival tissue is able to maintain the normal depth of the anterior chamber in front of a large scleral perforation and to drain the aqueous without filtration blebs.

INTRODUCTION

Practised for the first time in 1928 by Orlov (9), rediscovered by Smith (1) Sugar (4) and Coryllos (5), the trabeculectomy (T) actually exists in two main variants according to the wideness and postoperative aspect of the eye (Fig. 1): the Cairns' (4) variant (C.T) achieves an extirpation of a 3 mm long trabecular strip and the success is usually associated with macroscopic signs of filtration; the Vancea's (15,16) variant (V.T.) excises a trabecular strip of 10–11 mm in length (120°) and the macroscopic signs of filtration are usually lacking in case of durable compensation.

Our study tries to select in a quasi-experimental manner the main pathway of the aqueous flow amongst the four theoretical ones (Fig. 2). We have chosen the V.T. as the constant absence of blebs in cases with durable compensation suggests the preponderence of nonfistulating mechanisms.

We have started from the idea that if the main flow is not through the operatory wound, a V.T. with cyclodialysis and peripheral iridectomy performed without affecting the continuity of postschlemmal draining system (emissary veins-aqueous veins-episcleral veins) should succeed in an IOP equal or slightly superior to the episcleral veins pressure (9 mm Hg).

281

E.L. Greve, W. Leydhecker & C. Raitta (eds.), Second European Glaucoma Symposium, Helsinki 1984.
© *1985, Dr. W. Junk Publishers, Dordrecht. ISBN 978-94-010-8934-0*

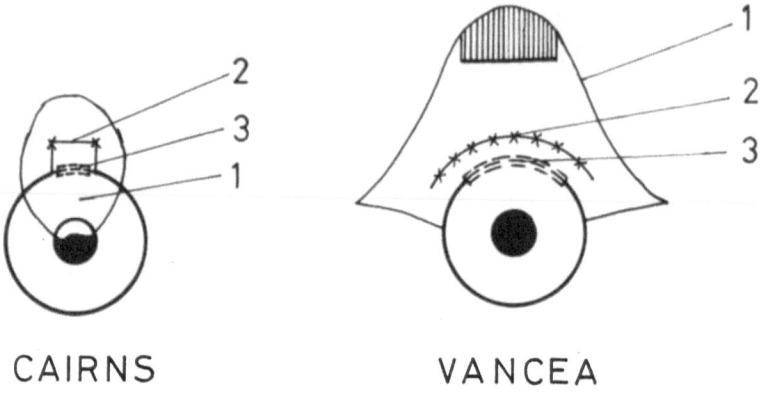

CAIRNS   VANCEA

Fig. 1. Two main variants of the trabeculectomy: 1) conjunctival flap; 2) scleral wound; 3) trabeculectomy.

SURGICAL PROCEDURE (Fig. 3)

A corneal non-perforating incision with a centripetal "biseau" is performed from 10 to 2, 1 mm in front of the conjunctival insertion, ended with 2 radial corneo-sclero-conjunctival incision slightly angulated in order to facilitate the dissection; posterior interlamellar dissection; posterior interlamellar dissection, up to 1 mm beyond the scleral spur located with Minsky's manoeuvre; 3 security threads; a 120°T including in the fragment 0.5 mm of scleral tissue beyond the scleral spur (cyclodialysis); 2 peripheral iridectomies;

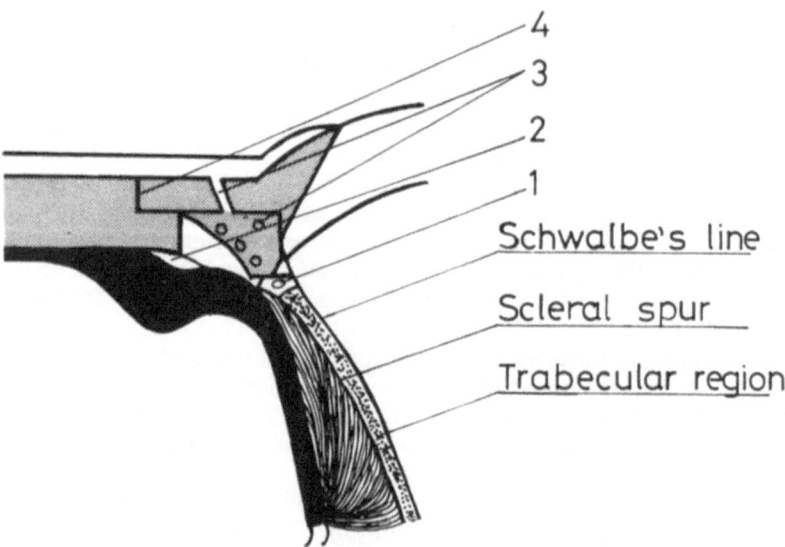

Schwalbe's line

Scleral spur

Trabecular region

Fig. 2. Four theoretical ways for the aqueous flow: 1) Schlemm's canal; 2) cyclodialysis slit; 3) emissary veins; 4) operatory wound.

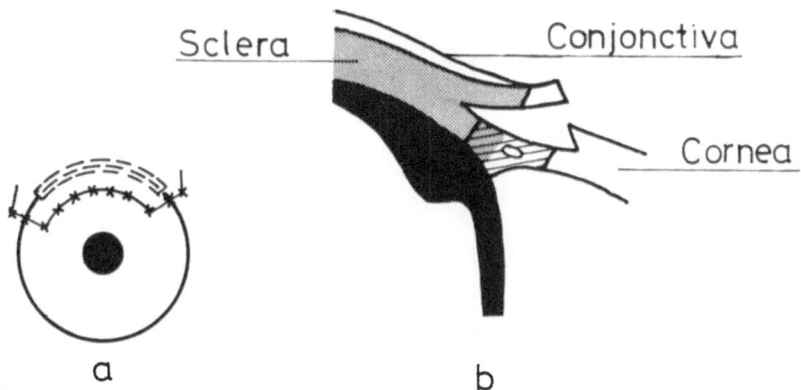

Fig. 3. Our surgical procedure: a) frontal view; b) saggital section.

a careful suture of the corneal wound and two-plane suture of sclerocon-
junctival radial incisions (usually 9 points of suture are sufficient, as shown
in the Fig. 3a) filling of the anterior chamber (A.C.) with serum; if there is
some leakage, the suture will be completed.

Antiseptic, anti-inflammatory and mydriatic eye drops. Binocular dressing
for 24 hours.

MATERIAL

We performed such an operation in 10 wide angle glaucomas (Table 1).

In 5 cases (1, 2, 8, 9, 10) a subconjunctival 4—6 mm long perforation on
the superficial flap occurred during the posterior interlammellar dissection; at
the end of the operation the A.C. was easily refilled with serum and it was
durably maintained.

In case no. 6 the radial incisions have not been sutured because of the
spontaneous reformation of the A.C. during the corneal wound suture.

RESULTS

The operation was unsuccessful when the preoperatory scheme was carried
out perfectly (case nos. 3, 4, 5, 7). The success was durably noted (24—36
months) only in cases with operatory incidents (case nos. 1, 2, 6, 8, 9, 10).
In all these cases, a filtration bleb occurred during the first days in 5 cases
and lasted permanently in a microcystic form in one case. In case no. 6 a
cataract extraction was performed 8 months later through an inferior corneal
incision "in inverse steps" (3). During the operating manoeuvre prior to the
opening of the eye two flat blebs appeared in the zone of the radial non-
sutured incision and rapidly disappeared afterwards. Five months later,
after a gonioscopy with Zeiss four mirror lens, the flat filtration reappeared
in the same zones.

Table 1.

No.	Name	Age	Evolutive stage (François[7])	Pi$_1$	Incidents	Bleb (days)	Pi$_2$	Interval (months)	Pi$_3$	Bleb
1.	B.I.	71	I	32p.	Perforation	5	18	22	19	—
2.	G.M.	66	V	45p.	Perforation	1	10	20	10	—
3.	B.C.	64	V	32p.	—	—	18	18	48p.	—
4.	U.E.	51	V	58p.	—	—	35	18	47p.	—
5.	B.M.	62	V	68	—	—	32	1	76	—
6.	U.E.	51	III	38p.	Incomplete suture	3	13	16	17	Occasional
7.	M.A.	41	0	40p.	—	—	35	16	45p.	—
8.	M.V.	64	IV	45	Perforation	3	6	16	7	—
9.	B.G.	55	0	30p.	Perforation	4	7	16	10	—
10.	P.M.	52	II	52	Perforation	Permanent	7	16	16	1.5 mm

284

In case 10 a traumatic tearing of the bleb occurred 16 months later.

After the excision of scarred tissues, a conjunctival covering was performed. A flat bleb reappeared but the IOP increased from 16 to 26 mm Hg, without medication.

COMMENTS AND CONCLUSIONS

1. From the physiopathological point of view there are at least four drainage ways after a successful T: the operatory wound, the ends of Schlemm's canal, the cyclodialysis slit and transscleral through the ends of emissary veins. During the early 70's the first hypothesis was almost unanimously accepted, supported by studies of histology (showing the closure of the ends of Schlemm's canal (13)), of experimental surgery (showing the same rate of success whether there was a trabecular or a purely corneal excision (13, 8) with or without cyclodialysis (8)) and by long-term follow-ups (showing the high rate of filtration blebs after a successful C.T.). Recent studies seem to complicate the situation by the resuscitation of the second (12) or of the fourth hypothesis (1, 2, 10, 12, 6); Vancea (15, 16) even describes a neo-trabeculum that would restore the physiological draining system.

In our study, the close connection between the success and the existence of some operatory incidents (subconjunctival perforation, incomplete suture of the scleral portions of the wound) prove that even when the macroscopic signs of filtration are lacking, the main pathway of the aqueous flow takes place through the scleral operation wound and that the role of other theoretical ways is unimportant. As a practical consequence any device that can ensure a permanent dehiscence of the scleral wound is salutary.

2. The evolution of the five cases with perforative incidents was surprisingly good. Though the superficial flap had a 5 mm long perforation placed in front of a large deep sclerectomy, the A.C. was always easily refilled with serum and it remained permanently deep.

In comparison with this, a flat chamber is not a rare finding in classical surgery that implies conjunctival dissection. That is why we believe that the resistance to distention of the intact or of slightly surgically damaged subconjunctival tissue is able to maintain the normal depth of the A.C. in front of a large scleral perforation.

3. The accidental parietal fistula achieved by us in six cases was restricted to a small area, 5 mm long, similar to that achieved in any fistulous classical device. Nevertheless, while a filtration bleb frequently accompanies the success of such a surgery including C.T., it had an ephemeral existence in 5 out of 6 cases. This fact proves that the intact or slightly surgically damaged subconjunctival tissue is more fitted to drain the humor without macroscopic signs of filtration. If Benedikt's (1, 2) conclusions are correct, we can suppose that such a tissue is more fitted than the damaged one to develop draining neovessels.

4. The evolution of the case no. 10 in which the subconjunctival dissection and covering resulted in a 10 mm. increase in IOP suggests that the intact or slightly damaged subconjunctival tissue is able to ensure lower levels of IOP.

285

REFERENCES

1. Benedikt, O. Zur Wirkungsweise der Trabekulektomie. Klin. Mbl. Augenheilk. 167:679–685 (1975).
2. Benedikt, O. Zur Wirkungsweise fistelbinder Operationen. Klin. Mbl. Augenheilk. 170:10–19 (1977).
3. Bordeianu, C. D. L'incision cornéenne, "en marche d'escalier" inverse dans l'opération de la cataracte. J. Fr. Ophthalmol. 10:589–594 (1980).
4. Cairns, J. E. Trabeculectomy: A preliminary report of a new method. Am. J. Ophthalmol. 66:673–679 (1968).
5. Koryllos, K.: Trabeculectomy, a new glaucoma operation. Delt. Hellin, Ophthal. Hetair 35:147–155 (1967).
6. David, R. and Sachs, U. Quantitative trabeculectomy. Br. J. Ophthalmol. 65:457–459 (1981).
7. Francois, J. and Neetens, A. Deterioration of the visual field in glaucoma and the blood pressure. Doc. Ophthalmol. 28:73–132 (1970).
8. Miles, A., Galin, Vivien Boniuk, R. M., Robbins. Surgical landmarks in trabecular surgery. Am. J. Ophthalmol. 80:696–700 (1975).
9. Orlov, K. H., 1927, in Rukovodstvo po glaznîm bolezniam Medghiz. Vol. 5. Moskva, 1960, p. 135.
10. Shields, M. B., Bradbury, M. J., Shelbourne, J. D. and Bell, S. W. The permeability of the outer layers of limbus and anterior sclera. Invest. Ophthalmol. Visual Sci. 16:866–869 (1977).
11. Smith, R. J. H. A new technique for opening the canal of Schlemm. Br. J. Ophthalmol. 44:370–374 (1960).
12. Spaeth, G. L., Effie Poryzees, A comparison between peripheral iridectomy with thermal sclerostomy and trabeculectomy, a controlled study. Br. J. Ophthalmol. 65:783–789 (1981).
13. Spencer, W. H. Histologic evaluation of microsurgical glaucoma techniques, Trans. Am. Acad. Ophthalmol. Otolaryngol. 76:389–397 (1972).
14. Sugar, H. S. Experimental trabeculectomy in glaucoma. Am. J. Ophthalmol. 51:623–627 (1961).
15. Vancea, P. P. and Schwartzenberg, T. Le traitement chirurgical des glaucomes par la technique de la trabéculectomie. Ann. d'occ. 207:563–581 (1974).
16. Vancea, P. P. and Schwartzenberg, T. La trabéculectomie, avec l'extraction du cristallin cataracté. Ann. d'occ. 207:337–351 (1974).

Author's address:
Dr. C.D. Bordeianu
15 Cameliei Street
Ploiesti, Romania

THE TRABECULO-KERATENCLEIZIS UNDER SCLERAL FLAP

C.D. BORDEIANU
(Ploiesti, Romania)

ABSTRACT

A corneotrabecular or a purely corneal strip is reflected posteriorly under a scleral flap; careful suture of the flap. By varying the shape and the dimensions of the scleral flap an intrascleral tunnel 4–10 mm long can be achieved, thus avoiding the conunctival zones compromised by surgery or burns and allowing the fistulizing surgery on internal and external limbal sectors. The displacement of the endothelial end of the fistula in full cornea diminishes the risks of closure in rubeotic glaucoma. The avascular paucicellular structure of the endothelialised strip increases the chances of success. Late good results in 18 out of 19 cases, without filtration bleb in 14.

INTRODUCTION

In a previous work (1) we proved that the main flow of the aqueous takes place through the dehiscences in the operatory wound and barely through other theoretical ways. If the fistula is all that matters in glaucoma surgery, any device that can ensure a permanent dehiscence of the wound is salutary. Various structures have been used: iris (6, 10), superifical (7) or profound sclera (5,11), muscle (3), artificial implants (4,8,9).

Our procedure – trabeculokeratencleizis under scleral flap (TK) – uses the corneotrabecular strip that in classical trabeculectomy is excised; this strip is reflected posteriorly over the thinned bed and is covered with the scleral flap. Through this intrascleral tunnel the aqueous can be drained in a zone of normal conjunctiva. There are three types of TK according to the length of the tunnel: TK_I (4 mm), TK_{II} (6 mm), TK_{III} (8 mm or more).

SURGICAL PROCEDURE

1. A classical conjunctival incision (TK_I) or a conjunctival limbal approach (TK_{II} and TK_{III}): Fig. 1.
2. A scleral nonperforating incision affecting 1/2–2/3 of scleral thickness

287

E.L. Greve, W. Leydhecker & C. Raitta (eds.), Second European Glaucoma Symposium, Helsinki 1984.
© *1985, Dr. W. Junk Publishers, Dordrecht. ISBN 978-94-010-8934-0*

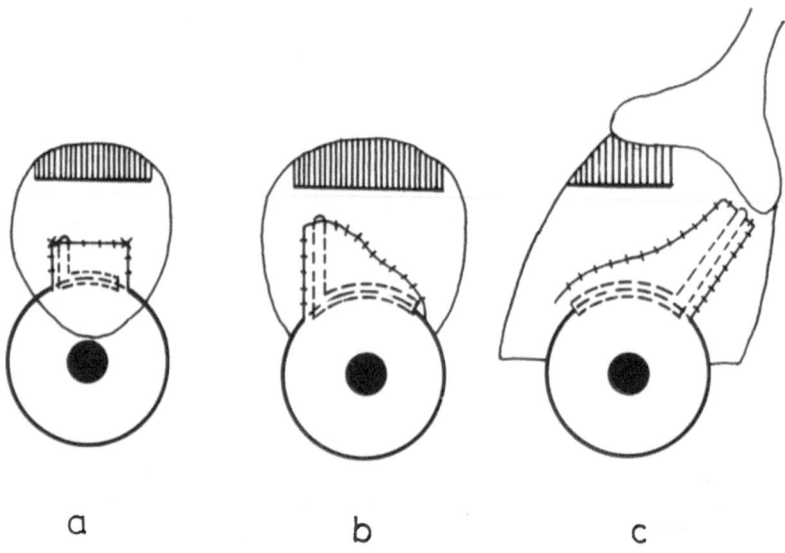

Fig. 1. Surgical procedure: a) TK$_I$, b) TK$_{II}$, c) TK$_{III}$.

permits the dissection of a superficial scleral flap. The dissection is pushed 2 mm in clear cornea. The dimensions of the scleral flap can vary from 4/6 mm (TK$_I$) to 6/8 mm (TK$_{II}$) and 8/6 mm with a perilimbal prolongation of 2/5 mm (TK$_{III}$). Two to five security threads are passed: Fig. 1.

3. Corneal puncture at 2 mm from the limbus prolongated with scissors. The same instrument cuts the other two incisions, delimiting a corneotrabecular (TK) or a purely corneal (keratencleizis) strip, nasally pedicled, 1–1.5 mm in width and with a length that can vary from 5 mm (TK$_I$), to 7 mm (TK$_{II}$) and to 9 mm (TK$_{III}$). Close to the pedicle the incisions will be curved towards the cornea, so that the endothelial end of the tunnel is placed in clear cornea, at distance from the mobile and vascularised elements of the anterior segment. The strip is reflected posteriorly and placed close to the postero-nasal angle of the scleral flap. When cataract extraction is intended, the wound is enlarged up to 180°.

4. 1–3 peripheral iridectomies, the largest being placed in front of the endothelial orifice.

5. Careful scleral suture until easy filling of the anterior chamber with serum and air is possible. When the serum leaks abondantly near the strip, another point of suture is added close to it, or even in its place, after its exteriorised end is cut off.

6. Conjunctival suture. Midriatic, antiseptic and antiinflammatory eye drops; binocular dressing for 24 hours.

MATERIALS

Nineteen eyes were operated according to this procedure, age varying between 4 months and 82 years. There were 4 TK$_I$ (1 associated with cataract

Table 1. Late results

Criteria		Trabeculo-keratencleizis						Total
		I		II		III		
		S	+ C	S	+ C	S	+ C	
Intraocular pressure	7–10 mmHg	–	–	2	1	–	–	3
	11–15	–	–	1	3	1	3	7
	16–20	3	–	1	3	–	–	7
	21–22	–	1	–	–	–	–	1
	23–	–	–	1	–	–	–	1
Gonio-sinochies	absent	3	–	4	4	1	2	15
	present	–	1	–	3	–	–	3
	imprecise	–	–	1	–	–	–	1
Signs of filtration	absent	–	–	3	6	1	2	12
	flat oedema	2	–	2	1	–	–	5
	microkistic oedema	–	1	–	–	–	–	1
	macrokistic oedema	1	–	–	–	–	–	1
Corneal alterations		–	–	1	1	–	1	3
Corneal astigmatism	–0.5 D	2	–	–	–	–	–	2
	– 1 D	1	1	1	–	–	–	3
	2–3 D	–	–	3	4	1	1	9
	4 D	–	–	–	3	–	1	4
	imprecise	–	–	1	–	–	–	–

S: simple; + C: cataract extraction associated

extraction), 12 TK_{II} (7 with cataract extraction) and 3 TK_{III} (2 with cataract extraction). More than half of our operations were practised on scarred tissues (1 following a severe alkalinous burn and 9 following the failure of other antiglaucomatous operations). In 2 cases with rubeotic glaucoma a pure keratencleizis I was practised. As postoperative complications, there were 2 cases with hiphema.

After 16–26 months, the final control revealed (Table 1): the high frequency of cases compensated without medication and with free angle, the scarceness of macroscopic signs of filtration and of corneal modifications, and an objective astigmatism that in TK_{II} and TK_{III} is more important than in classical techniques.

COMMENT

The advantages of our technique, as compared with the existing ones are:

I. The superficial end of the fistula can be displaced at a greater distance from the limbus, near (TK_{II}) or even beyond (TK_{III}) the muscular insertions of recti. Thus, our technique:

— can be practised on scarred conjunctival tissue: 9 of our cases were successful reinterventions on superior sector of the eye and one followed a severe alkalinous burn (at the final control: Pi = 25 mm $Hg_{(Schiotz)}$, C = 0.24).

— can be practised (TK_{II} and TK_{III}) on internal and external sectors of the eye, as it ensures a good protection for the filtration zone and as the filtration bleb is a rare finding.

II. The endothelial end of the fistula is placed in clear cornea, where the neovascularization of rubeotic glaucoma does not appear. The success of our operation (K_I) in 2 such cases enables us to hope that the pure keratencleizis could cure the neovascular glaucoma.

III. The corneotrabecular strip has an avascular, paucicellular structure and carries an endothelium that continues the corneal one. Thus the risks of blockade by fibrous proliferation (autochtonous or of a sanguine origin) are diminished.

The disadvantages of our techniques (TK_{II} and TK_{III}) are represented by bleeding during the scleral dissection, corneal alterations at the site of absent strip and a higher degree of astigmatism. However, we must stress that intraocular bleeding is rarely found (2/19) and that corneal alterations are rare (3/19) and without importance (discrete nephelioma covered by a localised epithelial oedema). When the suture is good, the anterior chamber is always deep.

CONCLUSIONS

1) The TK_I can be practised as a first operation in any form of glaucoma, excepting that provoked by the increase in venous pressure.

2) The displacement of the filtration zone towards the conjunctival fundi makes our technique more fitted than others when performed on scarred conjunctival tissues or on lateral sectors of the eye.

3) The displacement of the endothelial orifice in clear cornea increases the chances of success in rubeotic glaucoma.

4) The avascular structure of the endothelialized strip increases the chances of maintaining the fistulous traject.

REFERENCES

1. Bordeianu, C. D. Research on the mechanism of trabeculectomy: the main pathway of the aqueous humor. This volume.
2. Cernea, P. and Constantin, F. Glaucomal. Medicala, Bucureşti, 1979.
3. Chilaris, G. A. Goniomiostomy. A new glaucoma operation. Am. J. Ophthalmol. 58:373–377 (1964).
4. Etienne, R., Trepsat, C. and Roussille, N. Note preliminaire sur la technique d'implantation du drain en hydron: Bull. S.O. France 78:303–304 (1978).
5. Farnarier, G. and Mouly, A. Technique modifiée de l'iridocyclorétraction de Krasnov. Bull. S.O. France 76:1171–1173 (1976).
6. Holth, S. Eines neues Prinzip der operativen Behandlung des Glaukoms: Ber. Dtsch. Ophthal. Ges. Heidelberg 33:123–128 (1907).
7. Krasnov, M. M. Iridocycloretraction in narrow angle glaucoma. Br. J. Ophthalmol. 55:389–395 (1971).
8. Krupin, Th., Podos, S. M., Becker, B. and Newkirk, J. B. Valve implant in filtering surgery. Am. J. Ophthalmol. 81:232–235 (1976).
9. Molteno, A. C. B. New implant for drainage in glaucoma. Br. J. Ophthalmol. 53: 606–615 (1969).

10. Pacurariu, I. Iridectencleizis: cit. 2. (1955).
11. Yankova, L. Modification de l'opération d'iridocyclorétraction de Krasnov. J. Fr. Ophthalmol. 4:147–148 (1981).

Author's address:
Dr C.D. Bordeianu
15 Cameliei St.
Ploiesti, Romania

A MODIFICATION OF COHAN'S FILTERING CORNEAL TREPHINATION

I. TAKÁTS

(Pécs, Hungary)

ABSTRACT

At the IVth Microsurgical Symposium Cohan described an operation called "filtering corneal trephination". He had devised the operation for painful, blind eyes with primary or secondary glaucoma in order to avoid enucleation. In Cohan's operation the conjunctiva is incised and separated widely from the limbus. Then a curved incision is made in the cornea and half of its superficial part stripped off. The remaining cornea is trephined and an iridectomy performed through the hole. The conjunctiva is fixed to the corneal wound with sutures (Fig. 1, left side: front view and lateral view).

We have also employed Cohan's operation on four eyes, but it was successful only in one eye. We thought that the failure might have been due to adhesion of the conjunctiva to the cornea.

Therefore, we modified the operation. We cut out a strip of the cornea, sparing the most peripheral part of it (Fig. 1, right side; front view and lateral view). Our idea was that this part of the cornea, covered with epithelium, would prevent adhesion.

The steps of the operation are as follows. Dissection of the conjunctiva away from the limbus in the upper part of the temporal or nasal quadrant. Delivery of the conjunctiva towards the fornix. A central, curved incision in the cornea to about thirds of its depth made with a razor-blade fragment. A peripheral curve incision in the cornea. Ablation of the remaining part of the cornea. 1.0 or 1.5 mm trephination in the lamellar corneal bed. Iridectomy

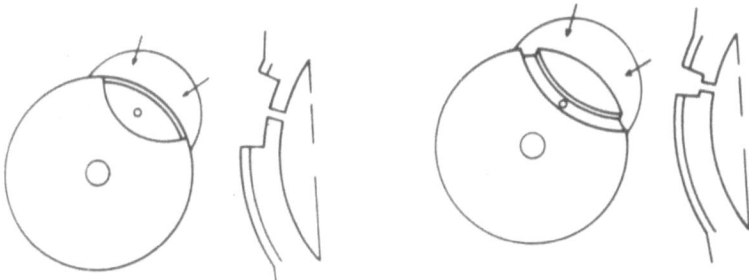

Fig. 1.

293

E.L. Greve, W. Leydhecker & C. Raitta (eds.), Second European Glaucoma Symposium, Helsinki 1984.
© *1985, Dr. W. Junk Publishers, Dordrecht. ISBN 978-94-010-8934-0*

Table 1. Data of operated eyes

Number of eyes: 16
Age: 18–76 yrs. (mean: 53 yrs)
Cause of absolute glaucoma:
Occlusion of the central retinal vein: 7
Diabetes: 5
Uveitis: 1
Primary glaucoma: 1
Inveterate retinal detachment: 1
Rieger's syndrome: 1
IOP prior to surgery: 35–82 mmHg (mean: 46 mmHg)
IOP after surgery: 8–35 mmHg (mean: 21 mmHg)
Enucleation: 4

through the trephination hole. Washing of the anterior chamber with cold Ringer solution, if necessary, in order to stop bleeding and remove the blood. Stitching of the conjunctiva to the edge of the central corneal wound with a continuous Ethilon 10/0 suture.

We have operated on 16 eyes in the same way during the past four years. The operation was successful in 12 cases (Table 1). There was no growth of epithelium into the anterior chamber. It seems interesting that although in some cases the intraocular pressure did not fall to normal values, the eyes became free from pain.

In the remaining four cases there was severe, rapidly developing rubeosis of the iris. On the days after the operation the anterior chamber was full of blood, the pain did not disappear and the eyes had to be removed.

On the basis of our experience we recommend our modified operation on blind, painful glaucomatous eyes.

REFERENCES

Cohan, B. E. Adv. Opthalmol. 30:327–328 (1975).

VARIATION IN ANTERIOR CHAMBER VOLUME DURING THE PILOCARPINE/PHENYLEPHRINE PROVOCATIVE TEST

CHARLES V. CLARK and ROY MAPSTONE
(Liverpool, U.K.)

ABSTRACT

Anterior chamber volume was measured by a photogrammetric technique during the course of a pilocarpine/phenylephrine provocative test. In eyes without a peripheral iridectomy, there was a significant decrease in the volume of the anterior chamber; if a peripheral iridectomy was present, anterior chamber volume significantly increased. The aetiology of dynamic changes in anterior chamber volume is discussed.

INTRODUCTION

The depth of the anterior chamber of the eye is not a static dimension and may show rapid and transient changes (1). Such alterations in depth are directly related to the pupil block force (2,3), itself a manifestation of autonomic activity in the anterior segment (Fig. 1). Contraction of the pupil may be resolved into a series of component forces, the net effect summating to increased iris/lens apposition (4). Pupil block is maximal if the pupil is fixed, as a result of relative parasympathetic and sympathetic activity, in mid-dilatation with the sphincter muscle contracting strongly. The magnitude of pupil block force has been calculated and shown to be maximal at a pupillary diameter between 3.8 and 4.2 mm (1,5). The only known method of maintaining pupillary diameter at mid-dilatation is to simultaneously maximally stimulate both sympathetic and parasympathetic nervous systems in the anterior segment, the basis of the pilocarpine/phenylophrine provocative test (6,7). The component forces determining the position of the iris/lens diaphragm at equilibrium are the production of aqueous, the facility of outflow, and the degree of pupil block (Fig. 2a). Assuming a constant production of aqueous, both pupil block and facility of outflow are increased during the pilocarpine/phenylephrine provocative test. As aqueous flow from the posterior to anterior chamber is less than the rate of outflow from the anterior chamber (8), the resultant pressure differential results in forward movement of the iris/lens diaphragm and consequently

295

E.L. Greve, W. Leydhecker & C. Raitta (eds.), Second European Glaucoma Symposium, Helsinki 1984.
© *1985, Dr. W. Junk Publishers, Dordrecht. ISBN 978-94-010-8934-0*

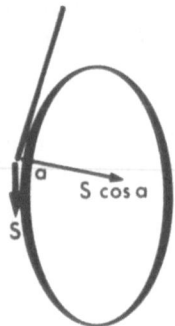

Fig. 1. Pupil block.

shallowing of the anterior chamber (Fig. 2b). the first stage of angle closure (i.e. iridocorneal contact) is thus facilitated (9,10). It has been clearly shown that axial anterior chamber depth may decrease significantly during provocative testing; however minimal changes in depth at the periphery of the

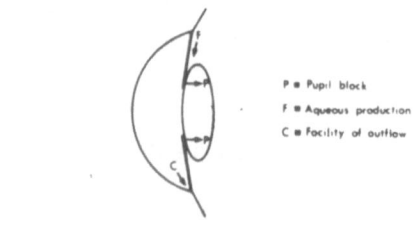

(a) Forces determining the position of the iris-lens diaphragm

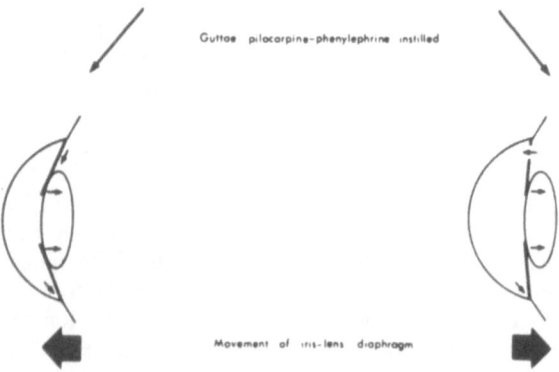

(b) Eyes without a peripheral iridectomy

(c) Eyes with a peripheral iridectomy

Fig. 2. Variation in anterior chamber volume volume during the pilocarpinephenylephrine provocative test.

anterior chamber are of much greater significance in the pathogenesis of angle closure (11,12). Reproducible documentation of this latter measurement is provided by the photogrammetric technique, in which the depth of the anterior chamber is measured at 0.5 mm intervals from the optic axis to the iridocorneal angle from a polaroid photograph, using a transparent optically-distorted curvilinear grid (13,14,15).

The presence of a peripheral iridectomy negates the effect of decreased aqueous flow via the pupil, and the vector force of pupil block without a pressure differential across the iris results in posterior displacement of the iris/lens diaphragm (Fig. 2c).

Rapid, accurate measurements of anterior chamber volume are thus possible during dynamic changes in the dimensions of the anterior chamber subsequent to autonomic provocation.

PATIENTS AND METHODS

Patients were selected on the basis of the following criteria:
1. Acute closed-angle glaucoma in the contralateral eye
2. Ocular hypertension in association with narrow angles
3. Ocular hypertension in association with wide angles

Fifty-six patients were included in the study. A pilocarpine 2%/phenylephrine 10% provocative test was performed according to the standard method. In addition, anterior chamber depth and volume were measured using a Zeiss photo slit-lamp and Polaroid camera attachment. With the slit illuminator set at 55° and magnification × 16, the slit was aligned vertically along the optic axis such that the upper border of the pupil and lower border of the cornea were visible. The photograph was taken ensuring maximum clarity of the iridocorneal angle. A transparent anterior chamber template was aligned with the posterior corneal curve, and the depth of the anterior chamber measured to an accuracy of 0.1 mm at 0.5 mm intervals from the optic axis. The depths were multiplied by an appropriate weighting factor and summated, resulting in the total anterior chamber volume.

The final experimental model involves two discrete stages:
1. Prior to provocation, the following baseline measurements were taken in both eyes: i. Intraocular pressure
        ii. Facility of outflow
        iii. Depth and volume measurement of anterior chamber
        iv. Gonioscopy
One drop of pilocarpine 2% and phenylephrine 10% instilled in one eye.
2. Two hours later all measurements were repeated. Test terminated with guttae thymoxamine 0.5% (plus acetazolamide 500 mg i.v. if necessary).
The anterior chamber depth and volume were calculated from the photographs on a single-blind basis, i.e. the observer was not aware of details relating to each photograph at the time of measurement.

Significance was assessed by Student's paired and unpaired 't' tests, and Kruskal-Wallis one-way analysis of variance by ranks.

Table 1. Variation in anterior chamber volume during the pilocarpine 2%/phenylephrine 10% provocative test (Group mean values ± SD)

	Volume of A/C before provocation (µl)	Volume of A/C 2 hours later (µl)	Change in volume of A/C (µl)	Significance
Pilocarpine 2%/phenylephrine 10% provocative test in eyes without a peripheral iridectomy				
All (n = 77)	98.31 ± 35.11	84.22 ± 32.41	14.09 ± 14.55	p < 0.001
Fellow eye of patients with closed-angle glaucoma (n = 15)	76.17 ± 10.94	61.15 ± 14.82	15.02 ± 13.37	p < 0.001
Ocular hypertension/narrow angles (n = 28)	77.68 ± 20.95	68.73 ± 21.13	8.95 ± 14.06	p < 0.01
Ocular hypertension/wide angles (n = 34)	125.09 ± 33.09	107.03 ± 30.77	18.06 ± 14.05	p < 0.001
Pilocarpine 2%/phenylephrine 10% provocative test in eyes with a peripheral iridectomy (n = 20)	92.93 ± 29.03	105.05 ± 28.46	12.12 ± 13.54	p < 0.001
Control group: eyes in which no drops were instilled (n = 12)	90.13 ± 27.01	89.26 ± 25.63	0.87 ± 3.98	p > 0.05

298

RESULTS

1. *Provocative test in eyes without a peripheral iridectomy*
There was a significant decrease ($p < 0.001$) in the volume of the anterior chamber during the test (Table 1). No significant differences ($p > 0.05$) were shown in comparisons between each of the three subgroups.

2. *Provocative test in eyes with a peripheral iridectomy*
There was a significant increase ($p < 0.001$) in the volume of the anterior chamber during the test (Table 1).

3. *Control group: eyes in which no drops were instilled*
This group exhibited no significant change in volume ($p > 0.05$) during the 2 hour period between commencement and termination of provocation in the contralateral eye.

DISCUSSION

Significant variation in the dimensions of the anterior chamber has been shown to occur during the course of a provocative test with pilocarpine and phenylephrine. The stimulation of both parasympathetic and sympathetic nervous systems in the anterior segment by the simultaneous administration of guttae pilocarpine and phenylephrine maintains the pupil in mid-dilatation by isometric contraction of the iris musculature, resulting in maximal pupil block. In eyes without a peripheral iridectomy, aqueous flow from the site of production (ciliary processes) to that of escape (trabecular meshwork and uveoscleral route) can only occur via the pupil. Increasing pupil block thus results in decreased aqueous flow from the posterior to the anterior chamber. The increased facility of outflow previously shown to occur in the early stages of a pilocarpine/phenylephrine provocative test (as a result of pilocarpine-induced contraction of the ciliary muscle opening trabecular meshwork via the scleral spur) produces shallowing of the anterior chamber as a direct consequence of the pressure differential across the iris/lens diaphragm.

The presence of a functioning peripheral iridectomy permits free transfer of aqueous. As no pressure difference exists between the posterior and anterior chambers, the direction and degree of displacement of the iris/lens diaphragm is controlled exclusively by the vector component of pupil block, i.e. posteriorly. The translational movement of the iris/lens diaphragm by autonomic provocation can only be explained on this basis.

Anterior chamber volume assessment by the photogrammatic technique permits accurate measurement of rapid changes in the dimensions of the anterior segment. The fact that significant changes in volume were observed in each of the three groups of patients examined suggests the possibility of a common aetiological factor. This is currently the basis of further investigation.

CONCLUSIONS

This study has established the degree to which variation in the dimensions of the anterior chamber contribute to angle closure, providing photographic evidence by an objective, reproducible, accurate technique. More significantly, quantification of changes in anterior chamber volume is possible in those cases in which angle closure does not occur and thus intraocular pressure remained unchanged. A negative provocative test merely indicates no significant increase in intraocular pressure; however significant changes in ocular dimensions may occur with consequent prognostic implications.

ACKNOWLEDGEMENTS

C.V. Clark is presently the Samuel Crossley Barnes Research Fellow in glaucoma, University of Liverpool, and in receipt of a Wellcome Trust Travel Scholarship.

REFERENCES

1. Mapstone, R. Acute shallowing of the anterior chamber. Br. J. Ophthalmol. 65: 446 (1981).
2. Mapstone, R. Mechanics of pupil block. Br. J. Ophthalmol. 52:19 (1968).
3. Mapstone, R. Closed-angle glaucoma in eyes with non-shallow anterior chambers. Trans. Ophthal. Soc. U.K. 101:218 (1981).
4. Mapstone, R. Autonomic effects on aqueous outflow. Res. Clin. Forums 3:35 (1981).
5. Mapstone, R. Glaucoma. In Davidson, S. I. (ed.) Recent Advances in Ophthalmology (6). Edinburgh: Churchill Livingstone, 1983:23.
6. Mapstone, R. Provocative tests in closed-angle glaucoma. Br. J. Ophthalmol. 60:115 (1976).
7. Mapstone, R. The role of provocative tests in closed-angle glaucoma. Res. Clin. Forums 2:67 (1980).
8. Mapstone, R. Outflow changes in positive provocative tests. Br. J. Ophthalmol. 61:634 (1977).
9. Mapstone, R. Partial angle closure. Br. J. Ophthalmol. 61:525 (1977).
10. Mapstone, R. One gonioscopic fallacy. Br. J. Ophthalmol. 63:221 (1979).
11. Coakes, R. L., Lloyd-Jones, D. and Hitchings, R. A. Anterior chamber volume. Trans. Ophthal. Soc. U.K. 99:78 (1979).
12. Hitchings, R. A. and Powell, D. J. Pilocarpine and narrow-angle glaucoma. Trans. Ophthal. Soc. U.K. 101:214 (1981).
13. Johnson, S. B., Coakes, R. L. and Brubaker, R. F. A simple photogrammetric method of measuring anterior chamber volume. Am. J. Ophthalmol. 85:469 (1978).
14. Brubaker, R. F. and Fontana, S. T. Volume and depth of the anterior chamber in the normal aging human eye. Arch. Ophthalmol. 98:1803 (1980).
15. Hitchings, R. A., Romano, J. and Clark, P. Measurements of axial and peripheral anterior chamber depth: accuracy of a photographic method. Br. J. Ophthalmol. 68:212 (1984).

Authors' address:
St. Paul's Eye Hospital
Old Hall St.
Liverpool L3 9PF
U.K.

UNILATERAL ANGLE CLOSURE GLAUCOMA:
A BIOMETRIC STUDY

G. STRASSER and W. HAUFF
(Vienna, Austria)

ABSTRACT

Keratometry and biometry were done on both eyes in 20 patients suffering from unilateral acute angle closure glaucoma. In the diseased eye the anterior chamber depth was significantly more shallow and the lens significantly thicker than in the fellow eye. Other data showed no significant differences.

INTRODUCTION

In patients with a unilateral acute angle closure glaucoma, an attack of the fellow eye sometimes may develop after a period of several years or even not at all (1). By means of comparative keratometry and biometry of both eyes in patients with unilateral angle closure glaucoma, possible differences between the diseased and the fellow eye were to be ascertained.

PATIENTS AND METHOD

In 20 patients suffering from unilateral acute angle closure glaucoma, the anterior chamber depth, thickness of the lens and length of the vitreous body were determined echographically in both eyes. For biometry, the set Ocuscan 400 with its corresponding biometry component DRB 400 was used; keratometry was done with the autokeratometer of Humphrey. The corneal diameter was measured with the scale of the fixation control of Goldmann's perimeter. During the examination, both eyes were free of any local medication.

RESULTS

The results of biometric and keratometric measurements of eyes after acute angle closure glaucoma as well as of their healthy fellow eyes are given in Table 1. In the diseased eyes a significantly more shallow anterior chamber

301

E.L. Greve, W. Leydhecker & C. Raitta (eds.), Second European Glaucoma Symposium, Helsinki 1984.
© *1985, Dr. W. Junk Publishers, Dordrecht. ISBN 978-94-010-8934-0*

Table 1. Echographic and keratometric data of both eyes in 20 patients with unilateral angle closure glaucoma (mm)

	Max.	Min.	Mean	S.D.
A1	2.48	1.61	2.00	0.258
F1	2.65	1.85	2.19	0.244
A2	6.19	5.00	5.41	0.329
F2	6.10	4.27	5.16	0.3809
A3	16.40	13.10	14.69	0.844
F3	17.84	13.49	14.85	0.999
A4	24.01	20.42	22.11	1.031
F4	25.59	20.73	22.41	1.175
A5	8.39	7.23	7.66	0.315
F5	8.26	7.26	7.67	0.274
A6	8.06	6.98	7.66	0.353
F6	8.01	6.78	7.62	0.341
A7	12.00	11.00	11.55	0.356
F7	12.00	11.00	11.58	0.323

A: diseased eye; F: fellow eye. 1: anterior chamber depth; 2: thickness of the lens; 3: length of the vitreous body; 4: axial length of the globe; 5, 6: radius of the cornea; 7: diameter of the cornea

($t_{15} = -5.39$; $p \ll 0.001$) on the one hand and a significantly thicker lens ($t_{15} = 3.01$; $p < 0.01$) on the other hand were found. No significant differences between both eyes could be detected as regards length of the vitreous body, entire length of the globe, keratometry and corneal diameter (Table 2).

DISCUSSION

As already stated by Törnquist (3), in unilateral angle closure glaucoma the anterior chamber of the diseased eye is significantly more shallow than that of the fellow eye. Since the anterior chamber depth is determined by the corneal radius and diameter, the entire length of the globe, the thickness and the position of the lens, a significant difference in one or more of these parameters can be expected when both eyes are compared. Ortlepp (2) could

Table 2. Differences between data of diseased eye and fellow eye in 20 patients with unilateral angle closure glaucoma (diseased eye minus fellow eye; mm)

	Max.	Min.	Mean	S.D.	Significance
D1	0.01	−0.68	−0.19	0.158	$p \ll 0.001$
D2	1.47	−0.09	0.25	0.374	$p < 0.01$
D3	0.60	−1.44	−0.16	0.494	n.s.
D4	0.85	−3.88	−0.30	0.959	n.s.
D5	0.24	−0.23	0.00	0.135	n.s.
D6	0.63	−0.21	0.04	0.199	n.s.
D7	0.00	−0.25	−0.03	0.088	n.s.

D1: anterior chamber depth; D2: thickness of the lens; D3: length of the vitreous body; D4: axial length of the globe; D5, D6: radius of the cornea; D7 diameter of the cornea.

not find significant differences of the corneal radii and diameter, respectively. The lens of the diseased eye, however, was significantly thicker than that of the fellow eye. The length of the globe as well as the length of the vitreous body showing no significant differences, as a rule the increasing thickness of the lens induces a flattening out of the anterior chamber.

ACKNOWLEDGEMENT

The authors thank P. Bauer for his statistical advice.

REFERENCES

1. Lowe, R. F. Acute angle-closure glaucoma. The second eye: An analysis of 200 cases. Br. J. Ophthalmol. 46:641 (1962).
2. Ortlepp, J. Messungen des Hornhaut durchmessers und-krümmungsradius als Beitrag zur Klärung der speziellen Struktur des Glaukomauges. Albrecht v. Graefes Arch. Klin. Exp. Ophthal. 169:194 (1966).
3. Törnquist, R. Chamber depth in primary acute glaucoma. Br. J. Ophthalmol. 40: 421 (1956).

Author's address:
2. Univ.-Augenklinik
Alserstr. 4
A-1090 Wien
Austria

LIMBAL AND AXIAL CHAMBER DEPTH. VARIATIONS. DETECTION OF PRIMARY ANGLE-CLOSURE GLAUCOMA*

P.H. ALSBIRK

(Copenhagen, Denmark)

ABSTRACT

In an unselected population sample of Greenland Eskimos, limbal chamber depth (LCD) was estimated according to van Herick et al. (1969), and axial chamber depth (ACD) was measured optically using Haag Streit pachymetry. The material comprised 541 persons, including 505 right eyes, a priori without glaucoma. For comparison, LCD was estimated in 308 Danes over the age of 40.

A marked naso-temporal asymmetry in LCD was found while no corresponding gonioscopic asymmetry was observed. Significant age, sex, and ethnic variations were demonstrated. Primary angle-closure glaucoma (PACG) detection was a main goal. Eight new cases were found. The final prevalence was 2% in men and 10% in women above age 40, including 13 previously known cases. LCD as well as ACD estimations were important primary steps in finding gonioscopically narrow angles.

The study emphasized the value of LCD estimation as an integral part of slitlamp examination in all elderly persons.

*To be published in Acta Ophthalmologica.

304

E.L. Greve, W. Leydhecker & C. Raitta (eds.), Second European Glaucoma Symposium, Helsinki 1984.
© *1985, Dr. W. Junk Publishers, Dordrecht. ISBN 978-94-010-8934-0*

VALUE OF ULTRASONOGRAPHIC BIOMETRY
IN CONGENITAL GLAUCOMA

AHTI TARKKANEN, RISTO UUSITALO and JERZY MIANOWICZ

(Helsinki, Finland/Warsaw, Poland)

ABSTRACT

We report the follow-up of the axial length measured by ultrasonographic biometry in 40 glaucomatous eyes of 24 children with congenital glaucoma. Whereas intraocular pressure measurements gave information on the situation at a given time, change in axial length gave information on a long-term course of the disease. Echographic measurements proved to be a supplement to the diagnosis and follow-up of children with congenital glaucoma. Axial length measurements made the indication for surgical intervention easier and helped to detect cases in which intraocular pressure was not satisfactorily regulated in spite of normal IOP values measured under general anaesthesia. Conclusions which derive from axial lengths for clinical assessment of the diagnosis are presented.

INTRODUCTION

Primary infantile glaucoma has a relative incidence of one in 10,000 births. Eighty per cent of cases are bilateral although significant asymmetry is frequently noticed between eyes involved. Males are affected in two-thirds of cases. This disease occurs in children up to two or three years of age. The diagnosis of primary infantile glaucoma is obvious in sufficiently advanced cases. It is interesting to remember that in 30% of cases it will present with a cloudy cornea at birth and in 80% of cases it will appear within first year. The diagnosis is based on clinical symptoms and intraocular pressure (IOP). The following symptoms are typical for infantile glaucoma which may already be noticed by the mother of the child: photophobia, epiphora and blepharospasm. The ophthalmologists will notice a corneal edema and usually at least some kind of asymmetry between two eyes, ruptures in Descemet's membrane, cupping of optic nerve and of course the basis for the diagnosis, elevated intraocular pressure.

In borderline cases the diagnosis of congenital glaucoma may be very difficult. Schiotz tonometry is very unreliable in children. We used hand-held applanation tonometres which are better although they have not been

305

E.L. Greve, W. Leydhecker & C. Raitta (eds.), Second European Glaucoma Symposium, Helsinki 1984.
© *1985, Dr. W. Junk Publishers, Dordrecht. ISBN 978-94-010-8934-0*

calibrated for infants' large and edematous corneas. When we suspect that the child has glaucoma he needs to be examined under general anaesthesia, which might affect IOP at the time of measurement. Daily tension curves are not obtained and visual fields cannot be examined. Only ophthalmoscopy provides us with reliable information of the elevated IOP as seen by cupping of the optic nerve. There is certainly need for additional parameters in congenital glaucoma cases. As such we have been using axial length measurements done by ultrasonography (1,2,4,6).

PATIENTS AND METHODS

We have studied 40 glaucomatous eyes of 24 children with congenital glaucoma. The patients were divided into two groups: those aged from 0.5 to 2 years (primary infantile glaucoma group) and those aged from 4 to 9 years (juvenile glaucoma group). As controls in the first group (Table 1) 20 eyes of 10 patients with non-glaucomatous megalocornea of the same age and three non-glaucomatous fellow eyes of the children in the glaucoma series were used. In juvenile glaucoma group (Table 2) the controls consisted of 5 fellow eyes of unilateral glaucoma patients. Method A ultrasonographic biometry was performed to all eyes at the time of examination. Anterior-posterior axis was measured either by using Lasertek equipment or STORZ Alpha 20/20 with soft probe. Lasertek has an echograph which is coupled to a polaroid camera and measurements were done exactly as described earlier (6). Storz Alpha has advanced microtechnology and inbuilt computer. It also has an audible axial alignment to recognize signals from cornea, from anterior and posterior capsule of the lens and from retina. Actually every measurement done by Storz Alpha is already a mean of 480 individual measurements done by computer.

Table 1. Echometry in normal and gluacomatous eyes in patients aged 0.5 to 2 years

Echometry (mm)	Normal eyes Mean ± SE	Glaucomatous Mean ± SE
N	23	27
AC	3.5 ± 0.1	4.0 ± 0.1
Lens	3.4 ± 0.2	3.4 ± 0.1
Vitr.	13.9 ± 0.1	15.2 ± 0.3
Ax.	21.0 ± 0.2	23.8 ± 0.3

Table 2. Echometry in normal and glaucomatous eyes in patients age 4 to 9 years

Echometry (mm)	Normal eyes Mean ± SE	Glaucomatous Mean ± SE
N	5	13
AC	4.1 ± 0.2	4.3 ± 0.1
Lens	3.1 ± 0.2	3.5 ± 0.1
Vitr.	15.5 ± 0.4	17.2 ± 0.4
Ax.	23.0 ± 0.5	25.7 ± 0.4

Echometry was carried out before surgery (trabeculectomy) and in the follow-up after the surgery 4 to 6 weeks and then depending on the IOP and the possible change in axial length of glaucomatous eyes. The axial length/age tables of Sampaolesi and Caruso (5) was used in plotting the findings of borderline cases for the decision on therapy. Increase of the axial length following surgery was an indication for very frequent measurements of the IOP and possible reoperation. At the time of examination the patients were anaesthetized, IOP was taken by hand-held Perkins applanation tonometer, corneal diameter were measured with a ruler, refraction with sciascope and the eyes were also studied with microscope and fundus with a direct and indirect ophthalmoscopy.

RESULTS

Tables 1 and 2 show means values and standard deviations of the anterior chamber depth (AC), lens thickness (lens), the length of vitreous body (vitr.) and the axial length (Ax) obtained in two different age groups both in control eyes and in those with congenital glaucoma (primary infantile glaucoma in Table 1 and juvenile glaucoma in Table 2). The axial length values are significantly higher ($p < 0.001$) in glaucomatous eyes of both these two groups as compared to controls. The increase of axial length in glaucomatous eyes is seen to be due to enlargement of the post-equatorial readings. It is notable that the depth of anterior chamber and the lens thickness are about the same in glaucomatous and their age matched control eyes.

We have followed our glaucoma patients now up to two years with ultrasonographic biometry. Two typical cases are presented in Figs. 1 and 2. Axial length value is decreased after the successful surgery as seen in Fig. 1. However, after about half a year the axial length returned to original level, which was followed by normal growth rate of the eyeball when IOP was equal to a maximum of 15 mmHg. The reversal of cupping of optic nerve was also seen in these successful cases. In some cases the patients were subjected to more than one operation (Fig. 2). After the first operation the axial length of the left eye was seen to grow abnormally as compared to the axial length/age tables of Sampaolesi and Caruso (5) although the IOP was not high (18 mmHg). Increase in the cupping of optic nerve was not seen but decision was done to reoperate because of disproportionate growth rate of the left eye (Fig. 2). The successfulness of this decision was seen as the axial length decreased postoperatively and after follow-up of $1\frac{1}{2}$ years the reversible of cupping was also seen in this patient.

DISCUSSION

The diagnosis of congenital glaucoma is based on clinical symptoms and intraocular pressure. When IOP is above 25 mmHg the diagnosis is easily confirmed. If small infants have symptoms with borderline pressures between

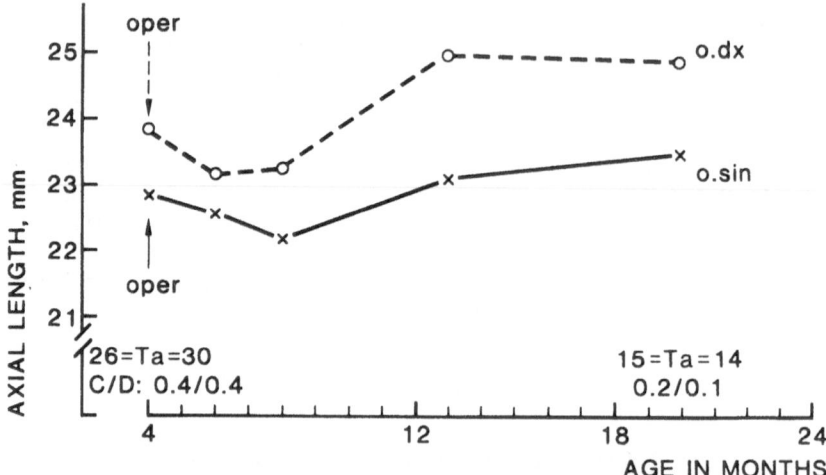

Fig. 1. Post-operative follow-up of axial length of a boy with primary infantile glaucoma. Diagnosis was done at the age of 4 months and both eyes were operated (trabeculectomy). Intraocular pressure (Ta) and cupping of optic nerve (C/D) are also given at the time of operation and after follow-up of 1.5 years.

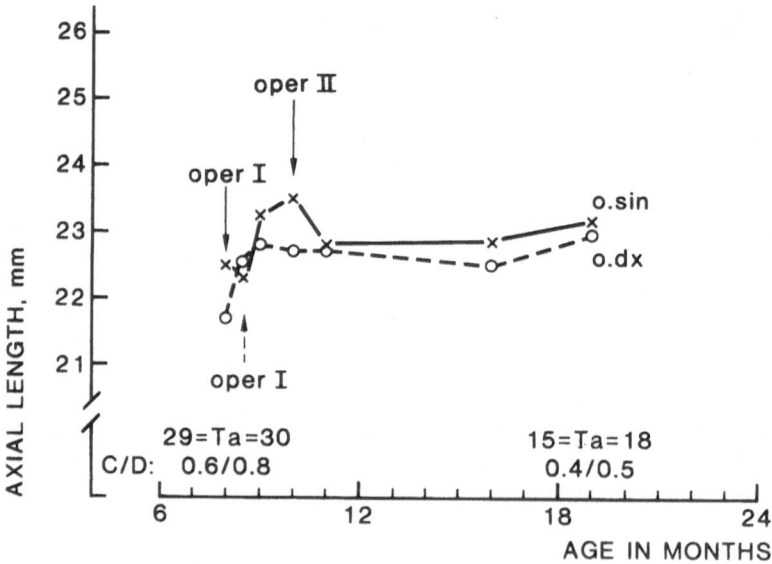

Fig. 2. Post-operative follow-up of axial length of a girl with primary infantile glaucoma. Same parameters are given as in Fig. 1. Diagnosis and operation was done at the age of 8 months. Postoperatively axial length of the left eye increased although IOP was not high (18 mmHg). A second operation was performed which resulted in stabilization of its axial length.

308

15 to 20 mmHg the diagnosis is usually very difficult and comes with the follow-up of the case with cupping of optic nerve. As the diagnosis is obvious only in advanced cases with high IOP and corneal edema, every additional parameter in these rare cases is most valuable. It should be also remembered that IOP by applanation is never measured more than once daily when general anaesthesia is needed to perform the measurement. The increased axial length in congenital glaucoma on the contrary reflects variations occurring during prolonged periods (day, months, or years) as a result of the increased mean IOP acting on a distensible eye. Thus it is quite evident that even one axial measurement might give more information of pathologically increased pressure than one applanation tonometry done under anaesthesia. To evaluate the meaning of axial length value it is necessary to know the corresponding values in the normal eye of that age group. The axial length/age tables done by several researchers can be used in plotting the finding of axial length similarly as comparing IOP values of glaucoma patients to normal values at that age group (3).

An important advantage of ultrasonographic biometry as compared to applanation tonometry when glaucoma is suspected is the use of advanced microtechnology and inbuilt computers in A-scan equipments. These enable audible axial alignment and by the use of soft probe make it possible to get reliable biometric values in infants' eyes even without using general anaesthesia. When we suspect that a child has glaucoma he needs to be examined under general anaesthesia for many reasons. It is, possible, however, that in the follow-up of these cases the need for examinations under anaesthesia is reduced when echographic values are possible to obtain by local anaesthesia.

Our results in ultrasonography biometry confirm earlier findings that it is a very valuable additional parameter in the diagnosis and especially in the post-operative follow-up of congenital glaucoma in infants under 3 years of age. Three most important parameters in the follow-up examinations are: 1. intraocular pressure measured by applanation tonometry, 2. axial length values measured by ultrasonographic biometry, and 3. cupping of optic nerve visualized by ophthalmoscopy.

REFERENCES

1. Buschmann, W. and Bluth, K. Regelmässige echographische Messung der Achsenlänge des Auges zur Kontrolle der Druckregulierung bei Hydrophthalmie. Klin. Mbl. Augenheilkd. 165:878 (1974).
2. Gernet, H. and Hollwich, F. Oculometrie des kindlichen Glaukoms. Ber. Zusammenkunft Dtsch. Ophthalmol. Ges. 69:341 (1969).
3. Goethals, M. and Missotten, L. Intraocular pressure in children up to five years of age. J. Pediatr. Ophthalmol. 20:49 (1983).
4. Sampaolesi, R. Ocular echometry in the diagnosis and follow-up of congenital glaucoma. Doc. Ophthalmol. Proc. Ser. 29:177 (1981).
5. Sampaolesi, R. and Caruso, R. Ocular echometry in the diagnosis of congenital glaucoma. Arch. Ophthalmol. 100:574 (1982).
6. Tarkkanen, A., Uusitalo, R. and Mianowicz, J. Ultrasonographic biometry in congenital glaucoma. Acta Ophthalmol. 61:618 (1983).

Authors' addresses:
Prof. A. Tarkkanen
Dr R. Uusitalo
Eye Clinic
University of Helsinki
Haartmaniakato HC
3F-00290 Helsinki 29
Finland

Dr J. Mianowicz
University Eye Clinic
Lindley AH
Warsaw, Poland

ASTIGMATISM AND AMBLYOPIA IN CONGENITAL GLAUCOMA

J. TSAMPARLAKIS, E. STAVRAKAS, T. KITSOS and A. AMARIOTAKIS

(Athens, Greece)

ABSTRACT

It is suggested that unexpected preventable visual loss among successfully treated children with C.G. is imposed by a series of amblyopia-inducing factors acting during the whole sensitive period.

We focused our attention on the high rate of astigmatism — mainly against the rule — which is very uncommon in the early formative years of healthy humans, and in the important bulk of knowledge on deprivation amblyopia accumulated since 1963, is known to be the cause of "meridional" amblyopia. Astigmatism probably plays a role in the establishment of low vision encountered so often in C.G.

If preserving vision is the ultimate goal, early regulation of I.O.P. is the first step. Intensive care to identify and minimize the complex of amblyopia inducing parameters must also be taken.

In the light of knowledge gained during the last decades on amblyopia, it is clear that the responsibility for this high risk group of patients must be shared by both the glaucoma and the orthoptic clinics.

INTRODUCTION

A high percentage of the successfully operated eyes suffering from Congenital Glaucoma (C.G.) never attain visual acuity consistent with the anatomical integrity of the affected eye. This is due to the ensuing amblyopia. Preventive measures are of paramount importance and must be applied correctly and in time. Of course the basic step for prevention is the control of I.O.P. at the earliest possible time.

In these patients, there are many factors inducing vision deprivation amblyopia in the early formative years, the "sensitive period". They stem either from the disease per se (corneal haze, Haabs striae, refractive errors) or its surgical treatment (patching of the operated eye, possible post-operative complications).

Amblyopia as a significant cause of poor vision in children with C.G. in spite of early control of I.O.P. is well known (1, 7, 8). In previous papers

311

E.L. Greve, W. Leydhecker & C. Raitta (eds.), Second European Glaucoma Symposium, Helsinki 1984.
© *1985, Dr. W. Junk Publishers, Dordrecht. ISBN 978-94-010-8934-0*

(9, 10, 11), we drew attention to the high incidence of a) astigmatism against the rule found in the operated eyes and b) amblyopia in unilateral cases.

In this paper a further attempt is made to show how astigmatism is a factor causing low vision in C.G. This is made in light of recent knowledge on visual deprivation amblyopia gained by experimental and clinical studies (3,6,12,13).

MATERIAL AND METHODS

We reviewed the files of successfully treated patients (goniotomies or filtering operations) suffering from C.G. and re-examined a non-selected series of 27 cases. There were 17 unilateral (15 simple C.G. and 2 Sturge-Weber syndrome) and 10 bilateral cases.

The criteria for the inclusion in this study were:

1) Age on examination at least 4 years old. Age ranged from 4 to 14 yrs. except one (20 yrs. old). Sufficient cooperation in examination.

2) Structures of the eye (cornea, retina, optic disc) consistent with potentially good visual acuity.

3) I.O.P. well within safe limits after one or more operations. Under regular follow-up in the glaucoma and orthoptic departments.

The standard examination included:

1) Visual acuity for far and near (Pigassou chart).

2) Retinoscopy under mydriasis — cycloplegia.

3) Keratometry (Javal keratometer). Attention was focused to an exact measurement of the refractive-astigmatic error.

4) Full orthoptic evaluation.

In all patients, measures against amblyopia were applied at the earliest possible time, including correction and oclusio therapy. Glasses and oclusio therapy were often not accepted by the patient or his parents in the unilateral cases, for obvious reasons.

Experience with V.A. screening in these children has shown the disparity between near and far V. acuities in many eyes, near vision always being the better, especially if high refractive effors and/or advanced corneal lesions characteristic of the disease are present (Fig. 1).

In this study only near vision was considered as the main index of functional amblyopia.

RESULTS

Distant V.A. as plotted against near V.A. is presented in Fig. 1. Cases attaining perfect acuity for near and far were rather few, including all with minimal corneal scarring and refractive error, which of course may signify a rather mild clinical expression of the disease.

Spherical and astigmatic refractive errors, state of binocular vision and visual acuity are present in Table 1 (unilateral cases) and Table 2 (bilateral

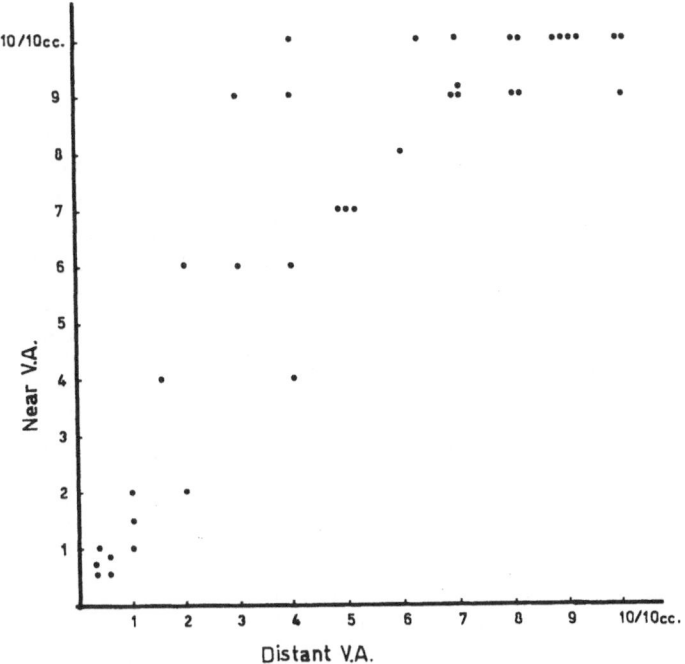

Fig. 1. Far and near V.A. in the 37 eyes examined.

cases). Note the high incidence of astigmatism against the rule – in about 50% and oblique astigmatism in 5 out of the 35 affected eyes.

The astigmatic component seems to be mainly corneal in origin, provided that both the degree and the axis – as found in retinoscopy – practically coincided with the ones found in keratometry. This is probably attributed to the peculiar corneoscleral distension in C.G. producing corneal toricity with a steeper horizontal meridian.

The impact on binocular vision seems interesting. In particular:

1. Only 7 out of 27 children has good V.A. and binocular vision within normal limits on both eyes (only 1 bilateral, 6 unilateral).

2. Bilateral cases developed strabismus but rarely amblyopia. In sharp contrast to the unilateral group in which 11 out of the 17 (64% of the affected eyes!) were amblyopic.

3. Binocular reflexes in bilateral group were poor, while in the unilateral group, if amblyopia was avoided, binocularity was rather well developed.

4. "Heavy eye phenomenon" was noticed in some of the unilateral amblyopic eyes.

DISCUSSION

There are three main conclusions from this study:

1. Disparity between far and near V.A. in many of the affected eyes.

313

Table 1. Refraction in unilateral cases

No.	Healthy eye			C.G.			Binoc. vision Status	V.A.
	Sph	Cyl	Axis°	Sph	Cyl	Axis°		
1)	−	−	−	−	− 4.50	30	Strabismus	Ambl.
2)	−	−	−	− 1.00	− 1.50	25	Orthoph.	Normal
3)	−	−	−	− 1.00	− 1.50	85	Strabismus	Ambl.
4)	−	−	−	− 1.50	− 2.00	45	Strabismus	Ambl.
5)	+ 2.50	−	−	+ 4.50	+ 1.75	180	Orthoph.	Normal
6)	−	− 1.00	15	−	− 8.00	160	Strabismus	Ambl.
7)	−	+ 5.50	5	−	− 1.75	15	Strabismus	Ambl.
8)	−	−	−	− 11.00	−	−	Strabismus	Ambl.
9)	− 2.00	− 1.50	90	− 1.50	− 1.00	15	Orthoph.	Normal
10)	−	−	−	− 5.00	− 3.50	45	Strabismus	Ambl.
11)	−	−	−	− 0.50	− 1.25	90	Orthoph.	Normal
12)	−	− 1.50	180	+ 1.50	+ 2.00	95	Strabismus	Ambl.
13)	−	−	−	−	− 1.00	10	Strabismus	Ambl.
14)	−	−	−	− 1.00	− 1.50	140	Straight eyed	Ambl.
15)	−	−	−	− 4.50	−	−	Orthoph.	Normal
16)	−	−	−	− 4.00	− 3.00	180	Strabismus	Ambl.
17)	+ 0.75	−	−	+ 0.75	−	−	Orthoph.	Normal

Astigmatism with   the rule: 3 eyes (Nos. 3,5,11).
Astigmatism against the rule: 8 eyes (Nos. 1,2,6,7,9,12,13,16).
Astigmatism oblique: 3 eyes (Nos. 4,10,14).

2. Astigmatism, usually against the rule to a considerable degree, is only exceptionally found in healthy eyes in comparable age group.

3. High incidence of amblyopia in unilateral, poor binocular vision but rarely amblyopia in bilateral cases.

Refraction by retinoscopy is practically impossible to perform on presentation of the patient with C.G. due to the corneal haze. Early detection of

Table 2. Refraction in bilateral cases.

No.	R.E.			L.E.			Binoc. Vision Status	V.A.
	Sph	Cyl	Axis°	Sph	Cyl	Axis°		
1)	− 1.50	− 3.50	110	+ 2.75	− 3.25	150	Strabismus	Normal
2)	− 10.50	−	−	− 4.00	− 1.00	70	Straight eyed	Ambl. RE
3)	− 2.00	− 1.00	140	− 7.00	− 1.50	180	Strabismus	Normal
4)	+ 3.00	− 5.00	5	− 7.00	− 2.00	155	Strabismus	Normal
5)	− 1.00	− 2.00	115	− 2.00	− 5.50	20	Strabismus	Ambl. LE
6)	− 6.00	−	−	− 6.00	− 1.00	130	Orthoph.	Normal
7)	− 3.00	− 3.00	180	− 2.50	− 2.50	180	Strabismus	Normal
8)	− 8.50	− 2.50	170	− 5.00	−	−	Strabismus	Normal
9)	−	− 3.00	90	− 4.00	− 1.50	90	Strabismus	Normal
10)	− 4.50	− 3.00	10	− 7.50	− 2.00	15	Strabismus	Normal

Astigmatism with   5 eyes (Nos. 1 RE, 2 LE, 5 RE, 9 RLE).
Astigmatism against the rule: 10 eyes (Nos. 1 LE, 3 LE, 4 RLE, 5 LE, 7 RLE, 8 RE,
    10 RLE).
Astigmatism oblique: 2 eyes (Nos. 3 RE, 6 LE).

visual defects is a basic step for the prevention of amblyopia, and this is easily overlooked if cosmetically obvious squint is not present (4). This well-known fact justifies refraction in early age as a reliable objective method, predicting amblyopia before V.A. can be assessed; this is highly necessary for the high risk group of infants with C.G.

Anisometropia during the sensitive period is statistically found to be a strong predisposing factor and the eye at risk is usually the more hypermetropic and/or astigmatic one. The role of defective accommodation is also well documented.

In accordance with modern views, the sensitive period of deprivation amblyopia begins with the second month of life and ends by the tenth year. Until the 24th month, susceptibility is very high; and coincides with the period when a) operation(s) are performed, b) tests to evaluate visual function are difficult to perform and are very often unreliable, and c) merely some days of stimulus deprivation suffice to establish amblyopia (or to regain normality under appropriate treatment).

On the development of refraction in early life of humans, we know that a high incidence of astigmatism is found in infants from birth to 1 year of age, and this is not so in children and adults (2). It is presumed that many individuals lose their astigmatism after the first year of life; there is a lack of evidence on when this occurs and whether infant astigmatism is due to developmental peculiarities of corneal or lens growth. We also know that astigmatism present in early age "with the rule" progresses to "against the rule" type in the elderly.

Persistence of this astigmatism during the sensitve period of early life has been supposed to lead, through selective neural development, to "meridional" or in a more complex form of "visual deprivation" amblyopia. What meridional (astigmatic) amblyopia means in clinical terms is not yet clear. We also do not know to what extent anisometropic amblyopia is aggravated in the presence of anisoastigmatism, as in our unilateral cases.

There is some evidence that astigmatism does not decline to adult levels until after the second year of life and that infantile astigmatism does not contribute to "meridional" amblyopia, the sensitive period of which is supposed to begin later (by the third year?) than that of the "form deprivation" amblyopia (5).

As a matter of fact, our sample of patients, among other well known amblyopia inducing factors, shows a high rate of astigmatism persisting during the presumed sensitive period, which must play some undetermined role in the visual disturbance.

The practical clinical usefulness of this study − at first glance suitable for a strabismological meeting − is to alert glaucoma specialists on the danger of finding later in infancy unexpected low vision despite early and successful control of I.O.P. And this is more so in the presumably relatively "benign" unilateral involvement.

REFERENCES

1. Clothier, C. M., Rice, N. S., Dobinson, P. and Wakefield, E. Amblyopia in congenital glaucoma.

2. Howland, H. C., Atkinson, J., Braddick, O. and French, J. Infant astigmatism measured by photorefraction. Science 202:331–332 (1978).
3. Ikeda, H. and Wright, M. J. Amblyopia due to incipropriate stimulation of the sustaired pathway during development. Br. J. Ophthalmol. 58:165–175 (1974).
4. Ingram, R. M. The possibility of preventing amblyopia. Lancet 585–587 (1980).
5. Mohindra, I., Held, R., Gwiazda, J. and Brill, S. Astigmatism in infants. Science 202 (1978).
6. Noorden, Von, G. Experimental amblyopia in monkeys. Further behavioral observations and clinical correlations. Invest. Ophthalmol. 12:721 (1973).
7. Rice, N. S. C. Management of infantile glaucoma. Br. J. Ophthalmol. 56:294 (1972).
8. Richardson, K. T., Ferguson, W. J. and Shaffer, R. N. Long-term functional results in infantile glaucoma. Trans. Am. Acad. Ophthalmol. Otolaryng. 71:883–837.
9. Tsamparlakis, J., Scouras, J., Gregoratos, N. et Kallipolitis, P. Le problème du strabisme dans le cadre du traitement du glaucome infantile. Bull. et Mém. S.F.O. Masson et Cie ed. p. 115, 1976.
10. Tsamparlakis, J., Alexakis, J. and Stavropoulos, A. Visual development in successfully treated cases of congenital glaucoma. Child Care, Health Devel. 5:431–438 (1979).
11. Tsamparlakis, J., Kallipolitis, P., Stavrakas, E. and Kitsos, T. Strabismus and amblyopia associated with congenital glaucoma. Strabismus. Proceeding of the Intern. Symp. C.E.S.S.D., Florence, 1982, p. 409.
12. Vaegan and Taylor, D. Critical period for deprivation amblyopia in children. Trans. Ophthalmol. Soc. U.K. 99:432, 1979.
13. Wiesel, T. N. and Hubel, D. H. Effects of visual deprivation on morphology and physiology of cells in the cat's L.G.B. J. Neurophys. 26:978 (1963).

Author's address:
Dr A. Amariotakis
Ophthalmiatrion Eye Hospital
Athens, Greece

316

HEREDITARY JUVENILE GLAUCOMA

OLAVI VALLE and TERO KIVELÄ
(Kotka, Finland)

ABSTRACT

A Finnish family is presented in which a mother and six of her eight children and one grandchild have juvenile glaucoma. The inheritance appears to be autosomally dominant with complete penetrance. The symptoms appeared at the age of 11 to 23 years with visual disturbances, coloured rings or headache. The initial IOP ranged between 36 to 81 mm Hg. The appearance of the chamber angle was characteristically anomalous. A fistulating operation was done at least once in each affected eye. Postoperatively the IOP has remained normal without any medication in four cases and with anti-glaucoma therapy in three patients. The prognosis of patients with juvenile glaucoma is good provided the diagnosis and a fistulating operation is made early enough when the visual fields are still intact.

INTRODUCTION

Juvenile glaucoma is a type of primary glaucoma occurring in children over three years of age and young adults up to 30 years of age. The age of three differentiates juvenile from infantile glaucoma, because after this age the eye no longer expands in response to elevated intraocular pressure (1, 2).

Most patients with juvenile glaucoma have an inborn predisposition to the disease and many of them also have other congenital anomalies, either in the eyes of elsewhere. The gonioscope appearance is characteristic with a high insertion of the iris root which forms a scalloped line in an open chamber angle (2). The course of the disease is usually similar to chronic open angle glaucoma (1,3).

Very often juvenile glaucoma is hereditary. Among the familial cases the most common type of inheritance is autosomal dominant (3,4,5), but recessive inheritance has also been reported (6).

Since glaucoma in this age group is rare and the subjective symptoms are not always clear cut, the diagnosis of juvenile glaucoma may be missed and the disease then progresses leading to severe visual field defects. An early diagnosis is important, as only an early operation to lower intraocular pressure can prevent the loss of visual fields (1).

E.L. Greve, W. Leydhecker & C. Raitta (eds.), Second European Glaucoma Symposium, Helsinki 1984.
© *1985, Dr. W. Junk Publishers, Dordrecht. ISBN 978-94-010-8934-0*

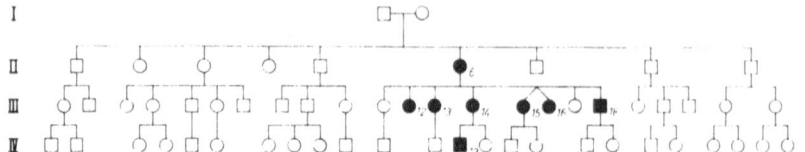

Fig. 1. Pedigree of the family studied.

● ■ = Glaucoma juvenile (bilateral)

○ □ = Healthy

CASE REPORTS

A Finnish family is described in which a mother and six of her eight children have juvenile glaucoma. An additional case of incipient juvenile glaucoma in an eight-year-old boy has been detected in her grandchildren (Fig. 1). To our knowledge, there are no consanquineous marriages in this family.

The gonioscopic picture in all affected was characteristically similar: an open chamber angle with a high insertion of the iris root near Schwalbe's line, partly hiding the trabecular meshwork. In addition to the members described, all other siblings and most of their offspring have been examined for juvenile glaucoma and found to be healthy. To the best of our knowledge, the first generation (Fig. 1) has not been affected with juvenile glaucoma. Detailed case reports of the affected family members are presented in Table 1.

DISCUSSION

The symptoms of juvenile glaucoma usually appear at the time of puberty (3). In the present family they were typically noticed at the age of 11 to 13 years simultaneously in both eyes. The initial intraocular pressures were high, on an average 50 to 60 mm Hg in both eyes (range: 36 to 81 mm Hg). The subjective symptoms were visual disturbances, halos around lights or headache, as has been reported previously (7). The gonioscopic appearance in all affected was similarly anomalous and typical of juvenile glaucoma (2, 5).

Juvenile glaucoma is often hereditary. There are two earlier reports also from Finland (3,7). Autosomally dominant juvenile glaucoma has been described in eight members in three successive generations in a family which is not the same as the one presented here. Dominant inheritance has also been noticed in seven members in four consecutive generations by Razemon et al. (5) in France. Similarly, in the present family juvenile glaucoma seems to be linked to a dominant gene with complete penetrance. It is noticeable that at present the members of the fourth generation in our family are so young that it cannot be definitively concluded who has inherited the glaucoma gene.

The screening and the follow-up of new generations in families with hereditary juvenile glaucoma is important. A thorough ophthalmological examination which includes ophthalmoscopy, tonometry and gonioscopy is essential, at the latest, when the child reaches the age of ten.

Table 1. Clinical data, treatment and results of eight patients with hereditary juvenile glaucoma

Generation, Case No., Date of birth	Age (years) at onset of visual deterior.	Subjective symptoms	Initial IOP (mm Hg) RE/LE	Operative treatment	Gonioscopic appearance	Discs	Visual fields	Follow-up time (years)	Present treatment
II₆ 25 04 16	17	visual deter. colored rings pain in eyes	60/60	Iridencleisis BE ICCE RE-81 ICCE LE-82	anom.	margin. excav.	central + temporal remnants	50	Timolol Acetazolamide
III₁₂ 19 01 45	11	headache visual deter. exotropia LE	68/81	Cyclodialysis BE Trepan. Elliot BE Enucleation LE	anom.	margin. excav.	large defect in RE	26	Pilocarpin
III₁₃ 11 06 46	13	colored rings for 2 years	60/60	Cyclodialysis RE Trepan. Elliot BE Revision ×2LE	anom.	slight margin. excav.	small paracentr. defects	23	No treatment
III₁₄ 13 10 51	23	periodical visual disturb. visual deter.	70/70	Cyclocryocoag. LE Trabeculectomy ×2 RE, ×1 LE	anom.	margin. excav.	temporal remnants only	8	Pilocarpin Epinephrine Timolol Acetazolamide
III₁₅ 14 12 52	12	headache for 1 month	42/50	Periferal iridencleisis BE	anom.	slight excav.	normal	18	No treatment
III₁₆ 14 12 52	12	headache for 6 days	36/36	Periferal iridencleisis BE	anom.	normal	normal	18	No treatment
III₁₈ 26 07 58	12	colored rings	46/46	Trepan. limb. a.m. Walser BE	anom.	normal	normal	12	No treatment
IV₁₃ 04 10 74	8	–	22–29/22–33	–	anom.	normal	normal	6	No treatment

RE = right eye; LE = left eye; BE = both eyes.

319

The treatment is operative (1,2,3,7). In young children, goniotomy, goniopuncture (1) or trabeculotomy (2) is preferred, in older children and in adults a fistulating operation (1,3,7) such as iridencleisis, limbal trephination or trabeculectomy is recommended. The response to operation is good in over 50% of patients (1,2,3) and satisfactory in most of the other cases, allowing control of intraocular pressure with medication (2).

In the present family, all affected members underwent a fistulating operation at least once in both eyes. The follow-up time so far in on average 22 years (range 8 to 50 years).

Four of the patients do not need any medical therapy and three of them have normal intraocular pressures with postoperative medication. The visual field defects have not progressed after the operations. The prognosis of juvenile glaucoma patients is good, provided the diagnosis and a fistulating operation to lower intraocular pressure is made early enough when the visual fields are still intact.

REFERENCES

1. Scheie, H. G. Infantile and juvenile glaucoma. Trans. Am. Acad. Ophthalmol. Otol. 67:458–466 (1963).
2. Shields, M. B. Primary congenital glaucoma. In: Schields, M. B. (ed). A Study Guide for Glaucoma. 1st edn. Baltimore, Williams & Wilkins, 1982, pp. 197–209.
3. af Ursin, K. V. The fate of infantile and juvenile glaucoma patients (in Finnish with English summary). Duodecim 63:52–68 (1977).
4. Duke-Elder, S and Jay, B. Glaucoma and hypotony. In: Duke-Elder, S (ed.) System of Ophthalmology. London, Kimpton, 1969, XI:397.
5. Razemon, M. M. P., Capier, M. J. and Couter, P. Le glaucome juvénile hérédo-familial. Bull. Soc. Ophthalmol. Fr. 74:471–474 (1974).
6. Beiguelman, B. and Prado, D. Recessive juvenile glaucoma. J. Genet. Hum. 12: 53–54 (1963).
7. Werner, S. Zur Kenntnis des erblichen juvenilen Glaukoms. Acta Ophthalmol. 7:162–168 (1929).

Authors' address:
Olavi Valle, M.D.
Eye Dept.
Central Hospital of Kotka
48210 Kotka 21
Finland

CHRONIC OPEN-ANGLE GLAUCOMA WITH EXFOLIATION SYNDROME. LONG-TERM FUNCTIONAL PROGNOSIS OF TREATED AND REGULARLY FOLLOWED PATIENTS

P. DEMAILLY and D. GRUBER

(Paris, France)

ABSTRACT

The long-term prognosis of patients (35 eyes), with open angle glaucoma with exfoliation syndrome was studied, over a mean follow-up period of $7\frac{1}{2}$ years. The minimal follow-up was 4 years. Each eye was examined twice a year. The evolution of the visual field was quantified. The evolution characteristics were computerized. The respective evolution of the visual field in glaucoma with exfoliation syndrome and in glaucoma simplex were compared on matched group.

Analysis of the results showed that the severity of the campimetric evolution in glaucoma with exfoliation is related to age of onset: the younger the patient, the more severe the evolution. The evolution of the visual field of regularly treated and followed eyes with glaucoma with exfoliation syndrome is not worse than that of eyes with glaucoma simplex.

INTRODUCTION

The aim in treating chronic open angle glaucoma (OAG) is to avoid perimetric deficits or stop their progression, whatever method is used.

Its success implies that the glaucoma patient accepted the proposed treatment and the strain often imposed by medical treatment and regular life-long follow-up. Success also implies that the physician have rigorous and reproducible means of control, both perimetric and tonometric.

The perimetric follow-up of a patient with glaucoma can be quantitative and allow comparison from one examination to the next. This kind of follow-up can easily be done with Friedmann's quantitative perimetric analyser, which quantifies visual field loss by the notion of "visual capability" (VC) (2).

The visual capability of one of Friedmann's points is defined as the ratio of the value of the filter with which a point is seen (N) to that of the filter with which it should have been seeen according to the age (R): $VC = N + 2/R + 2$. Total visual capability (TVC) is thus compared as the sum of the VC of each of the 47 points on Friedmann's standard plaque. Its maximal value is therefore 47 for one eye.

E.L. Greve, W. Leydhecker & C. Raitta (eds.), Second European Glaucoma Symposium, Helsinki 1984.
© *1985, Dr. W. Junk Publishers, Dordrecht. ISBN 978-94-010-8934-0*

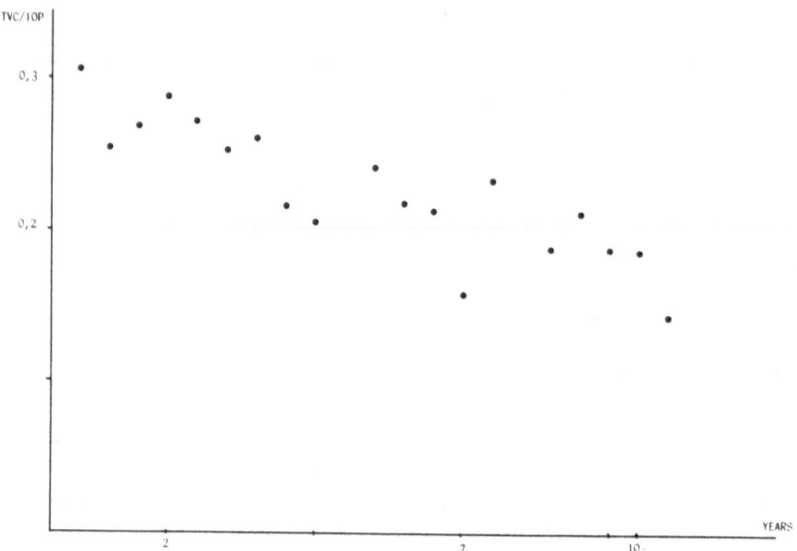

Fig. 1. Linear variation of TVC/IOP over time. Example of an eye followed for 10½ years. Mrs M., 60 years old; Sg = −1.00399848.

Even if the chronic glaucoma patient is correctly treated and regularly followed, there is a progressive and irreversible decrease of the visual field, easily conceived if one draws the curve of TVC over time for each glaucomatous eye. This curve is a straight line whose slope is almost always negative and with exception horizontal.

In a preceding work we have shown by statistical analysis that for a given eye the variations in intraocular pressure alone could not explain the worsening of the vision, and that these two parameters were only very weakly correlated: despite apparent control of the intraocular pressure, the visual field steadily worsened. Instead, it appeared that the worsening of TVC was a function of time. A linear relationship of TVC/IOP/time could therefore be drawn for each eye (Fig. 1): TVC/IOP = at + b, t being the follow-up interval for each eye; a and b being highly correlated, it was deemed possible to consider the slope a (evolution slope) as the main parameter giving the results of the various examination (1). The more negative the slope, the more severe the evolution. The aim of the treatment would therefore be to avoid a too steep evolution slope (a).

Using rigorous follow-up and Friedmann's quantitative analyser. we have decided to retrospectively study the evolution of the visual capability of patients with OAG with exfoliation syndrome, whose prognosis is reputedly severe and compare this evolution with that of a matched group of patients with OAG simplex.

MATERIAL

1) Thirty-five eyes were studied in 28 patients with OAG with exfoliation syndrome. There were 13 mean (17 eyes) and 15 women (18 eyes). All these

patients were seen at least twice a year. Mean initial age was 66.4 ± 7.2 years (52–79 years). At each examination, the best possible tonometric result was sought, using a pragmatic method associating medical and surgical procedures as required. In the more difficult cases, the quality of tonometric control was checked by a nycthemeral IOP variation study. All patients were followed for at least 4 years. Mean follow-up was $7\frac{1}{2}$ years (maximum $11\frac{1}{2}$ years).

(2) A control population of 35 eyes was selected among the patients with OAG simplex, similarly treated and followed for at least 4 years. They were matched with the study group according to age, sex, and eventual surgical treatment.

METHODS

At each examination, the following were recorded: visual acuity. IOP by aplanation, state of the cristal lens, central visual field (Friedmann) completed by a kinetic perimetry (Goldmann), state of the optic disc.

The cristal lens was subjectively placed in one of the five following classes: 0) clear lens; 1) lens opacity without influence on visual acuity; 2) lens opacity slightly decreasing visual acuity; 3) mild cataract; 4) clear-cut cataract with a significant decrease of close vision.

The state of the optic disc was appreciated by the cup/disc ratio subjectively measured by binocular biomicroscopy. We used the cup/disc surface ratio.

Central visual field was assessed by TVC measured with Friedmann's analyser. For each eye the data concerning the visual field were condensed into the slope of the TVC/IOP over time curve. To better approximate the clinical evolution, we used the severity gradient (= evolution slope −1). The first examination data were not taken into account for the determination of the severity gradient to avoid bias related to the first IOP measurement (with or without treatment).

All the information concerning these eyes seen every six months was coded and stocked in a Iris 80 computer for later analysis.

RESULTS

The mean severity gradient for the 35 eyes with OAG with exfoliation syndrome was −0.997149. There was a statistically significant relationship between the severity gradient and the initial subject age ($r = 0.515$; $n = 35$; $p < 0.01$). The younger the patient, the more severe the evolution (Fig. 2).

The other studied parameters did not have a significant relationship with the severity gradient: sex (e\ 0.281; $n = 35$ Wilcoxen test), state of the cristal lens ($H = 2.76$; $n = 31$; Kruskall wallis test); initial (before treatment) IOP ($r = 0.385$; $n = 18$); initial cup/disc ($r = 0.162$; $n = 28$) eventual associated diabetes ($\epsilon = 0.156$; $n = 30$; Mann Withney). Partial correlation analysis confirmed the relationship between severity gradient and age with

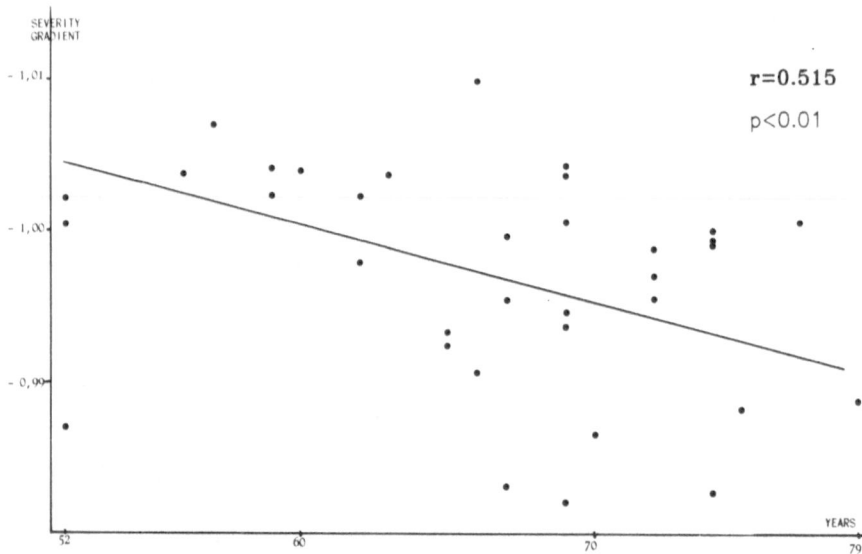

Fig. 2. Regression curve of the severity gradient, related to initial age, of the 35 eyes with OAG with exfoliation syndrome.

constant C/D (r = 0.568; n = 28), as well as the severity gradient–age relationship with constant initial IOP (r = 0.595; n = 18).

Aphakia did not significantly change the severity gradient. Aphakic patients did not have a better severity gradient, despite their having no cristal lens opacities (ϵ = 0.376; n = 35, Wilcoxon).

There was no significant difference between the severity gradient of the patients with OAG with or without exfoliation syndrome (ϵ = 0.448; n = 35; Wilcoxon paired test) (Fig. 3).

DISCUSSION

Only age of the different clinical parameters noted at the initial examination has any influence on the evolution of these open angle glaucomatous eyes: the younger the patient, the more severe the evolution and therefore the prognosis.

The age effect in open angle glaucoma with exfoliation syndrome could be explained by two different mechanisms: goniodysgenesis form the glaucoma itself, and pigment and exfoliation material accumulation in the angle due to the exfoliation syndrome.

Jerndal (4) has suggested that the goniodysgenesis appears earlier when severe, explaining the severity of early onset glaucoma. Also, as in pigmentary glaucoma (3), pigmentation decreases with age, limiting its hypertensive effect in older patients. We have no gonioscopic evidence supporting these theories in this study, however.

Our two patient populations, OAG with exfoliation syndrome and OAG simplex, appear perfectly comparable: Age, sex and eventual surgical

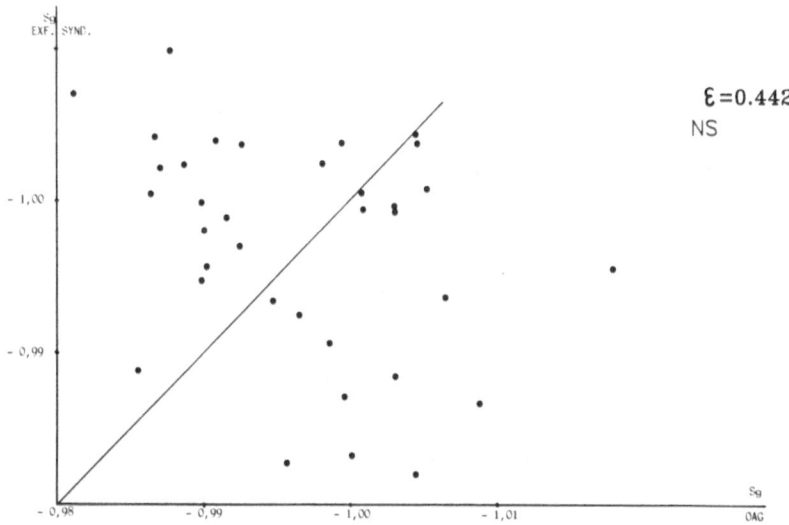

Fig. 3. Paired severity gradient: OAG with exfoliation syndrome/OAG simplex (n = 35). Homogeneous repartition of the 35 points around the bissectrix.

treatment were the matching parameters. Both the initial state of the cristal lens ($\chi_c = 2.97$; n = 35) and the initial cup/disc ($\epsilon = 1.36$; n = 9; Wilcoxon paired test) were similar between the two groups as well as the follow-up.

This goes against the classical notion of increased severity of OAG with exfoliation syndrome compared to OAG simplex. We think this apparent discrepancy with the common belief can be explained by identical regular and precise follow-up and treatment in both groups. It thus appears that a well treated and often followed OAG with exfoliation syndrome need not have a worse prognosis than a matched open angle glaucoma simplex.

REFERENCES

1. Demailly, Ph. and Papox, L. Long term study of visual capability in relation to intra-ocular pressure in chronic open angle glaucoma. Second international field symposium, Tubingen 1976, Vol. 14. Dr Junk Publishers, The Hague.
2. Demailly, Ph., Papoz, L. and Wencker-Brisset, B. L'analyseur périmétrique quantitatif de Friedmann. Son intérêt dans le dépistage des altérations périmétriques débutantes du glaucome chronique à angle ouvert. Arch. Ophtal, (Paris) 33:109–22 (1973).
3. Demailly, Ph., Plane, C., Limon, S. and Luton, J. P. Glaucome pigmentaire. Rapport annuel Bull. Soc. Ophtalmol. Fr., 1979, Numéro spécial, 225 pp.
4. Jerndal, T., Hansson, H. A. and Bill, A. Goniodysgenesis. A new perspective on glaucoma. Scriptor Copenhagen 1978, 211 pp.

Authors' address:
Dr D. Gruber
Hôpital Saint-Joseph
7 rue Pierre Larousse
75674 Paris Cédex 14
France

BARING OF THE OPTIC DISC CIRCUMLINEAR VESSELS IN OCULAR HYPERTENSION AND GLAUCOMA

M. ROLANDO, G.P. PESCE and G.A. CALABRIA

(Genoa, Italy)

ABSTRACT

The authors evaluate the incidence of baring of circumlinear vessels in optic disc of normal, hypertensive and glaucomatous eyes. Baring of circumlinear vessels was present in 10% of normal, in 39.3% of hypertensive and in 87.6% of glaucomatous eyes. Baring of circulinear vessels was present in 10% of normal, in 39.3% of hypertensive and in 87.6% of glaucomatous eyes. The observation of the condition of circumlinear vessels seem to be useful system for the early detection of optic nerve damage in the glaucoma suspect.

INTRODUCTION

The study of optic disc morphology is universally recognized as useful in the assessment of glaucoma (4, 5). Most of the traditional signs of optic disc deterioration (rim notching; C/D ratio; thinning of the rim; focal saucerization; overpass of the vessels) are present together with a visual field defect detectable by routine kinetic and static perimetry.

Quigley (6, 7) has shown that a loss of at least 30% of nerve fibers is necessary in glaucomatous eyes before initial perimetric defects could be shown. Motolko and Drance (2) have demonstrated that an increase of C/D ratio occurs before the appearance of a visual field defect in 31% of cases. Recently Herschler and Osher (1) have studied the rate of baring of optic disc circumlinear vessels in eyes with ocular hypertension.

As circumlinear vessels are identified the little vessels which come from the bottom of the disc cup and that bind to follow the rim of the physiological cup to aim towards the macula, overpassing the disc rim (Fig. 1). They are often a useful hint to define the edges of the disc cup. At the ophthalmoscopic observation these vessels are usually dimmed by a thin sheet of glia. During the process of baring, the vessels gradually lose their glial cover and contrast against the pinker neural tissue of the disc and appear outlined by a thin white border (Fig. 2). When the process is advanced their anatomical property of outlining the optic cup edge is lost.

327

E.L. Greve, W. Leydhecker & C. Raitta (eds.), Second European Glaucoma Symposium, Helsinki 1984.
© *1985, Dr. W. Junk Publishers, Dordrecht. ISBN 978-94-010-8934-0*

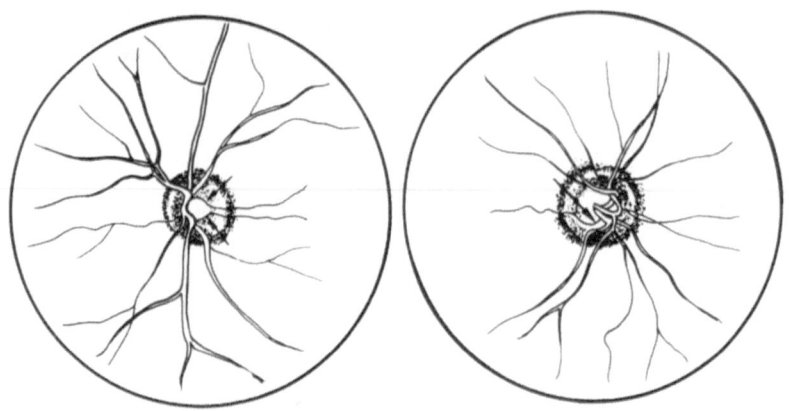

Fig. 1 *(left)*. Circumlinear vessl in a normal eye.
Fig. 2 *(right)*. Bared circumlinear vessel in a glaucomatous eye.

We have evaluated the rate of baring of circumlinear vessels in normal, hypertensive and glaucomatous eyes to assess the precocity and specificity of this sign in the assessment of optic disc damage in glaucoma.

MATERIALS AND METHODS

Three groups of patients between 20 and 90 years of age, showing a circumlinear vessel on the optic disc have been studied.

1. The first group included 46 normal subjects.
2. The second group included 40 subjects with ocular hypertension (intraocular pressure over the statistical average but without detectable visual field defects). Eleven did not receive any topical or general medication, the rest were under medical therapy because of the high degree of I.O.P. or because of the presence of risk factors such as anaemia, increased blood pressure, diabetes, high myopia, etc.
3. The third group included 38 subjects with primary open angle glaucoma and characteristic visual field defects.

For every subject, refraction, gonioscopy, ophthalmoscopy and Goldmann perimetry was performed. Optic disc examination was done in stereoscopy after pupil dilation at the slit-lamp with Goldmann or Hruby lens.

In every eye the presence and the condition of the circumlinear vessels was checked by two observers (M.R., G.P.P.) in order to decrease the influence of subjective assessment.

Each group was divided into three arbitrary classes of age (less than 40; between 40 and 60; over 60) to evaluate the correlation between age and the incidence of the baring of circumlinear vessels.

RESULTS

Group 1: The baring of the circumlinear vessels was present in 9 out of 90 eyes (10%) (Table 1A)

328

Table 1.

Circumlinear vessels	Age: < 40		Age: > 40 ⩽ 60		Age: > 60		Total	
	No. eyes	%	No. eyes	%	No. eyes	%	No. eyes	%
A. Normals (46 patients)								
Not bared	20	95.2	50	86.2	11	100	81	90
Bared	1	4.8	8	13.8	–	–	9	10
B. Ocular hypertension (40 patients)								
1. Not bared in patients without medical therapy	4	100	9	64.2	–	–	13	72.2
2. Bared in patients without medical therapy	–	–	5	35.8	–	–	5	27.8
3. Not bared in patients under medical therapy	5	50	25	58.2	5	62.5	35	57.4
4. Bared in patients under medical therapy	5	50	18	41.8	3	37.5	26	42.6
Total – groups 1 & 3 (not bared)	9	64.3	34	59.6	5	62.5	48	60.7
Total – groups 2 & 4 (bared)	5	35.7	23	40.4	3	37.5	31	39.3
C. Glaucoma (38 patients)								
Bared	11	84.6	17	100	36	83.7	64	87.6
Not bared	2	15.4	–	–	7	16.3	9	12.4

Group 2: The baring of circumlinear vessels was present in 31 out of 79 eyes (39.3%). In the eyes with ocular hypertension without any medical therapy (n = 18), the baring was present in 27.8% of the cases, while in the eyes with ocular hypertension under medical antiglaucomatous therapy (n = 61), the baring was present in 42.6% of the cases (Table 1B).

Group 3: The baring of the circumlinear vessels was present in 64 out of 73 (87.6%) glaucomatous eyes (Table 1C).

DISCUSSION

The assessment of the circumlinear vessels can sometimes be difficult for an untrained observer (8). It should be emphasized that in a high percentage of normal eyes (56%) the circumlinear vessels are absent (1). Stereoscopic examination is important to evaluate the entity of their glial cover on the optic disc. The baring of the circumlinear vessels in our subjects was also present without ocular hypertension or glaucoma; this is in good agreement with the data of Herschler and Osher (1) who report a 11.1% rate of baring in normal eyes. The same authors report the presence of baring of these vessels during neurologic or ischemic diseases involving the optic nerve.

We have not been able to correlate the presence of baring to the different groups of age.

Baring of the circumlinear vessels is more frequent in eyes with ocular hypertension than in normals. Particularly interesting is the finding that in our subjects with ocular hypertension and presence of baring, the first circumlinear vessel to be bared was the one in the inferior temporal sector of the optic disc. This agrees with the finding that the initial increase in glaucomatous cupping is often in the lower temporal sector of the disc.

The difference in baring incidence between the hypertensive eyes under antiglaucomatous therapy and without any therapy has to be considered. The need for therapy in those patients was a consequence of the presence of risk factors associated to the increase in I.O.P. The higher rate of baring of circumlinear vessels seems to demonstrate the real sensitivity of the disc to the increased intraocular pressure in these eyes.

The high percentage of baring of circumlinear vessels in the disc of glaucomatous eyes with visual field defect emphasizes the fact that the sign is the result of optic disc sufference and is linked to the phenomenon of glaucomatous cupping. In this group of patients the sign loses its forecasting characteristic since in this phase of the disease other more specific signs are present.

The observation of the circumlinear vessels seems to be an important examination method due to the peculiar position of the vessel as under lineators of physiological papillary cupping. Any change between the position of the vessel and the edge of the excavation would indicate an increase of cupping which has been demonstrated (2) to be an early sign of glaucomatous damage. The possibility of proving the baring allows us to identify, within confines of our results, a group of ocular hypertensive patients with a higher risk of visual field damage.

The loss of glial shading of this vessels indicates an initial sufference of the optic nerve and possibly a loss of nervous fibers not yet detectable by perimetry.

REFERENCES

1. Herschler, J. and Osher, R. H. Baring of the circumlinear vessel. An early sign of optic nerve damage. Arch. Ophthalmol. 98:865–869 (1980).
2. Motolko, M. and Drance, S. M. Features of the optic disc in preglaucomatous eyes. Arch. Ophthalmol. 99:1992–1994 (1981).
3. Osher, R. M. and Herschler, J. The significance of baring of the circumlinear vessel. Arch. Ophthalmol. 99:817–818 (1981).
4. Quigley, H. A. Miller, N. R. and George, T. Clinical evaluation of nerve fiber layer atrophy as an indicator of glaucomatous optic nerve damage. Arch. Ophthalmol. 98:1564–1571 (1980).
5. Quigley, H. A., Addicks, E. M. and Green, W. R. Optic nerve damage in human glaucoma. II–The site of injury and susceptibility to damage. Arch. Ophthalmol. 98:635–649 (1981).
6. Quigley, H. A. and Addicks, E. M. Quantitative studies of retinal nerve fiber layer defects. Arch. Ophthalmol. 100:807–814 (1982).
7. Quigley, H. A., Addicks, E. M. and Green, W. R. Optic nerve damage in human glaucoma. III–Quantitative of nerve fiber loss and visual field defect in glaucoma, ischemic neuropathy, papilledema, and toxic neuropathy. Arch. Ophthalmol. 100:135–146 (1982).
8. Sutton, G. E., Motolko, M. A. and Phelps, C. D. Baring of a circumlinear vessel in glaucoma. Arch. Ophthalmol. 101:739–744 (1983).

Authors' address:
University Eye Clinic
Viale Benedetto XV, 5
16132 Genoa
Italy

GLAUCOMATOUS ALTERATIONS OF THE OPTIC DISC IN HIGH MYOPIA

M. MIGLIOR, R. RATIGLIA, G. CAPITANI and S. MIGLIOR

(Milan, Italy)

ABSTRACT

The incidence of chronic glaucoma in high myopia is elevated. The myopic alterations of the optic disc disguise its typical glaucomatous changes.

The authors examine some cases of high myopia associated with chronic glaucoma and point out the early morphological glaucomatous changes of the optic disc. These alterations can confirm the diagnosis of glaucoma particularly in cases without elevated intraocular pressure.

INTRODUCTION

The rate of chronic glaucoma in high myopes is anything but negligible, being far more frequent than the total percentage of glaucoma in the general population. Furthermore, sensitivity to the provocation test with corticosteroids is far higher (at least 6 times) in myopes over 5 diopters than in the general population. This means that myopia represents a risk factor of glaucoma.

Considering that a diagnosis of chronic glaucoma rests on peculiar alterations in the optic disc and the visual field — in addition to depending on intraocular pressure (IOP) — a diagnosis becomes very difficult when glaucoma is associated with high myopia, also characterized, among other things, by serious lesions in both the optic disc and the visual field. In such cases morphological and functional alterations could overlap each other, thus hiding their origin and causing delays in diagnosing the glaucomatous disease either primarily or in the follow-up.

Of all the problems created by this association, the pathogenetic ones should be emphasized, connected with possible concomitant responsibility of ocular hypertension, owing to reduced scleral rigidity of the myopic eye, in the development of the posterior staphyloma.

Our study is designed to examine the various morphological and functional aspects of optic damage in both glaucoma and high myopia, with the purpose of proposing reliable criteria of clinical discrimination between the two diseases.

333

E.L. Greve, W. Leydhecker & C. Raitta (eds.), Second European Glaucoma Symposium, Helsinki 1984.
© *1985, Dr. W. Junk Publishers, Dordrecht. ISBN 978-94-010-8934-0*

PHYSIOPATHOLOGICAL ASPECTS OF THE OPTIC DISC

The optic disc may be examined and studied either by direct ophthalmoscopy, by using the slit-lamp and the Goldmann lens or constant-enlargement photography so as to measure the diameter of the papillary surface and that of the cup and to follow the biometrical and morphological values of the optic disc itself over time; further, greatly enlarged stereoscopic photographs can be used, in order to carry out planimetric or photogrammetric measurements.

Lesions at the optic nerve head are often indirectly demonstrated by a perimetrical examination.

Normal optic disc

A normal optic disc is pink, flat, clear-edged and slightly excavated in the centre.

The horizontal diameter in emmetropic subjects varies from 1.2 to 1.9 mm and is altered in ametropic subjects. Its surface varies from 1.2 to 3 mm^2.

The cup/disc ratio varies from 0.2 to 0.5 (in any case less than 0.7); this value increases in direct relation to the disc's size.

In the area of the excavation the distance between the retinal level and that of the lamina cribrosa is 0.7 mm on average.

Between the two eyes there is a certain symmetry in both the optic disc and the physiological excavation; the maximum physiological value accepted as a differential index for the cup's diameter between the two eyes is 1/5 of the papillary diameter.

The optic disc in high myopia

In high myopia there may be both exclusively papillary alterations and peripapillary ones. The optic disc may present an oval shape with vertical major axis, a bag-shaped physiological excavation with nasal supertraction and a nasal sickle of the choroid and the sclera, hiding the optic nerve.

Around the optic disc it is possible to identify a temporal scleral sickle or "myopic conus", a juxtapapillary staphyloma or the congenital peripapillary staphyloma, either isolated or associated with a tilted disc (tilted disc syndrome).

From a biometric point of view, an important fact in high myopia is the distance between the retinal level and that of the lamina cribrosa, which varies from 0.2 to 0.5 mm. This means that the evident glaucomatous excavation in myopes is about half as deep as that normally observed in glaucomatous emmetropic subjects, as explained below.

The optic disc in chronic glaucoma

A morphological examination of a glaucomatous emmetropic subject's optic disc reveals a rather deep excavation which tends to become undermined, with a shift in the emergence of retinal vessels towards the nasal sector of the optic disc itself; the excavation is oval-shaped on the surface, due to its supporting the prelaminar vessels. This ovalization begins on the level of the vertical or oblique diameter, both upwards and downwards (90°–270°; 45°–225°; 135°–215°). Furthermore, a localized reduction in the peripheral ring, a nick in the edge of the physiological excavation and a particular angle of the smallest vessels – which can be especially noticed in a normally coloured territory – are observable. The observation of microhaemorrages along the peripheral ring, especially at 12 and 6, is less frequent.

The glaucomatous optic disc turns pale after the establishment of the excavation.

From a biometric point of view, a cup/disc ratio higher than 0.7 can be observed, with a differential value of the diameter of the papillary excavation between the two eyes with 1/5 larger papillary diameter.

OPTIC DAMAGE IN MYOPIA-GLAUCOMA ASSOCIATION

In the cases of glaucoma–high myopia association, optic damage may show particular morphological aspects which may often result in complicated perimetrical findings.

Morphological reports

Papillary damage due to the emergence of chronic hypertension in a myopic eye (which is the most frequent occurrence in the association we are dealing with, as shown below in the cases we observed) develops very slowly. It does not always show the characteristics of clinical chronic glaucoma.

Reduced scleral activity, peculiar to myopic eyes, can compensate for some time the effects of a difficult outflow on the level of ocular pressure, thus delaying the establishment of optic lesions.

The two most typical aspects of glaucomatous optic damage (excavation and pallor) tend, in such cases, to fade so that they can be confused with pre-existent myopic lesions. Firstly, the depth and extension of the excavation – whose edge is not always easily defined – appear to be very limited, even in advanced glaucoma. The papillary rim, concentric with the excavation, which in glaucoma is typically pink, in the case of concomitant high myopia is diffusely pale.

On the other hand the pallor of the cup, which is usually the concomitant of glaucoma, under these circumstances is often mixed up with decolourization phenomena involving the whole optic disc and, moreover, the surrounding area.

The typical indicator of both papillary edge and papillary excavation degree, represented in glaucoma by vessel inflections, is often missing, too, the vascularization in a myopic optic disc being very rarefied.

Perimetrical reports

The perimetrical alterations which may lead the observer to wrong considerations about their dubious pathogenesis (either myopic or glaucomatous) are primarily placed in the central area and in the pericentral sectors of the visual field.

It is on this level that absolute or relative scotomas can be identified, due to atrophic macular alterations of myopic origin, more or less related to physiological scotoma (often enlarged). In the same way, peripapillary staphylomatous areas too, either localized (tilted disc) or widespread, may originate perimetrical defects in pericentral sectors with the enlargement of the physiological scotoma; for this very reason these staphylomatous areas are to be assessed by perimetrical examination by adding lenses for correcting possible relative scotomas.

On the other hand, the islands of absolute or relative scotomas of the Bjerrum areas — typical of the eye affected by glaucoma — are localized in the paracentral sectors of the visual field. Furthermore, at developed stages, these scotomatous areas tend to join the "blind spot" and reach it at last to form the bow-shaped scotoma.

Personal observations

The cases of high myopia and glaucoma observed by us during the last 5 years, concern 17 subjects aged between 18 and 85, totalling 31 eyes.

Myopia was higher than 15 diopters in all but one case.

The types of glaucoma were distributed as follows: primary open angle glaucoma in 28 eyes (3 of which affected by "exfoliation syndrome" and 8 affected by pigmentary glaucoma), hyatrogenic open angle glaucoma in 2 eyes; malformative glaucoma in 1 eye. Eight were thought to have low-tension glaucoma.

In an indeterminable number of cases, despite the absence of a clinical history for glaucoma, it was reasonable to suspect, especially on the basis of perimetrical reports, a very developed stage of glaucomatous disease.

Diagnostic criteria

A correct clinical interpretation of perimetric data is obtained by comparing them with the optic disc's morphological and biometric data.

If the optic disc is normally coloured and shows neither alterations in the optic fibres nor glaucomatous alterations, the perimetrical alterations which may be present must be examined with a critical eye. On the contrary, if alterations are present in the optic disc, perimetrical alterations have to be scanned attentively.

Papillary alterations precede perimetrical alterations. Nevertheless, the progression of the optic disc's excavation not followed by perimetrical changes can sometimes be observed.

The green-light observation of the optic can also give indications about the lesions in the bottom, which must necessarily correspond with perimetrical alterations.

In the myopic eye all these semeiological elements are more difficult to emphasize, so the search for perimetrical lesions must be more accurate.

The progression of perimetrical alterations — despite the normalization of ocular tension — poses large diagnostic problems as far as the normal eye is concerned, and even more problems as far as the myopic eye is concerned.

The occurrence may be correlated with:
- inadequate control of ocular tension which may result, even though within physiological limits, in lesions for the optic fibres (low critical IOP);
- pathological IOP variations, especially at night-time, which have been ignored for a long time;
- variations in the optic disc's arterial flow;
- variations of scleral rigidity inadequately taken into account, especially on the occasion of ocular tonmetry by using the Schiotz.

These diagnostic problems will inevitably tend to increase for obvious reasons in the case of high myopia associated with low-tension glaucoma.

CONCLUSION

The cases studied by us illustrate the diagnostic problems of chronic glaucoma associated with high myopia.

In these cases neither morphological changes in the optic disc nor perimetric defects make an early diagnosis of the glaucomatous disease possible, especially because of the high frequency of "low" tension that we have found in about 1/3 of the cases observed.

A correct diagnosis of the glaucomatous disease must be confirmed by the provocation test and by a pathological outflow index.

Finally, a different progression of the visual field's defects in the two eyes, without important morphological alterations of the optic disc, could confirm the glaucomatous disease.

REFERENCES

1. Airaksinen, P. J., Mustonen, E. and Alanko, H. I. Optic disk hemorrhages. Analysis of stereophotographs and clinical data of 112 patients. Arch. Ophthalmol. 99:1795 (1981).
2. Becker-Shaffer. Diagnosis and Therapy of the Glaucomas. Mosby, St. Louis, 1983.
3. Bengston, B. The variation and covariation of cup and disk diameter. Acta Ophthalmol. 59:1 (1981).
4. Bengston, B., Holmin, C. and Alanko, H. J. Disk haemorrage and glaucoma. Acta Ophthalmol. 54:804 (1976).
5. Betz, P., Camps, F., Collignon-Brach, J. and Weekers, R. Photographie stereoscopique photogrammetrie de l'excavation de la papille. J. Fr. Ophtalmol. 4:193 (1981).
6. Betz, P., Camps, F., Collignon-Brach, J., Lavernge, G. and Weekers, R. Biometric study of the disk-cup in open-angle glaucoma. Gr. Arch. Clin. Exp. Ophtalmol. 218:70 (1982).
7. Gloster, J. Vertical ovalness of glaucomatous cupping. Br. J. Ophthalmol. 59:721 (1975).
8. Heilmann and Richardson. Glaucoma. Conception of a Disease. G. Thieme Publ., (1978.
9. Kirsch, R. E. and Anderson, D. R. Clinical recognition of the glaucomatous cupping. Am. J. Ophthalmol. 75:442 (1973).

Authors' address:
Istituto di Clinica oculistica
i Dell Universita' di Milano
Milan, Italy

ORBITAL HAEMODYNAMICS AND AQUEOUS HUMOUR DYNAMICS IN DISEASES OF THE CAROTID-CAVERNOUS AND VERTEBRO-BASILAR SYSTEMS

MARGIT VARGA, PIROSKA FOLLMANN, I. GÁBRIEL, L. REMENÁR
and MÁRTA HAJDA

(Budapest, Hungary)

ABSTRACT

Orbital arterial and venous circulation and aqueous humour dynamics were studied in 23 cases of diseases of the carotid-cavernous and vertebro-basilar systems and in intermittent exophthalmos. Observations are based on different kinds of cerebral angiographies, ophthalmodynamography, ophthalmodynamometry, measurement of intraocular pressure and tonography. The effect of the alterations of the orbital haemodynamics was studied on the intraocular pressure and the outflow of the aqueous humour.

INTRODUCTION

Ophthalmic artery pressure and orbital arterial pulse volume have been investigated by means of ophthalmodynamometry and ophthalmodynamography in intracranial vessel malformations, especially in carotid-cavernous fistula (2, 5, 6, 8, 9, 10, 12, 17, 18, 21, 23). Elevated intraocular pressure has been known to occur in patients with carotid-cavernous fistula since the last century (13), which has been attributed to elevated episcleral venous pressure (19, 20). The outflow resistance was found increased, which was reported to return to normal after the successful surgical intervention against the fistula (8, 15). Rarely was angle closure observed in these cases (7, 11). On the basis of pathological observations, Sugar (16) believed that in later stages of the disease the disturbance of the aqueous humour dynamics was aggravated by the hypoxia of the eye tissues. This latter pressure elevation appears in the clinical picture of neovascular glaucoma (22). Intraocular pressure elevation was described to occur in cases with extraocular venous hypertension (13). Also, a decrease in the originally elevated intraocular pressure after the relief of the venous hypertension was experienced (1).

The aim of the present study was to investigate the orbital arterial and venous circulation and the aqueous humour dynamics in various forms of intracranial vessel malformations.

339

E.L. Greve, W. Leydhecker & C. Raitta (eds.), Second European Glaucoma Symposium, Helsinki 1984.
© *1985, Dr. W. Junk Publishers, Dordrecht. ISBN 978-94-010-8934-0*

Table 1. Composition of material

Diagnosis		Patient no.
1. Carotid-cavernous fistula	traumatic	6
	spontaneous	6
2. Orbital cavernous haemangioma	without communication into	2
	with the cavernous sinus	4
3. Intracranial arteriovenous angioma	in the territory of the carotids	3
	in the territory of the vertebrobasilar system	2
Total		23

MATERIALS AND METHODS

The composition of the material is summarized in Table 1. The diagnosis was based on skull and orbital radiology, carotid and vertebral angiography, in some cases on orbital phlebography.

The ophthalmodynamography (ODG) was performed in a reclined position with the modified pressure chamber (4). The mean and diastolic ophthalmic artery pressure compared with the brachial blood pressure, the orbital pulse volume and pulse shape, the pulse wave propagation velocity in the internal carotids were evaluated. The ophthalmodynamometry (ODM) was performed using Bailliart's ophthalmodynamometer in a seated position. The results were evaluated according to Weigelin and Lobstein (21). The intraocular pressure was measured with the Goldmann applanation tonometer in a seated position. The scleral rigidity coefficient was determined with a Schwarzer electric tonometer using two plunger weights. Leydhecker's tonographic test was performed following the rigidity determination.

Gonioscopy revealed open chamber angles with no vessel neoformations in the angle.

RESULTS

1. *Carotid-cavernous fistula*

In the traumatic cases of young persons the amplitudes of the orbital oscillations in the course of ODG were the highest among the patients studied. Usually the so-called "post-diastolic spindle" (6, 18) commenced from the diastolic ophthalmic pressure and the amplitudes of the ophthalmodynamogram remained high until the end of the curve. The ophthalmic artery pressure was decreased both with ODM and ODG. Otherwise the parameters of the ophthalmodynamogram were normal. The scleral rigidity coefficient slighly decreased in the diseased eyes, the amplitude of the intraocular pressure pulse waves increased (Fig. 1a, b). Sometimes the pressure pulse waves resembled the arterial pulsations. The outflow resistance increased in all of the cases. Surprisingly, we could not find intraocular pressure elevation in any of these patients.

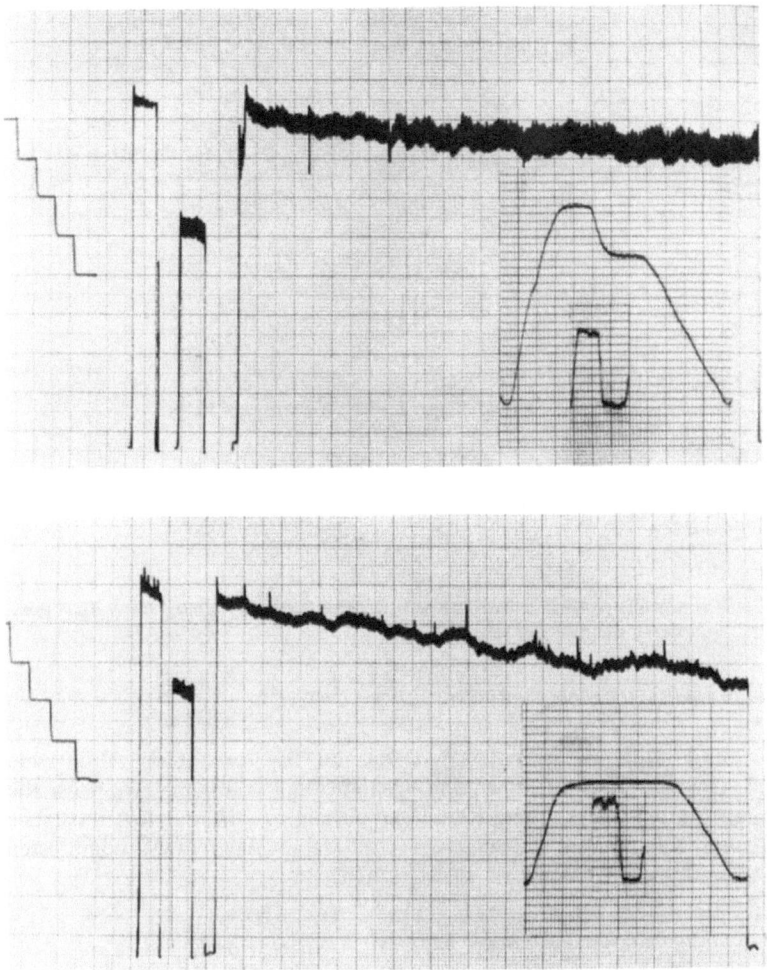

Fig. 1a. Traumatic carotid-cavernous fistula. Diseased eye. Rigidity determination with the 5.5 g and 10.0 g plunger weights. Leydhecker's tonographic test with the 5.5 g plunger weight. Insert: ocular pressure pulse wave with 0.2 SR calibration.
Fig. 1b. Traumatic carotid-cavernous fistula. Healthy eye. Rigidity determination with the 5.5 g and 10.0 g plunger weights. Leydhecker's tonographic test with the 5.5 g plunger weight. Insert: ocular pressure pulse wave with 0.2 SR calibration.

In the spontaneous cases, mainly elderly women in our material, the arterial circulatory disturbance was less expressed than in the traumatic cases. The "post-diastolic spindle" commenced at significantly lower chamber pressures than the diastolic ophthalmic artery pressure (Fig. 2). The ophthalmic artery pressure measured with ODG and ODM was normal or only slightly decreased. The scleral rigidity coefficient decreased, the amplitude of the pressure pulse waves and the outflow resistance increased in the diseased eyes. The intra-ocular pressure was moderately elevated in these eyes (25 to 35 mmHg).

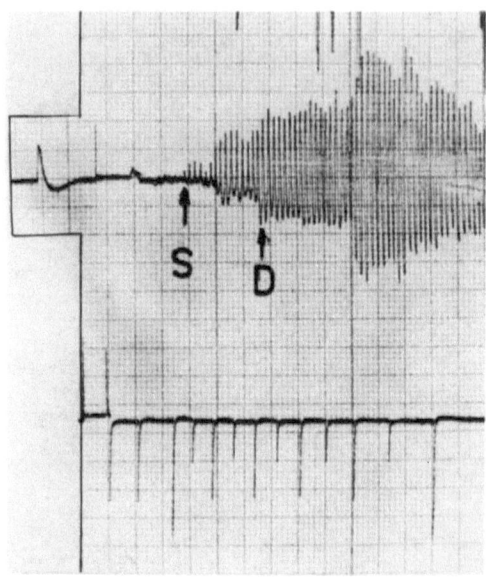

Fig. 2. Spontaneous carotid-cavernous fistula. Ophthalmodynamogram with "post-diastolic" spindle on the diseased side.

2. Orbital cavernous haemangioma

In circumscript cases the ODM, ODG and the tonometric values were normal. On the contrary, when the haemangioma communicated with the cavernous sinus, i.e. in intermittent exophthalmos, the outflow resistance increased in the diseased eye when the ipsilateral jugular vein was compressed (Figs. 3a and 3b).

3. Intracranial arteriovenous angioma

The intracranial arteriovenous haemangioma situated in the territory of the carotids as well as in the territory of the vertebro-basilar system influenced the investigated parameters. A distinct "post-diastolic spindle" was observed in the former cases when the angioma communicated with the cavernous sinus (Fig. 4), and a "post-diastolic spindle" could be guessed in the latter cases. The values of the ophthalmic artery pressure were divergent. The scleral rigidity coefficient slightly decreased in the diseased eye with angiomas in the territory of the carotids and remained unchanged with angiomas in the territory of the vertebro-basilar system. The outflow resistance in the diseased eyes increased in both instances (Figs. 5a, b). The amplitudes of the pressure pulse waves were higher in the discussed eyes than in the healthy ones in the case of angiomas in the territory of the carotids, while they were equal on both sides with the angiomas of the vertebro-basilar system.

342

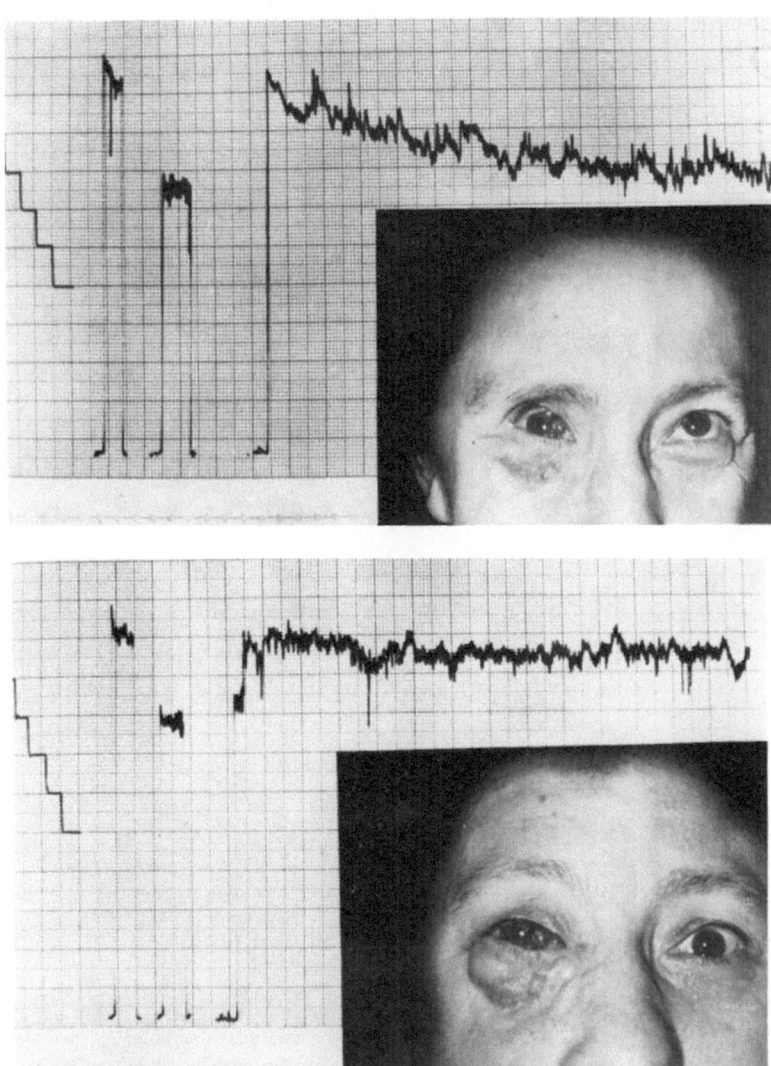

Fig. 3a. Intermittent exophthalmos. Leydhecker's tonographic test with the 5.5 g plunger weight in the diseased eye and photograph of the patient's eye at rest.
Fig. 3b. Intermittent exophthalmos. Leydhecker's tonographic test with the 5.5 g plunger weight in the diseased eye and photograph of the patient's eye during ipsilateral jugular compression.

DISCUSSION

There are no data in the literature on the comparison of ODM and ODG with the outcome of intraocular pressure measurements and tonography in the cases studied.

343

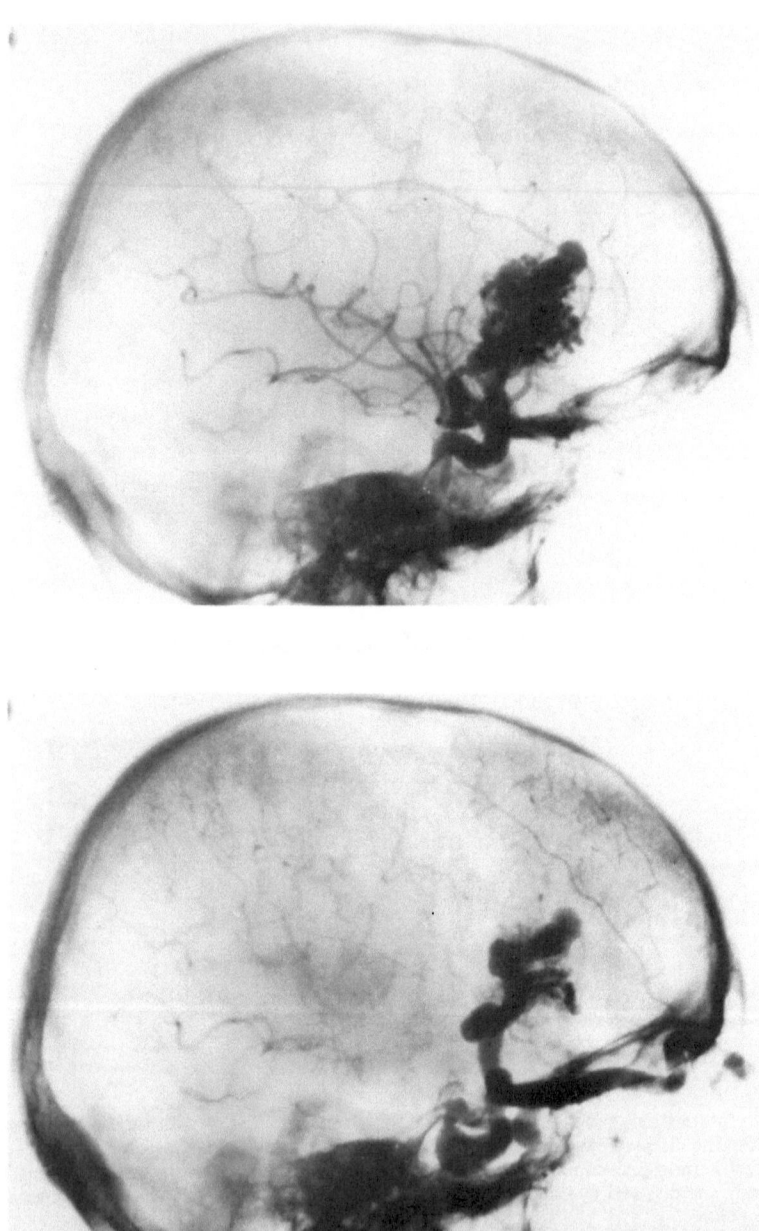

Fig. 4. Carotis angiogram of the patient with the arteriovenous angioma in the territory of the right middle cerebral artery (top). The angiogram in the late arterial phase shows the communication with the cavernous sinus, the orbital and frontal veins (bottom).

344

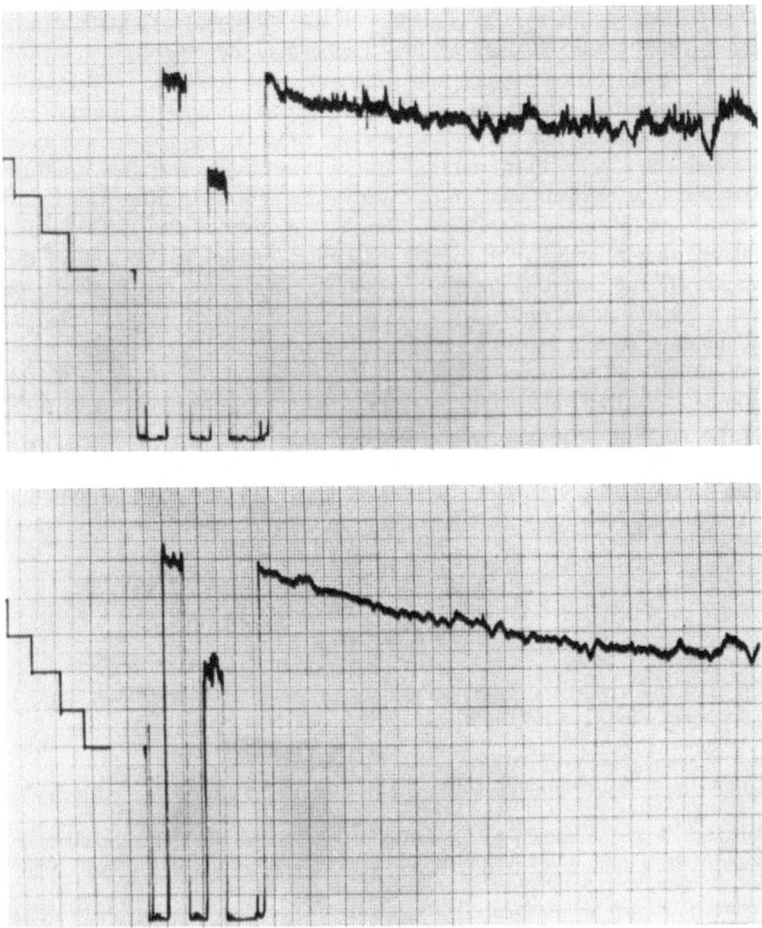

Fig. 5a. Arteriovenous angioma in the territory of the right middle cerebral artery. Diseased eye. Rigidity determination with the 5.5 g and 10.0 g plunger weights. Leydhecker's tonographic test with the 5.5 g plunger weight.

Fig. 5b. Arteriovenous angioma in the territory of the right middle cerebral artery. Healthy eye. Rigidity determination with the 5.5 g and the 10.0 g plunger weights. Leydhecker's tonographic test with the 5.5 g plunger weight.

In traumatic carotid-cavernous fistula, where the orbital haemodynamic changes were more serious than in the spontaneous cases, the intraocular pressure was not elevated as seen in the latter group. The outflow resistance increased in both groups of patients. One can speculate that the lower intraocular pressure was caused in the traumatic cases by the arterial circulatory deficiency which was shown by the lower ODM and ODG pressures. In the traumatic cases the increase of the outflow resistance could be partly due to the elevation of the venous pressure and to the homeostatic reflex regulation of intraocular pressure. In contrast, in spontaneous carotid-cavernous

345

fistula of elderly women, the increase of the episcleral venous pressure together with hypoxic changes of the tissues may be responsible for the increase of the outflow resistance and the intraocular pressure. The situation may be aggravated in these cases by the age related changes in the outflow pathways.

As seen in the cases with intracranial ateriovenous angiomas, the formation of intracranial arteriovenous "pools" can bring about similar ODG and tonographic symptoms as found in the case of carotid-cavernous fistula. Very likely, the intensity of the orbital heamodynamic changes and of the disturbance of the aqueous humour dynamics influences the presence or absence of the individual signs.

The increase of the outflow resistance with the ipsilateral jugular compression in intermittent exopthalmos is more evidence for the role of the elevation of the episcleral venous pressure in the development of the disturbance of the aqueous humour dynamics in these cases.

Of course, the investigation of several more cases is needed to understand the exact relationship between the orbital and intracranial-haemodynamic changes and the disturbance of the aqueous humour dynamics in the diseases examined.

REFERENCES

1. Alfano, J. E. Glaucoma following ligation of the superior vena cava. Am. J. Ophthalmol. 60:412–414 (1965).
2. Bettelheim, H. Zur Hämodynamik des Carotis-Sinus cavernosus-Aneurysmas. Klin. Mbl. Augenheilk. 153:329–338 (1968).
3. Bettelheim, H. Ophthalmodynamographische Befunde bei orbitalen und palpebralen Gefässanomalien. Klin. Mbl. Augenheilkd. 157:793–800 (1970).
4. Follmann, P. Methodische und apparative Verbesserungen der Ophthalmodynamographie. In: Finke, J. ed.: Ophthalmodynamographie. Proc. II. Internat. Symp. F.K. Schattauer Verl., Stuttgart-New York, 1974, pp. 43–47.
5. Follmann, P. and Remenár, L. Ophthalmodynamometrische und ophthalmodynamographische Befunde bei intrakraniell bedingten Durchblutungsstörungen der Augenhöhle. Acta chir. Acad. Sci. Hung. 12:337–350 (1971).
6. Hager, H.: cit. Bettelheim, 1970.
7. Harris, G. J. and Rice, P. R. Angle closure in carotid-cavernous fistula. Ophthalmology (Rochester, Minn.) 86:1521–1529 (1979).
8. Konstas, P., Minas, B. and Papoulis, A. A case of pulsating exophthalmos. Arch. Soc. Ophthalmol. Grece Nord 15:179–183 (1966).
9. Mapelli, G., Verzella, F. and Sebastiani, A. Clinical significance of ophthalmodynamography in the diagnosis of the carotid-cavernous fistula. Rass. Ital. Ottal., N.S. 1:178–200 (1971).
10. Martelli, A. and Caramazza, R. La oscillometria delle arterie oftalmice e temporali nello studio delle fistole arterovenose del distretto cefalico. Riv. oto-neuro-oftal. 37:473–484 (1962).
11. Mühlbacher, I. and Hanselmayer, H. Carotis-sinus-cavernosus Fistel. Klin. Mbl. Augenheilkd. 163:442–447 (1973).
12. Nizankowska, H. Ophthalmodyanmography in vascular anomalies of the orbit. Klin. Oczna 47:25–26 (1977).
13. Nordmann, J., Lobstein, A., Gerhard, J. P. and Lévy, J. P. A propos de 14 cas de glaucome par hypertension veineuse d'origine extraoculaire. Ophthalmologica (Basel 142, Suppl. 113:501–506 (1961).

14. Sattler, C. H. In Handbuch der gesamten Augenheilkunde. Ed. by A. von Graefe and E. T. Saemisch. Leipzig. W. Engelmann. Vol. 6, 1880, p. 745.
15. Sokolova, O. N., Zakhidov, B. A. and Serbinenko, F. A. Specificity of secondary glaucoma in patients with carotid-cavernous anastomoses. Vest. Oftal. (Mosk). 5:20–23 (1973).
16. Sugar, H. S. Neovascular glaucoma after carotid-cavernous fistula formation. Ann. Ophthalmol. 11:1667–1669 (1979).
17. Taptas, J., Chilaris, G. and Katsiotis, P. Arteriovenous aneurysm (carotis-sinus cavernous) without exophthalmos. Arch. Soc. Ophthalmol. Grece Nord. 14:165–167 (1965).
18. Verzella, F. Pathophysiogenese des Ophthalmodynamogrammes. Klin. Mbl. Augenheilkd. 158:49–58. 1971.
19. Weekers, R. and Delmarcelle, Y. Pathogenesis of intraocular hypertension in cases of arteriovenous aneurysm. A.M.A. Arch. Ophthalmol. 48:338–343 (1952).
20. Weekers, R. and Delmarcelle, Y. Pathogénie et traitement de l'hypertension oculaire dans l'exophtalmie par anévrysme artérioveineux. Arch. Ophtalmol. (Paris) 16:380–387 (1965).
21. Weigelin, E. and Lobstein, A. Ophthalmodynamometrie. S. Karger, Basel, 1962.
22. Weiss, D.I., Shaffer, R.N. and Nehrenberg, T.R. Neovascular glaucoma complicating carotid-cavernous fistula. A.M.A. Arch. Ophthalmol. 69:304–307 (1963).
23. Zanetti, R. Atti del simposio sulla diagnosi e semeiologia delle affezioni cerebro-vascolari con particolare riguardo alla oftalmodinamometria. Modena. 1965. Atti Italseber. 350. 1965. cit. Bettelheim, 1968.

Authors' addresses:
Prof. Dr M. Varga, Dr P. Follmann and I. Gábriel
I. Eye Clinic of the Semmelweis University Medical School
Tömő u. 25–29
1083 Budapest
Hungary

Dr L. Remenár and M. Hajda
Eye Department
Neurosurgical Research Institute
Amerikai ut 57
1145 Budapest
Hungary

PANRETINAL PHOTOCOAGULATION TREATMENT OF SEVERE, COMPLICATED GLAUCOMA

N.S. SCHIØDTE, O.I. NISSEN and S.V. KESSING

(Copenhagen, Denmark)

ABSTRACT

It was shown by Schiødte et al. (1980) that normotensive diabetic eyes with no sign of neovascular glaucoma, treated with panretinal photocoagulation, reacted with a long-term (half a year) reduction in IOP. Consequently, 12 severe, complicated glaucomas, otherwise untreatable surgically or medically, were given panretinal photocoagulations.

Short-term effect (one month): In all cases a reasonable IOP level of less than 20 mmHg was obtained. Two (range: 1–3) photocoagulation treatments were needed and in most cases the effect had to be stabilized with cyclo-cryothermia to obtain long-term ($2\frac{1}{2}$ years, range 1–3 years) normalization of IOP. Most patients were given cyclocryothermia before photocoagulations without lasting effect. The photocoagulations probably anaemitize the ciliary body, resulting in an increased vulnerability of the secretory epithelium to later applied cryotherapy.

348

E.L. Greve, W. Leydhecker & C. Raitta (eds.), Second European Glaucoma Symposium, Helsinki 1984.
© 1985, Dr. W. Junk Publishers, Dordrecht. ISBN 978-94-010-8934-0

HEMORRHAGIC GLAUCOMA AFTER INTRAOCULAR OPERATIONS

G. IMRE, G. SALACZ and JULIA BÖGI

(Budapest, Hungary)

The causes of rubeosis iridis and hemorrhagic glaucoma are well known. The most frequent are diabetic proliferative retinopathy, central retinal vein occlusion and carotid occlusion. It is also known that in cases of rubeosis iridis there are widespread retinal areas with obliterated capillaries (4, 8) or in cases of carotid occlusions hypoxy is present in every tissue of the eye.

According to our investigations lactic acid produced by hypoxic tissues and accumulated by deteriorated venous circulation is responsible for neo-vascularizations (5, 7). The lactic acid diffuses from the hypoxic retinal fields into the aqueous humour and in cases of rubeosis iridis there is a significantly increased lactic acid concentration in the aqueous humour (6). For this reason new vessels develop on the surface of the iris and chamber angle. But the aqueous lactic acid concentration may increase expressively only if the rate of aqueous flow is decreased. According to our investigations the aqueous formation of the eyes with rubeosis iridis may be considered as decreased in spite of the well known errors of the tonographic method of its determination (Table I). It is also a known fact that after intraocular operations there may be a prolonged decrease of aqueous production (3, 10, 11).

We report here on cases in which rubeosis iridis or hemorrhagic glaucoma developed after intraocular operation.

Between 1981 and 1983 nine patients were observed with rubeosis iridis or with hemorrhagic glaucoma arising after intracapsular cataract extraction or after filtering operation. All these operations were without complication. In both eyes of every patient an open chamber angle could be found and before the operation no new vessels could be observed either in the chamber angle or on the iris.

Four patients were diabetics with bilaterally the same retinopathy. After an average of 61 days following unilateral cataract extraction rubeosis iridis developed in three cases with hemorrhagic glaucoma and in one case without

Table 1. Tonographic values of 28 eyes with rubeosis . iridis. Mean ± SD

C: 0.09 ± 0.09	F: 0.61 ± 0.72 µl/min
in 20 eyes < 0.15	in 21 eyes < 1.0
in 8 eyes > 0.15	in 7 eyes > 1.0

E.L. Greve, W. Leydhecker & C. Raitta (eds.), Second European Glaucoma Symposium, Helsinki 1984.
© *1985, Dr. W. Junk Publishers, Dordrecht. ISBN 978-94-010-8934-0*

it. In one case a pan-retinal cryocoagulation was performed combined with cyclocryocoagulation. The intraocular pressure was normalized from the third postoperative day and the new vessels of the iris regressed rapidly from the seventh day. A year later no rubeosis could be found and the intraocular pressure was normal.

Three patients had bilateral open angle glaucoma and in one eye central retinal vein occlusion with moderate ischaemic areas. On both eyes of one patient and on one eye with vein occlusion of the other two patients filtering operation was performed. In the eyes with vein occlusion rubeosis iridis developed after an average of 83 days following operations. On the second patient a panretinal photocoagulation was performed and after 14 days the rubeosis totally regressed without reappearance. On the third patient the pan-retinal photocoagulation had been performed on the second postoperative day but 160 days later a moderate rubeosis developed. The intraocular pressure remained normal and the last examination a year later showed that rubeosis did not increase.

Two patients were not diabetics and their fundus was intact. After 60 and 30 days following the unilateral cataract extraction rubeosis developed in the same eye. One of the patients also had a hemorrhagic glaucoma. In both patients the ODM pointed to carotid occlusion, confirmed by ultrasound-doppler investigation and proved by carotid angiography.

Before the operations there were in all cases widespread areas of poor perfusion in the retina or in the whole eye and the operations promoted the development of the rubeosis iridis by decreasing the aqueous production. If these eyes had not had to be operated the rubeosis would have developed much later or not at all.

If there is a retinopathy or a vein occlusion a pan-retinal photocoagulation should be done before or after the intraocular operation to prevent the rubeosis iridis and goniorubeosis.

Rubeosis very frequently occurs after vitrectomy (1, 2, 9, 13), especially if it is combined with lensectomy. We believe that there may be a prolonged decrease in aqueous formation after this operation, and that a pan-retinal photocoagulation must also be done to prevent the development of the hemorrhagic glaucoma.

If the hemorrhagic glaucoma develops and the chamber angle is closed by fibrovascular tissue, the pan-retinal coagulation in itself will not always be sufficient. Therefore, the pan-retinal coagulation must be combined with other treatments, e.g. with goniophotocoagulation (12) or with an aqueous production reducing treatment. But the latter can be applied only if the causes of the rubeosis can be stopped; otherwise they are contra-indicated because decreasing the aqueous formation they promote the neovascularization.

REFERENCES

1. Blumenkranz, M. S. and Hernandez, E. Rubeosis iridis and vitrectomy. Invest. Ophthal. Vis. Sci. 22 (Suppl.): 344 (1982).
2. Ghartey, K. N., Tolentino, F. I., Freeman, H. M., McMeel, J. W., Schepens, C. L. and Aiello, L. M. Closed vitreous surgery. XVII. Results and complications of pars plana vitrectomy. Arch. Ophthal. (Chicago) 98:1248 (1980).

3. Goldmann, H. Über die Wirkungsweise der Cyclodialyse. Ophthalmologia 121:94 (1951).
4. Hasunama, T., Hashimoto, K., Ida, R., Numaga, T. and Horiuchi, T. Treatment of rubeosis iridis as a complication of diabetic retinopathy. Jap. J. Clin. Ophthalmol. 34:131 (1980).
5. Imre, G. Neovascularization of the eye. In: Contemporary Ophthalmology Honoring Sir St. Duke-Elder, Ed: J.G. Bellows, p. 88, William and Wilkins, Baltimore (1972).
6. Imre, G. Rubeosis iridis. In: 5th Congress of the Europ. Ophthalmol. Soc. Hamburg, 1976, p. 267, Enke, Stuttgart (1978).
7. Imre, G. and Bögi, J. Corneal vascularization. Internat. Congr. and Symp. Series 40:233 (1981).
8. Laaitakainen, L. and Kohner, E. M. Fluorescein angiography and its prognostic significance in central retinal vein occlusion. Br. J. Ophthalmol. 60:411 (1976).
9. Laqua, H. Rubeosis iridis nach Pars plana-Vitrektomie. Klin. Mbl. Augenheilk. 177:24 (1980).
10. Lee, P. F. and Trotter, R. R. Tonographic and gonioscopic studies before and after cataract extraction. Arch. Ophthal. (Chicago) 58:407 (1957).
11. Miller, J. E., Keskey, G. R. and Becker, B. Cataract extraction and aqueous outflow. Arch. Ophthal. (Chicago) 58:401 (1957).
12. Simmons, R. J., Deppermann, S. R. and Dueker, D. K. Laser prophylaxis of neovascular glaucoma: By goniophotocoagulation alone or in combination with panretinal photocoagulation. Doc. Ophthalmol. Proc. Series 22:203 (1980).
13. Syrdalen, P. One hundred consecutive cases of pars plana vitrectomy with the vitreous stripper. Acta Ophthal. (Kbh.) 57: 1039 (1979).

Authors' address:
2nd Dept. of Ophthalmology
Semmelweis University of Medicine
Mária U. 39
H-1085 Budapest
Hungary

BLOOD AND PLASMA VISCOSITY MEASUREMENTS IN GLAUCOMA PATIENTS

J.H.J. KLAVER, E.L. GREVE, H. GOSLINGA, H.C. GEIJSSEN and
J.H.A. HEUVELMANS

(Amsterdam, The Netherlands)

ABSTRACT

Blood viscosity at ten shear rates, plasma viscosity, haematocrit, plasma
fibrinogen, serum α_2-macroglobulin and serum proteins were measured
in 83 patients with low tension glaucoma (LTG) and 23 patients with "high
tension glaucoma" (HTG: at least one IOP reading above 40 mm Hg) and
compared with 50 controls.

Blood and plasma viscosity values and haematocrit were significantly
higher than controls in the LTG group. The HTG and the LTG groups differed
only in plasma viscosity, but smoking and drinking habits in the HTG patients
were greatly different from those in LTG patients and controls, thus preventing interpretation of data in the HTG group.

Within the LTG group viscosity values were highest in a subgroup designated earlier by us as focal ischaemic LTG, whereas another subgroup, senile
sclerotic LTG, did not show significant differences compared with controls.
These findings may indicate a factor in the pathogenesis of visual field defects
and disc cupping in some patients with LTG.

352

E.L. Greve, W. Leydhecker & C. Raitta (eds.), Second European Glaucoma Symposium, Helsinki 1984.
© *1985, Dr. W. Junk Publishers, Dordrecht. ISBN 978-94-010-8934-0*

SECONDARY GLAUCOMA IN REACTIVE LYMPHOID HYPERPLASIA OF THE CONJUNCTIVA AND UVEAL TRACT

Z. KULJAČA, V. LJUBOJEVIĆ and P. BOJIĆ

(Belgrade, Yugoslavia)

ABSTRACT

A 72-year-old man had reactive lymphoid hyperplasia of the conjunctiva and uveal tract, associated with secondary glaucoma. Histological and ultra-sonographical examinations revealed the nature of the disease. This report shows that significant complications may occur in reactive lymphoid hyperplasia of the conjunctiva and uveal tract.

INTRODUCTION

Reactive lymphoid hyperplasia may involve almost any part of the eye or ocular adnexa (1,3,4). Reactive lymphoid hyperplasia is of importance in the differential diagnosis of lymphosa and leukemia, particularly when associated with clinical findings, including glaucoma, uveitis or retinal detachment (3). The purpose of this report is to show the relatively unusual association of secondary open angle glaucoma and reactive lymphoid hyperplasia.

CASE REPORT

A 72-year-old man was examined because of redness and pain in his left eye of two weeks' duration. The patient was treated for scleritis with corticosteroids. The red-colored lesion on the superior bulbar conjunctiva (Fig. 1) showed immediate regression. Systemic medical work-up was normal. Six months later, similar lesion appeared in the same place. There was a moderate sero-fibrinous reaction in the anterior chamber. Posterior synechiae were found at that time. Open angle glaucoma with a tension of 30 mmHg was observed.

The biopsy specimens of the conjunctival lesions were taken, and it was found to be involved by reactive lymphoid hyperplasia.

Low-power microscopy demonstrated a portion of the conjunctiva and subconjunctival tissue that contained a dense infiltration of deeply basophilic cells (Fig. 2). High-power microscopy demonstrated that the lesions were composed primarily of mature lymphocytes and occasional plasma cells (Fig. 3).

353

E.L. Greve, W. Leydhecker & C. Raitta (eds.), Second European Glaucoma Symposium, Helsinki 1984.
© 1985, Dr. W. Junk Publishers, Dordrecht. ISBN 978-94-010-8934-0

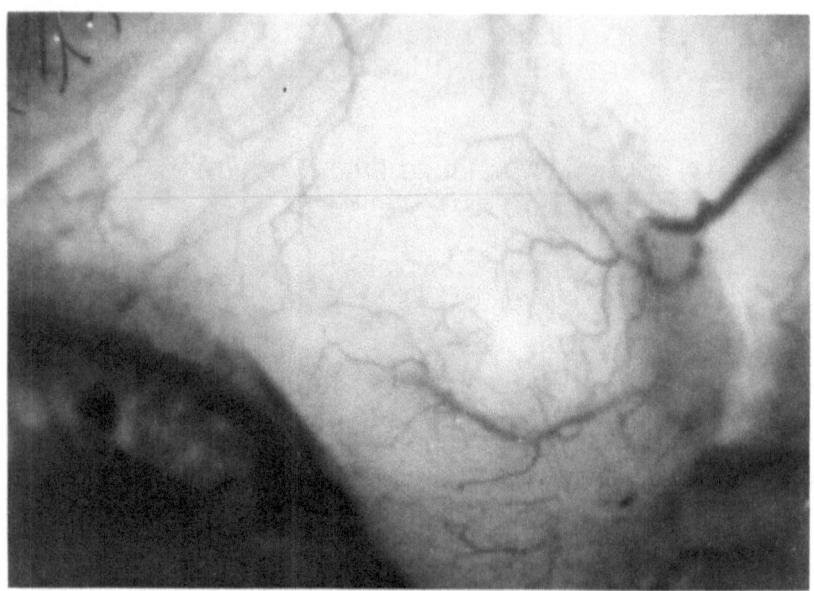

Fig. 1. Red-colored mass involving bulbar conjunctiva. Histopathologically, lesions were reactive lymphoid hyperplasia.

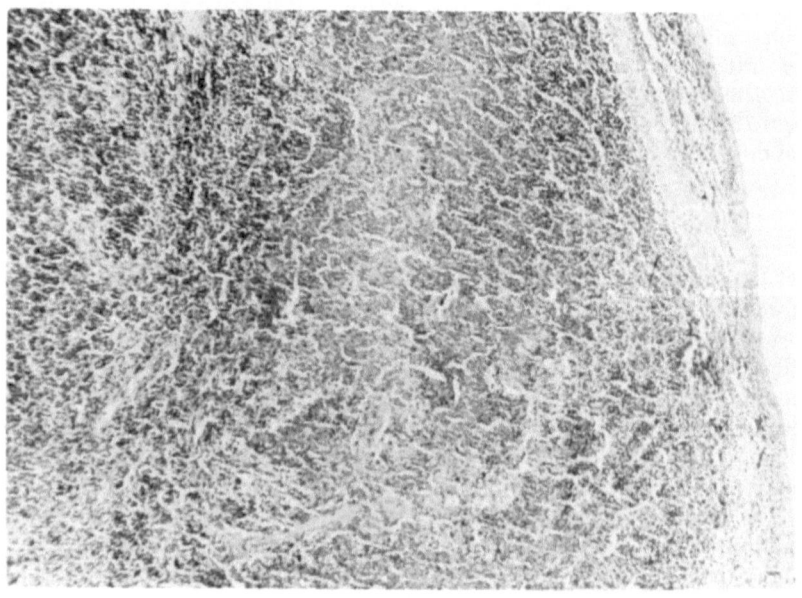

Fig. 2. Low-power microscopy. Diffuse reactive lymphoid hyperplasia (hematoxylin-eosin x60).

354

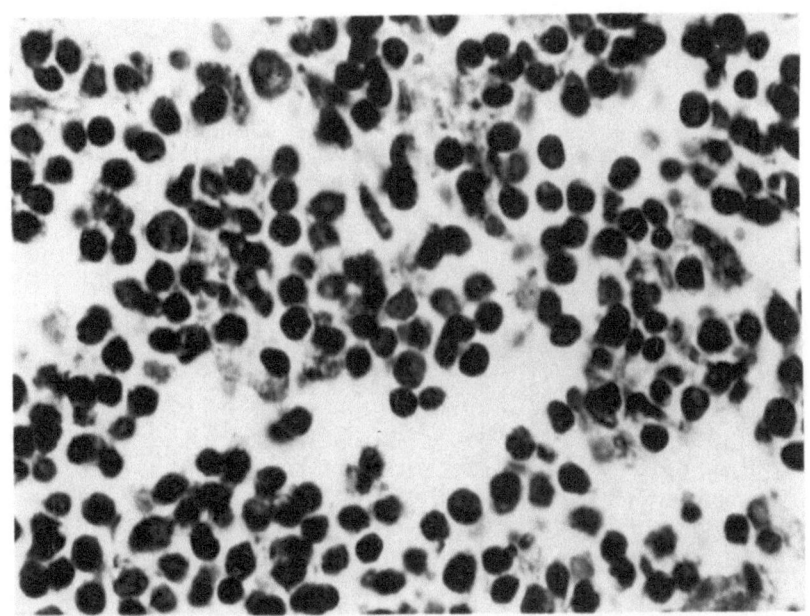

Fig. 3. High-power microscopy. Mature lymphocytes and occasional plasma cells (hematoxylin-eosin x600).

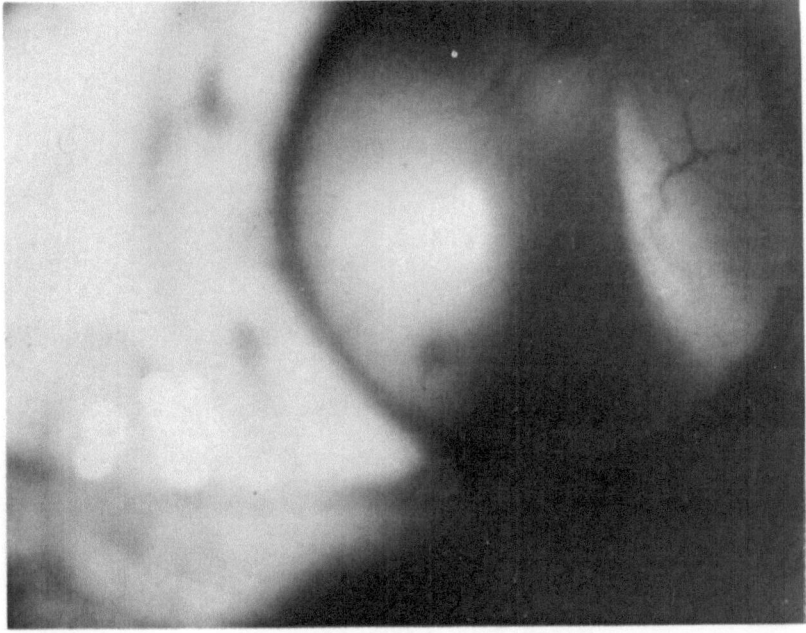

Fig. 4. Exudative retinal detachment.

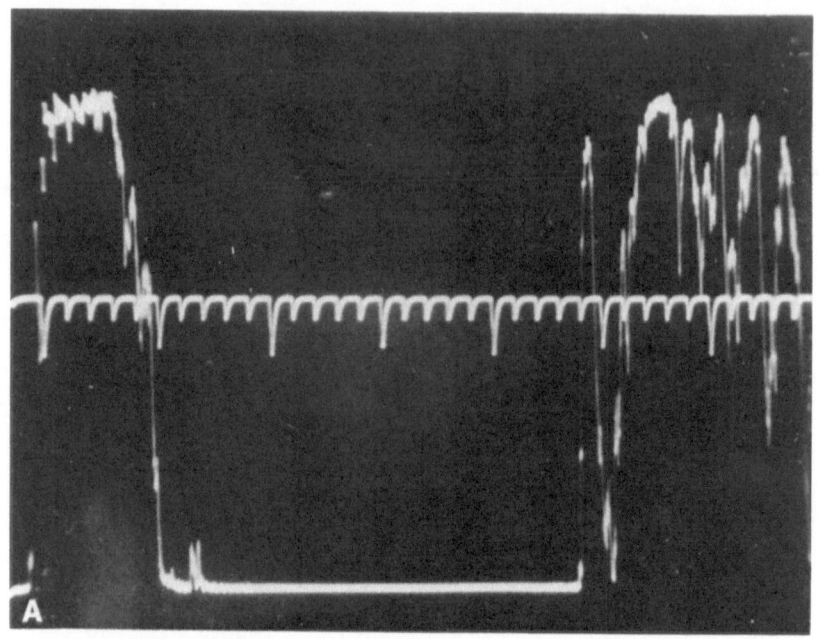

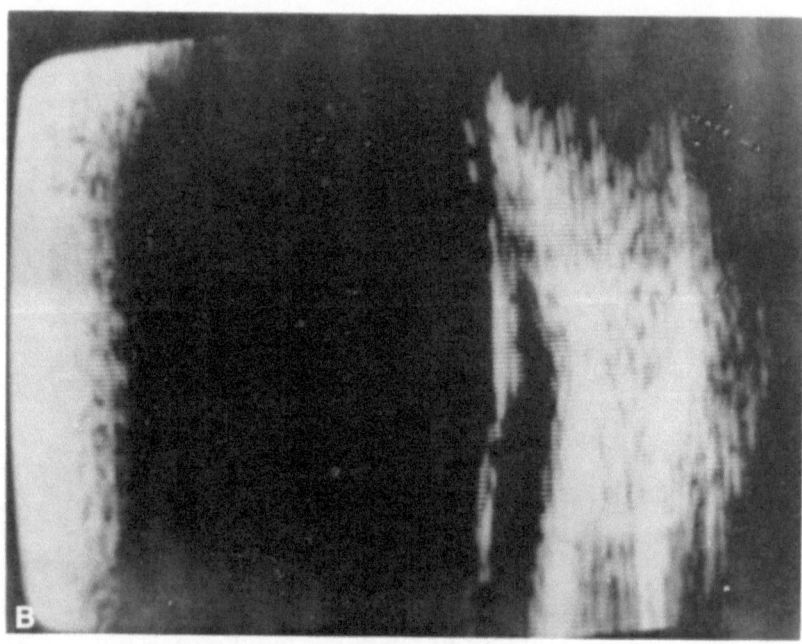

Fig. 5(a,b). A and B scan ultrasonography. Retinal detachment and diffuse thickening within the uveal tract.

Results of laboratory investigation, including a complete blood cell count, determination of electrolytes, liver enzyme levels, cells dependent immunity test (quantitative T and B lymphocytes by rosete with sheep erythrocytes) were normal. Inflamation and glaucoma were controlled with corticosteroids and timolol 0.5%.

Nearly one year later, visual acuity of the left eye was reduced to counting fingers. A massive exudative retinal detachment was found temporally (Fig. 4). A and B scan ultrasonography revealed a retinal detachment and diffuse thickening within the uveal tract (Fig. 5a,b).

When irradiation was administered, immediate partial regression of the conjunctival lesions resulted. Shallow retinal detachment and secondary glaucoma were persistent after radiation therapy.

Secondary glaucoma and inflammatory reaction were controlled with timolol 0.5% and occasionally steroids when exudation was present. Medical therapy was effective in maintaining the intraocular pressure at a level that prevents optic nerve or visual field damage. The clinical picture was unchanged when the patient was last observed, three years after onset of symptoms.

DISCUSSION

Benign lymphoid lesions of conjunctiva are too often misdiagnosed and overtreated (6). Our findings suggest that initial histopathologic evaluation is required for proper diagnosis.

Histopathologic features of benign reactive lymphoid hyperplasia were classified according to Jakobiec in monoclonal lesions, group 1 (well differentiated) (2). There are a number of clinical features of benign lymphoid hyperplasia which can be of assistance prior biopsy (5).

This case had many of them, and emphasizes another condition on the list of lymphoid lesions, which can be clinically confused with malignant melanoma. Secondary glaucoma is usually associated with reactive lymphoid hyperplasia of uvea, mostly of the closed angle type (3).

In the present case uveal involvement led to the chronic inflammatory reaction, which was probably responsible for trabecular damage and permanent open angle glaucoma. This type of secondary glaucoma is best managed medically with the combined use of steroids and timolol or acetazolamide, conjoined with local radiotherapy of the benign lymphoid lesion.

REFERENCES

1. Haddad, R., Slezak, H. and Till, P. Intra-und peribulbare reaktive lymphoide Hyperplasie. Klin. Mbl. Augenheilk. 176:334–336 (1980).
2. Jakobiec, F. A., Iwamoto, T. and Knowles, M. D. Ocular adnexal lymphoid tumors. Correlative ultrastructural and immunologic marker studies. Arch Ophthalmol. 100:84–99 (1982).
3. Ryan, S. J., Zimmerman, L. E. and King, F. M. Reactive lymphoid hyperplasia. An unusual form of intraocular pseudotumor. Trans Am. Acad. Ophthalmol. Otolaryngol. 76: 652–671 (1972).

4. Shields, A.J., Augsburger, J.J., Gonder, R.J. and MacLeod, D. Localized benign lymphoid tumor of the iris. Arch Ophthalmol. 99:2147–2148 (1981).
5. Sigelman, J. and Jakobiec, F. A. Lymphoid lesions of the conjunctiva. Relation of histopathology to clinical outcome. Ophthalmology 85: 818–843 (1978).·
6. Zimmerman, L. E. Lymphoid tumors. In Boniuk, M., Ocular and Adnexal Tumors: New and Controversial aspects. St. Louis, CV Mosby Co, pp. 429–446 (1964).

Authors' addresses:
Dr Z. Kuljača
Dr V. Ljubojević
Institute of Ophthalmology
Clinic-Hospital Center
Baje Sekulića 172
11000 Belgrade
Yugoslavia

Dr P. Bojić
Dept. of Pathology
Clinic-Hospital Center
Baje Sekulića 172
11000 Belgrade
Yugoslavia

THE NATURAL COURSE OF OPEN ANGLE GLAUCOMA
(POSTER EXHIBITION)

TORD JERNDAL

(Gothenburg, Sweden)

ABSTRACT

Open angle may take a hypertensive or normotensive course characterized by continuous nerve fiber loss. The hypertensive glaucoma comprises early and late congenital glaucoma, exfoliation glaucoma, pigmentary glaucoma and simple glaucoma. Most of these glaucomas have goniodysgenesis as a primary hypertensive factor. The normotensive glaucoma comprises low-tension glaucoma and to a certain extent simple glaucoma where goniodysgenesis is rare. The prognosis is poorer in the normotensive group, but also treated hypertensive glaucoma may lead to blindness with inadequate strategy. Strict perimetric strategy will change treatment only in retrospect and thus too late. A prospective strategy including early surgery is recommended.

INTRODUCTION

Every attempt to handle open angle glaucoma as a clinical or genetic entity has failed because open angle glaucoma is a mixed group. Within this group there are striking and well-known characteristics that subdivide the cases into different classes. Surprisingly enough, even recent papers on this subject may be vague on the very definition of what subgroup is actually referred to.

Since the poster illustrates in a schematic form the natural course of open angle glaucoma it is imperative to start with a definition of the various classes of glaucoma involved.

Two different patterns of natural course are outlined: the *hypertensive* pattern (Diagram I, Fig. 1) that includes early and late congenital glaucoma, exfoliation glaucoma, pigmentary glaucoma, and simple glaucoma; and the *normotensive* pattern (Diagram II, Fig. 2) includes low-tension glaucoma and to a certain extent simple glaucoma.

About simple glaucoma: This group is defined merely by negative criteria: absence of congenital or acquired abnormalities in the anterior segment. Thus it is greatly reduced in size and importance by the skilled use of detailed gonioscopy. A recent figure for the percentage of simple glaucoma in an

359

E.L. Greve, W. Leydhecker & C. Raitta (eds.), Second European Glaucoma Symposium, Helsinki 1984.
© *1985, Dr. W. Junk Publishers, Dordrecht. ISBN 978-94-010-8934-0*

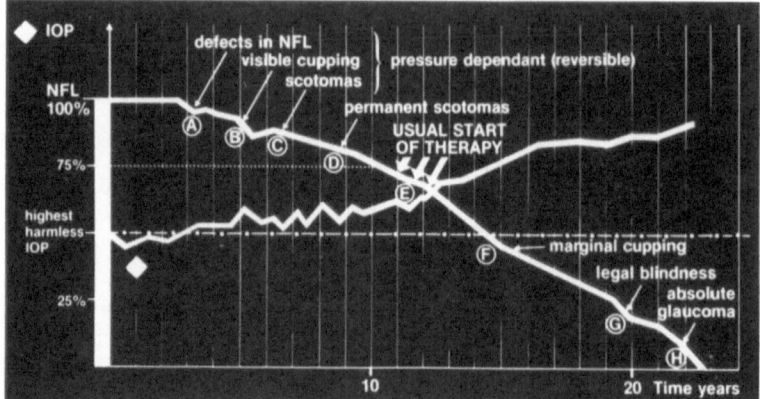

1.

Chronic glaucoma accounts for
a high proportion of blindness
which is preventable . . .
existing knowledge is not applied
as it should . . .

2.

The condition is frequently
insidious and advanced before
being identified . . .

3.

When diagnosed,
the management of glaucoma
is frequently inadequate . . .

R. Pitts Crick. Brit J Ophthal 59 236 1975

I Open angle glaucoma (schematic diagram)
Loss of nerve fibres determined by IOP

Fig. 1. The natural course of hypertensive open angle glaucoma. This graph illustrates
schematically the advancing defects of the nerve fiber layer (NFL) when the IOP gradually passes and rises high above the (theoretical) highest harmless level. As indicated,
start of therapy usually lags behind a couple of years.

outpatient service is 9.8 and in a surgical material 5.2 calculated on the total
glaucoma in each category (1).

DIAGRAM I

The hypertensive glaucoma course is followed by early and late congenital
glaucoma, exfoliation glaucoma, pigmentary glaucoma, and simple glaucoma,
all of which except the latter usually display goniodysgenesis as a primary
glaucoma factor (1).

The proposed etiology of reversible and irreversible field defects in hypertensive glaucoma is put forward by Hayreh (2).

Selective vulnerability to pressure-induced hypoxemia at the optic nerve
head will lead first to characteristic focal nerve fiber dysfunction and eventually to fiber death. As shown in the diagram (Fig. 1), the highest harmless
level of IOP is thought to be individual and dependent on age, sex, systemic
blood pressure, corticosteroid level, etc. In untreated open angle glaucoma
blindness intervenes after 10–25 years (3), sooner with an early start of the
elevated IOP and a steeper curve. The long-term tensional curve (Fig. 1)
makes a gradual and hesitating start with remissions to normal IOP before a
steady elevation takes over and nerve damage becomes permanent. Early
diagnosis is seldom achieved because of the lack of symptoms and the labile
IOP.

360

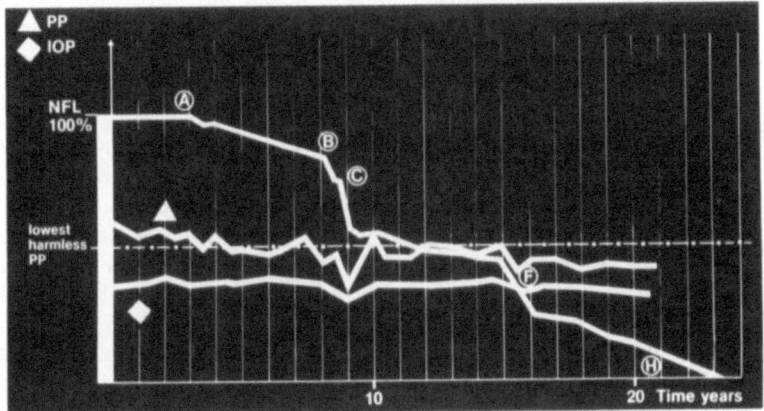

Many glaucomas are a mixture of I and II.

II Low tension glaucoma (schematic diagram)
Loss of nerve fibres determined by primary hypoxemia.

Perfusion Pressure   QUESTIONS: a) When does the glaucoma start?
                                 b) When should therapy start?
                                 c) Why is "ocular hypertension" a dangerous concept?
                                 d) Which therapy has best prognosis — medical or surgical?

Fig. 2. The natural course of normotensive open angle glaucoma. In spite of a normal IOP a gradual but more uneven loss of nerve fibers occurs here caused by focal hypoxemia-ischemia in the optic nerve head. This yielding circulation is symbolized by the sloping course of the perfusion pressure (PP). When PP falls below the theoretic harmless level a hypoxemic situation occurs.

The natural course of open angle glaucoma, i.e. long-term observation without treatment is seldom available for ethical reasons, but also the post-therapeutic course gives valuable information. During a period of 10—30 years it is evident that an escalation of the therapeutic efforts is necessary to meet the rising IOP. Therefore, an early combination of surgical and pharmacological therapy gives the best results. The fact that many glaucoma cases in old age seem to burn their hypertension out is of no comfort, since at that stage the nerve fibers are long lost.

The semantic trap of the term "ocular hypertension" (OH) should be pointed out here. Since most hypertensive glaucomas pass through a prolonged stage of OH on their way to definite glaucoma, repeated high (4) readings of IOP are not to be neglected. The prognosis becomes easier to assess after a meticulous search of the anterior segment for goniodysgenesis or exfoliative and pigmentary deposits.

DIAGRAM II (Fig. 2)

This diagram demonstrates the schematic course of normotensive glaucoma. This course is followed by low-tension glaucomas and to a certain extent by simple glaucomas. Impaired outflow is not the critical factor in this group and goniodysgenesis is rare. For the sake of simplicity the IOP has been

361

plotted at a steady normal level and the decisive factor for the development of nerve fiber defects is low perfusion pressure at the optic nerve head according to Hayreh (2), or "factor V" according to Levene (4), i.e. vascular changes from other causes then IOP. The steep drops of the curve depicting the nerve fiber layer symbolize segmental optic infraction minor drops splinter haemorrhages on the disc.

For the normotensive open angle glaucomas in contrast to the hypertensive ones (6) a reduction of the IOP has little value, although a limited benefit of subnormal IOP has been proposed. However, the natural course of normotensive glaucoma is mainly unaffected by medical and surgical efforts in the long run. In this context it is most important to point at the poster's warning sign "Many glaucomas are a mixture of I and II", i.e. a combination of "hypertensive" and "normotensive" factors.

The mixture is seldom discussed and will often deceive the therapist, particularly if the "normotensive glaucoma factor" is superimposed upon the hypertensive glaucoma years after the latter diagnosis was established. This insidious doubling of the glaucoma factors is certain to worsen the prognosis.

THERAPY

The continuous but twofold threat to the optic nerve described leads to a consideration of current therapeutic strategies.

The text of the poster starts with a sentence by Crick (7) "Chronic glaucoma accounts for a high proportion of blindness which is preventable . . . existing knowledge is not applied as it should . . ." and he goes on "The condition is frequently insidious and advanced before being identified." This is a real eye-opener. What can be done about a) early diagnosis, and b) efficient treatment?

The glaucomatous loss of the first 25% of the nerve fiber layer is often difficult to ascertain even with sophisticated perimetry, which gives the glaucoma a lead of several years. Cricks' third sentence is even more discouraging than the first two and reads "When diagnosed the management of glaucoma is frequently inadequate . . .", but it is true provided that the therapeutic strategy is guided by the confirmation of advancing field loss. The glaucoma pulls away and leaves the nerve fibers crumbling.

In innumerable top level discussions on glaucoma it has been suggested that we should base our therapeutic strategy, not on the level of IOP, but on the results of accurate perimetry and/or the cupping of the disc. Rational and sophisticated as this may seem, the result will be that after damage is done and confirmed, the treatment is changed to fight a situation already passed. In other words the strategy is based on hindsight and does not indicate possibilities of foresight. The following suggestions will outline an imaginative and prospective strategy:

1. Make a careful classification of the individual glaucoma! Congenital glaucoma of all ages, pigmentary glaucoma and exfoliation glaucoma are all progressively hypertensive and from the start candidates to surgical treatment. Meticulous gonioscopy is the tool of classification.

2. Follow the IOP graphically in a long-term tensional curve. The level as

well as the inclination of the curve and any peaks are important clues as to the potential threat of the glaucoma.

3. Heavy medication invites cheating and leads to unnecessary field loss. Early operation as an alternative has all the advantages, particularly with the introduction of laser trabeculopuncture. The patients live longer nowadays and should have a fair chance of visual ability as long as they live. Blindness in hypertensive glaucoma is usually preventable.

Finally a word on the screening possibilities in open angle glaucoma. Tonometric screening has somewhat unjustly received a tarnished reputation and some centers have even abandoned routine tonometry unless disc or field changes are evident (8). IOP mass screening is usually not worthwhile, but screening of target groups should be encouraged. Thus:

a) families with hereditary glaucoma where a dominant goniodysgenesis entails a theoretical risk of 50% for the development of glaucoma (often before 40 years of age). This screening program should also include gonisocopy.

b) In co-operation with the paediatricians all children with a distinct malformation of the anterior ocular segment (macrocornea, microcornea, aniridia, congenital cataract, congenital lens subluxation etc.). In addition children with a systemic malformation, e.g. neurofibromatosis, Sturge-Weber's syndrome, Rieger's syndrome, ectodermal dysplasia, chromosomal aberrations etc. Because of the risk of associated goniodysgenesis.

c) The group of individuals found to have the stigmata of the exfoliation and the pigmentary dispersion syndromes. These changes precede the hypertension by several years and can in fact contribute to give the ophthalmologist the upper hand in fighting early glaucoma.

Since goniodysgenesis is the only well-established genetic factor for the development of glaucoma open angle (1), a screening program that includes gonioscopy is rewarding because goniodysgenesis is congenital and static, whereas an elevated IOP is acquired and fluctuating.

REFERENCES

1. Jerndal, T., Hansson, H.-A. and Bill, A. Goniodysgenesis – a new perspective on glaucoma. Scriptor, Cobenh. (1978).
2. Hayreh, S. S. Optic disc changes in glaucoma. Br. J. Ophthalmol. 56:175 (1972).
3. Dake, C. L. Glaucoma simplex – long-term clinical study. van Gorcum, Assen (1967).
4. Goldmann, H. Open-angle glaucoma. Br. J. Ophthalmol. 56:242 (1972).
5. Levene, R. Z. Low tension glaucoma: a critical review and new material. Surv. Ophthalmol. 24:621 (1980).
6. Jerndal, T. and Lundström, M. 330 trabeculectomies – a long time study (3–5 1/2 years). Acta Ophthalmol. 58:947 (1980).
7. Pitts Crick, R. Prevention from blindness from glaucoma using the King's College Hospital computerized problem orientated medical record. Br. J. Ophthalmol. 59:236 (1975).
8. Bengtsson, B. Aspects of the epidemiology of chronic glaucoma. Acta Ophthalmol. Suppl. 146 (1981).

Author's address:
Dr Tord Jerndal
Vasa Kyrkogata 1
S-411 27 Gothenburg
Sweden

GONIODYSGENESIS IN ELDERLY GLAUCOMA AND NON-GLAUCOMA PATIENTS. A MASKED BIOMICROSCOPIC STUDY OF THE ANTERIOR SEGMENT*

B. SVEDBERGH, A. ALM, B. AMÉR, T. JERNDAL and W. THORBURN

(Uppsala/Visby/Gothenburg/Hudiksvall, Sweden)

ABSTRACT

The aim was to elucidate if goniodysgenesis is more frequently observed in elderly patients with glaucoma, and furthermore what signs of dysgenesis are important and most unanimously detected. Thus, three observers evaluated dysgenesis of the anterior segment in a masked fashion in 21 glaucoma patients compared to those of 19 non-glaucoma patients. Gonioscopy, slitlamp examinations and measurements of the corneal and pupillary diameters were performed, in all 28 variables. In the glaucoma patients there was significantly ($P < 0.05$) more frequent occurrence of an abnormal corneal diameter, scleral overriding, hypopolasia of the pupillary seam, abnormal Schwalbe's line and an opaque pretrabecular membrane (one observer). Significantly less frequent were a peripupillary yellow ring and pigmented "stars" on the lens. Interobserver variation was small regarding e.g. corneal diameter but rather large regarding e.g. the occurrence of pretrabecular membranes. We conclude that signs of dysgenesis in the anterior segment including goniodysgenesis are more frequently seen in glaucoma than in non-glaucomatous patients.

*To be published in Acta Ophthalmol. (Kbh).

364

E.L. Greve, W. Leydhecker & C. Raitta (eds.), Second European Glaucoma Symposium, Helsinki 1984.
© 1985, Dr. W. Junk Publishers, Dordrecht. ISBN 978-94-010-8934-0